T0229284

Cough: An Interdisciplinary Problem

Guest Editors

KENNETH W. ALTMAN, MD, PhD
RICHARD S. IRWIN, MD

OTOLARYNGOLOGIC CLINICS OF NORTH AMERICA

www.oto.theclinics.com

February 2010 • Volume 43 • Number 1

SAUNDERS an imprint of ELSEVIER, Inc.

W.B. SAUNDERS COMPANY
A Division of Elsevier Inc.

1600 John F. Kennedy Boulevard • Suite 1800 • Philadelphia, Pennsylvania 19103-2899

http://www.theclinics.com

OTOLARYNGOLOGIC CLINICS OF NORTH AMERICA Volume 43, Number 1
February 2010 ISSN 0030-6665, ISBN-13: 978-1-4377-1849-2

Editor: Joanne Husovski

Otolaryngologic Clinics of North America (ISSN 0030-6665) is published bimonthly by Elsevier, Inc., 360 Park Avenue South, New York, NY 10010-1710. Months of issue are February, April, June, August, October, and December. Business and Editorial Offices: 1600 John F. Kennedy Blvd., Suite 1800, Philadelphia, PA 19103-2899. Customer Service Office: 6277 Sea Harbor Drive, Orlando, FL 32887-4800. Periodicals postage paid at New York, NY and additional mailing offices. Subscription prices is $290.00 per year (US individuals), $527.00 per year (US institutions), $142.00 per year (US student/resident), $382.00 per year (Canadian individuals), $662.00 per year (Canadian institutions), $429.00 per year (international individuals), $662.00 per year (international institutions), $219.00 per year (international & Canadian student/resident). Foreign air speed delivery is included in all *Clinics*' subscription prices. All prices are subject to change without notice. **POSTMASTER:** Send address changes to *Otolaryngologic Clinics of North America*, Elsevier Health Sciences Division, Subscription Customer Service, 3251 Riverport Lane, Maryland Heights, MO 63043. **Telephone: 1-800-654-2452 (U.S. and Canada); 314-447-8871 (outside U.S. and Canada). Fax: 314-447-8029. E-mail: journalscustomerservice-usa@elsevier.com (for print support); journalsonlinesupport-usa@elsevier.com (for online support).**

Reprints. For copies of 100 or more of articles in this publication, please contact the Commercial Reprints Department, Elsevier Inc., 360 Park Avenue South, New York, NY 10010-1710. Tel.: 212-633-3812; Fax: 212-462-1935; E-mail: reprints@elsevier.com.

Otolaryngologic Clinics of North America is also published in Spanish by McGraw-Hill Interamericana Editores S.A., P.O. Box 5-237, 06500 Mexico D.F., Mexico.

Otolaryngologic Clinics of North America is covered in *MEDLINE/PubMed (Index Medicus), Current Contents/Clinical Medicine, Excerpta Medica, BIOSIS, Science Citation Index,* and *ISI/BIOMED.*

Printed and bound by CPI Group (UK) Ltd, Croydon, CR0 4YY

Transferred to Digital Print 2011

Contributors

GUEST EDITORS

KENNETH W. ALTMAN, MD, PhD
Director, Eugen Grabscheid MD, Voice Center, Associate Professor, Department of Otolaryngology—Head and Neck Surgery, Mount Sinai School of Medicine, New York, New York

RICHARD S. IRWIN, MD
Professor of Medicine and Nursing, Division of Pulmonary, Allergy, and Critical Care Medicine, University of Massachusetts Medical School; Chair, Critical Care Operations, UMass Memorial Medical Center, Worcester, Massachusetts

AUTHORS

MUHANNED ABU-HIJLEH, MD
Assistant Professor of Medicine, Division of Pulmonary and Critical Care Medicine, Warren Alpert Medical School of Brown University; Division of Pulmonary, Sleep and Critical Care Medicine, Rhode Island Hospital, Providence, Rhode Island

KENNETH W. ALTMAN, MD, PhD
Director, Eugen Grabscheid MD, Voice Center, Associate Professor, Department of Otolaryngology—Head and Neck Surgery, Mount Sinai School of Medicine, New York, New York

MILAN R. AMIN, MD
Assistant Professor, Department of Otolaryngology/Head and Neck Surgery, New York University School of Medicine, NYU Voice Center, New York, New York

PETER C. BELAFSKY, MD, MPH, PhD
Associate Professor, Department of Otolaryngology/Head and Neck Surgery, University of California, Davis, California

ROBERT G. BERKOWITZ, MBBS, MD, FRACS
Professor of Otolaryngology, Department of Otolaryngology, Royal Children's Hospital, Parkville, Melbourne, Victoria, Australia

DONALD C. BOLSER, PhD
Professor, Department of Physiological Sciences, College of Veterinary Medicine, University of Florida, Gainesville, Florida

SIDNEY S. BRAMAN, MD
Professor of Medicine, Division of Pulmonary and Critical Care Medicine, Warren Alpert Medical School of Brown University; Division of Pulmonary, Sleep and Critical Care Medicine, Rhode Island Hospital, Providence, Rhode Island

CHRIS E. BRIGHTLING, MBBS, MRCP, PhD
Professor, Department of Infection, Inflammation and Immunity, University of Leicester, Institute for Lung Health, Glenfield Hospital, Leicester, United Kingdom

STUART M. BROOKS, MD
Professor of Medicine and Public Health, Colleges of Medicine and Public Health, University of South Florida, Health Sciences Center, Tampa, Florida

BRENDAN J. CANNING, PhD
Associate Professor of Medicine, Department of Medicine, Division of Allergy and Clinical Immunology, Johns Hopkins Asthma and Allergy Center, Baltimore, Maryland

ANNE B. CHANG, MBBS, FRACP, PhD
Professor, Queensland Children's Respiratory Centre, Children's Medical Research Institute, Royal Children's Hospital, Brisbane, Queensland; Child Health Division, Menzies School of Health Research, Charles Darwin University, Northern Territory, Australia

KENT L. CHRISTOPHER, MD, FCCP, FAARC
Associate Clinical Professor of Medicine, University of Colorado Health Sciences Center, Denver, Colorado

DHAN DESAI, MBBS, MRCP
Clinical Research Fellow, Department of Infection, Inflammation and Immunity, University of Leicester, Institute for Lung Health, Glenfield Hospital, Leicester, United Kingdom

JENNIFER ELDER, MB, MRCP
Specialist Registrar in Respiratory Medicine, The Royal Group Hospitals, Belfast, Northern Ireland, United Kingdom

SCOTT M. GREENE
The Department of Otolaryngology—Head and Neck Surgery, The University of Texas Health Science Center at San Antonio, San Antonio, Texas

RICHARD S. IRWIN, MD
Professor of Medicine and Nursing, Division of Pulmonary, Allergy, and Critical Care Medicine, University of Massachusetts Medical School; Chair, Critical Care Operations, UMass Memorial Medical Center, Worcester, Massachusetts

JOHN H. KROUSE, MD, PhD
Professor and Chairman, Department of Otolaryngology—Head and Neck Surgery, Temple University School of Medicine, Philadelphia, Pennsylvania

J. MARK MADISON, MD
Professor of Medicine and Physiology, Division of Pulmonary, Allergy and Critical Care Medicine, University of Massachusetts Medical School, Worcester, Massachusetts

LORCAN P.A. MCGARVEY, MD, MRCP
Consultant Physician and Senior Lecturer in Respiratory Medicine, Respiratory Medicine Research Group, Centre for Infection and Immunity, The Queen's University of Belfast; The Royal Group Hospitals, Belfast, Northern Ireland, United Kingdom

ALBERT L. MERATI, MD, FACS
Associate Professor and Chief, Laryngology, Department of Otolaryngology—Head and Neck Surgery, School of Medicine, St Louis, Missouri; Adjunct Associate Professor, Department of Speech and Hearing Sciences, College of Arts and Sciences, University of Washington, Seattle, Washington

MICHAEL J. MORRIS, MD, FCCP
Pulmonary Disease/Critical Care Service, Department of Medicine, Brooke Army Medical Center, Fort Sam Houston, Texas

THOMAS MURRY, PhD
Professor of Speech Pathology in Otolaryngology, Department of Otorhinolaryngology, Weill Cornell Medical College, New York, New York

BRUCE K. RUBIN, MEngr, MD, MBA, FRCPC
Jessie Ball duPont Professor and Chair, Department of Pediatrics; Professor of Biomedical Engineering, Virginia Commonwealth University School of Medicine, Richmond, Virginia

CHRISTINE SAPIENZA, PhD
Professor and Chair, Department of Speech and Hearing Science, University of Florida, Gainesville, Florida

C. BLAKE SIMPSON, MD
The Department of Otolaryngology—Head and Neck Surgery, The University of Texas Health Science Center at San Antonio, San Antonio, Texas

JACLYN A. SMITH, MRCP, PhD
Respiratory Research Group, University of Manchester, University Hospital of South Manchester, Manchester, United Kingdom

Contents

Cough is a common and important respiratory symptom that can produce significant complications for patients and be a diagnostic challenge for physicians. An organized approach to evaluating cough begins with classifying it as acute, subacute, or chronic in duration. Acute cough lasting less than 3 weeks may indicate an acute underlying cardiorespiratory disorder but is most commonly caused by a self-limited viral upper respiratory tract infection (eg, common cold). Subacute cough lasting 3 to 8 weeks commonly has a postinfectious origin; among the causes, *Bordetella pertussis* infection should be included in the differential diagnosis. Chronic cough lasts longer than 8 weeks. When a patient is a nonsmoker, is not taking an angiotensin-converting enzyme inhibitor, and has a normal or near-normal chest radiograph, chronic cough is most commonly caused by upper airway cough syndrome, asthma, nonasthmatic eosinophilic bronchitis, or gastroesophageal reflux disease alone or in combination.

Bronchopulmonary C fibers and acid-sensitive, capsaicin-insensitive mechanoreceptors innervating the larynx, trachea, and large bronchi regulate the cough reflex. These vagal afferent nerves may interact centrally with sensory input arising from afferent nerves innervating the intrapulmonary airways or even extrapulmonary afferents such as those innervating the nasal mucosa and esophagus to produce chronic cough or enhanced cough responsiveness. The mechanisms of cough initiation in health and in disease are briefly described.

A variety of mucoactive medications are used to treat chronic lung disease. When evaluating the role of the cough, it must be considered as an important protective mechanism. Therefore, it may be more important to improve the effectiveness of cough than to suppress or eliminate a chronic cough in patients with chronic lung disease. This article discusses the composition of mucus and phlegm, the process of mucin

eliminate the symptoms and improve overall quality of life in patients who have these diagnoses.

Occupational, Environmental, and Irritant-Induced Cough **85**

Stuart M. Brooks

Occupational and environmental irritants play a role in the pathogenesis of chronic cough. An irritant is a non-corrosive chemical, which causes a reversible inflammatory change on living tissue by chemical action at the site of contact. The clinical and pathologic spectrum of chemically induced respiratory tract irritation ranges from neurogenically mediated alterations in regional blood flow, mucus secretion, and airway caliber to the initiation of cough. In an evolutionary perspective, two types of cough reflexes were created for different protective purposes, but each type used the same anatomic and physiologic neural and muscular structures. The mechanosensory type evolved as human ancestors adapted phonation over olfaction and the larynx moved in close proximity to the esophageal opening. The chemosensory type evolved to protect against an injured lung from a respiratory tract infection or after inhaling high levels of irritant gases and particulates that accumulated in confined quarters of early times. For this latter type of cough reflex, normally quiescent transient receptor potential (TRP) cation channels TRPV1(vanilloid) and TRPA1 (ankyrin) become activated or hyperactivated after lung injury, with lung inflammation, or in response to chemicals. Although animal and laboratory investigations support the possibility of human TRPpathies, further investigations are essential for the further elucidation of the role of TRP cationic channels in instigating chronic cough in humans.

Reflux and Cough **97**

Albert L. Merati

Reflux is a significant contributor to cough in otolaryngology practice; cough is just one marker of its many negative effects on the upper aerodigestive tract. Reflux causes cough both by direct irritation/inflammation and by increasing sensitivities to other noxious agents. Detailed and diligent clinical evaluation, including laryngoscopy, is useful in advancing the working diagnosis of reflux-associated cough. Supplemental testing, including impedance monitoring of esophageal refluxate, can be important to evaluate for both acidic and nonacidic reflux exposure. The mainstay of treatment continues to be dietary and other lifestyle interventions and drug therapy. Although proton-pump inhibitor therapy is effective in most patients, especially those with acid reflux disease, prokinetic therapy is probably very important with those with combined acid and nonacid disease and those with pure nonacid disease. It is likely that failure to improve can be due to behavioral and drug compliance issues. Antireflux surgery can yield long-lasting positive outcomes in carefully selected patients despite the lower efficacy of treatment for primary upper aerodigestive tract symptoms (cough, hoarseness, sore throat) compared with heartburn and regurgitation.

Rhinogenic Laryngitis, Cough, and the Unified Airway **111**

John H. Krouse and Kenneth W. Altman

Over the past 10 years, there has been increasing recognition of the interaction between the upper and lower airways in patients with a variety of infectious and inflammatory illnesses, including allergic rhinitis, rhinosinusitis, and asthma. Epidemiologic and mechanistic links have been proposed to demonstrate these relationships and to offer possible etiologic explanations to account for these observations. Among patients with upper respiratory illnesses, cough can be seen as a common symptom, both from the direct influences of upper airway inflammation, which incite reflex changes and bronchospasm, and from the exacerbation of associated pulmonary processes, such as asthma. Despite this increasing awareness of interaction between the upper and lower airways, the influence of both upstream and downstream respiratory inflammatory processes on laryngeal pathophysiology has not been extensively studied. Research suggests, however, that both direct stimulatory effects on the larynx and secondary effects of mucus production and mucus trafficking can create a range of laryngeal symptoms, including cough. This review discusses the interaction of the upper and lower airway in respiratory disease, and focuses on the effect of these respiratory processes on laryngeal inflammation, function, and symptoms.

Cough Due to Asthma, Cough-Variant Asthma and Non-Asthmatic Eosinophilic Bronchitis 123

Dhan Desai and Chris E. Brightling

Among the most common causes of chronic cough are asthma (25%) and nonasthmatic eosinophilic bronchitis (10%). In asthma, cough may present as an isolated symptom, in which case it is known as cough variant asthma. Variable airflow obstruction and airway hyper-responsiveness are cardinal features of asthma, which are absent in nonasthmatic eosinophilic bronchitis. The presence of eosinophilic airway inflammation is a common feature of asthma and is a diagnostic criterion for nonasthmatic eosinophilic bronchitis. At a cellular level, mast cell infiltration into the airway smooth muscle bundle, narrowing of the airway wall, and increased interleukin-13 expression are features of asthma and not nonasthmatic eosinophilic bronchitis. In most cases, the trigger that causes the cough is uncertain, but occasionally occupational exposure to a sensitizer is identified, and avoidance is recommended. In both conditions, there is improvement following treatment with inhaled corticosteroids, which is associated with the presence of an airway eosinophilia and increased exhaled nitric oxide. Generally, response to therapy in both conditions is very good, and the limited long-term data available suggest that both usually have a benign course, although in some cases fixed airflow obstruction may occur.

The Spectrum of Nonasthmatic Inflammatory Airway Diseases in Adults 131

Sidney S. Braman and Muhanned Abu-Hijleh

When the airways are overwhelmed by noxious particles, gases, or microorganisms, inflammatory and immune responses occur that may cause permanent structural changes. One consequence may be an overproduction of mucus and this may overwhelm mucociliary clearance mechanisms and cause a chronic cough phlegm syndrome. The expectorated mucus is usually clear or white (mucoid) but when it becomes infected, the mucus may become purulent and have a yellow or green color. Diseases associated with chronic productive cough discussed in this article include chronic bronchitis, bronchiectasis, and infectious and noninfectious bronchiolitis and their diagnosis and treatment.

Pharmacologic Management of Cough 147

Donald C. Bolser

This review is an update of recent advances in our understanding of cough suppressants and impairment of cough. Low-dose oral morphine has recently been shown to significantly suppress chronic cough, but the side effect profile of this opioid may limit its widespread utility. Several studies have demonstrated a dissociation between the efficacy of antitussives in some metrics of pathologic cough and their effects on cough sensitivity to inhaled irritants. The relevance of widely used inhaled irritants in understanding pathologic cough and its response to antitussives is questionable. A recent advance in the field is the identification and measurement of an index of sensation related to cough: the urge to cough. This measure highlights the potential involvement of suprapontine regions of the brain in the genesis and potential suppression of cough in the awake human. There are no new studies showing that mucolytic agents are of value as monotherapies for chronic cough. However, some of these drugs, presumably because of their antioxidant activity, may be of use as adjunct therapies or in selected patient populations. The term dystussia (impairment of cough) has been coined recently and represents a common and life-threatening problem in patients with neurologic disease. Dystussia is strongly associated with severe dysphagia and the occurrence of both indicates that the patient has a high risk for aspiration. No pharmacologic treatments ae available for dystussia, but scientists and clinicians with experience in studying chronic cough are well qualified to develop methodologies to address the problem of impaired cough.

Assessing Efficacy of Therapy for Cough 157

Jaclyn A. Smith

An antitussive agent should reduce the amount of coughing experienced by the patient sufficiently for the patient to appreciate an improvement in cough severity and regard the improvement as sufficient to outweigh any adverse effects or risks associated with the treatment. In recent years the development of objective cough counting devices and cough-specific quality of life tools have vastly improved our ability to appropriately assess the effectiveness of anti-tussive agents and hopefully will lead to the development of safe and effective treatments in the future. This article summarizes current knowledge of methodologies available for assessing cough therapies, the patient groups to study, and the design of clinical trials.

Unexplained Cough in the Adult 167

Richard S. Irwin

Unexplained cough is a diagnosis of exclusion that should not be made until a thorough validated diagnostic evaluation is performed, specific and appropriate validated treatments have been tried and failed, and uncommon causes have been ruled out. When chronic cough remains troublesome after the initial work up, determine that a protocol has been used that has been shown to lead to successful results. If such a protocol has been used, next consider whether or not pitfalls in management have been avoided. If they have been, the frequency of truly unexplained chronic cough usually should not exceed 10%. While patients with truly unexplained coughs have an overly sensitive cough reflex, the mere presence of an overly sensitive cough reflex does not by itself explain why they do not get better, because most patients with chronic cough, even those who respond to treatment and get better, have demonstrable heightened cough sensitivity. Management options include referral to a cough clinic with interdisciplinary expertise, speech therapy, and self-limited trials of drugs, preferentially with those shown to be effective in randomized, double-blind placebo-controlled trials in patients with unexplained chronic cough.

Cough in the Pediatric Population **181**

Anne B. Chang and Robert G. Berkowitz

Children with cough, in particular chronic cough, are sometimes referred to otolaryngologists for assessment, diagnosis, and management. Although the likely diagnoses encountered by otolaryngologists are rhinosinusitis, foreign body aspiration, and tracheomalacia, otolaryngologists should be cognizant of the many other possible diagnoses and the evidence for and against their association. This article highlights and focuses the discussion on the cough issues relevant to otolaryngologists.

Future Directions in Treating Cough **199**

Lorcan P.A. McGarvey and Jennifer Elder

Cough is a common and troublesome symptom that can be difficult to treat. New therapeutic options that are safe and more effective than those currently available are needed. In this article, the authors offer opinion on future directions in the treatment of cough, with a particular emphasis on the clinical syndrome associated with cough reflex hypersensitivity. In addition, the article provides an overview of some of the diagnostic technologies and promising drug targets likely to emerge from current clinical and scientific endeavor.

Index **213**

FORTHCOMING ISSUES

Thyroid and Parathyroid Surgery
Ralph Tufano, MD, and Sara Pai, MD,
Guest Editors

Rhinology: Evolution of Science and Surgery
Rodney Schlosser, MD, and
Richard Harvey, MD, *Guest Editors*

Meniere's Disease: Current Diagnostic and Treatment Methods
Jeffrey Harris, MD, and
Quyen Nguyen, MD,
Guest Editors

Prevention and Management of Complications in Sinus and Skull Base Surgery
Sam Becker, MD, and Alexander Chiu, MD,
Guest Editors

Head and Neck Ultrasound
Joseph Sniezek, MD, and
Robert Sofferman, MD,
Guest Editors

RECENT ISSUES

December 2009
Sialendoscopy and Lithotripsy
Michael H. Fritsch, MD, *Guest Editor*

October 2009
Technologic Innovations in Rhinology
Raj Sidwani, MD, *Guest Editor*

August 2009
Radiosurgery and Radiotherapy for Benign Skull Base Tumors
Robert A. Battista, MD, *Guest Editor*

RELATED INTEREST

Immunology and Allergy Clinics, August 2008
Environmental Factors and Asthma: What We Learned from Epidemiological Studies
M. Eisner, MD, *Guest Editor*

Cough Specialists Collaborate for an Interdisciplinary Problem

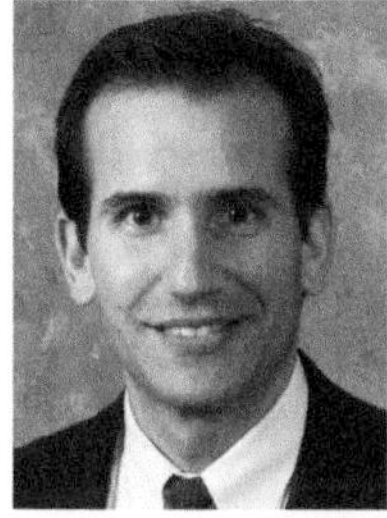

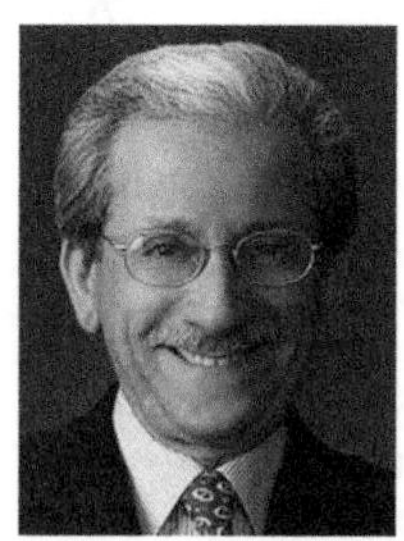

Kenneth W. Altman, MD, PhD Richard S. Irwin, MD
Guest Editors

Both acute and chronic cough are responsible for a significant portion of ambulatory medical visits annually (about 3%),[1] over-the-counter self-medication expenses in excess of $3.6 billion in the United States,[2] and impaired quality of life. The diagnosis of cough can be simple or profoundly challenging. This ranges from a solitary cause such as allergic rhinitis, to multifactorial and synergistic contributions, to a physiologic mystery that may ultimately impair respiratory function and hinder one's way of life. One unique aspect of this chronic cough is that it is an *indicator* of underlying disease, rather than being a disease itself.

Thus, as clinicians we consider cough as a manifestation of disease; yet, as scientists, we think of cough as a product of physiologic mechanisms. These diseases and mechanisms involve the spectrum of adult medical and pediatric disciplines, including otolaryngology, pulmonology and chest physicians, allergy and immunology, gastroenterology, neurology, cardiology, infectious disease, speech and swallowing pathologists, as well as psychiatry. It is particularly timely for this discussion of cough as a true interdisciplinary problem, since we now consider both "macrophysiologic" (interplay of diseases) and "microphysiologic" perspectives (interplay of mechanisms).

The list of diseases that may induce cough is growing, along with an appreciation of the inter-relatedness of these diseases, as described in **Fig. 1**. For example, emerging evidence now supports our long-held observation that the upper and lower airway diseases are closely related as an unified airway, and that allergy plays an important role in exacerbating both upper and lower airway disease. There is also a spectrum of both asthmatic and non-asthmatic lower airway inflammatory disease that often has overlapping clinical signs. Asthmatic, allergic, infectious and other irritant and inflammatory processes in the nose and lung similarly have complex and synergistic physiologic relationships.

Otolaryngol Clin N Am 43 (2010) xv–xix
doi:10.1016/j.otc.2009.12.004 **oto.theclinics.com**

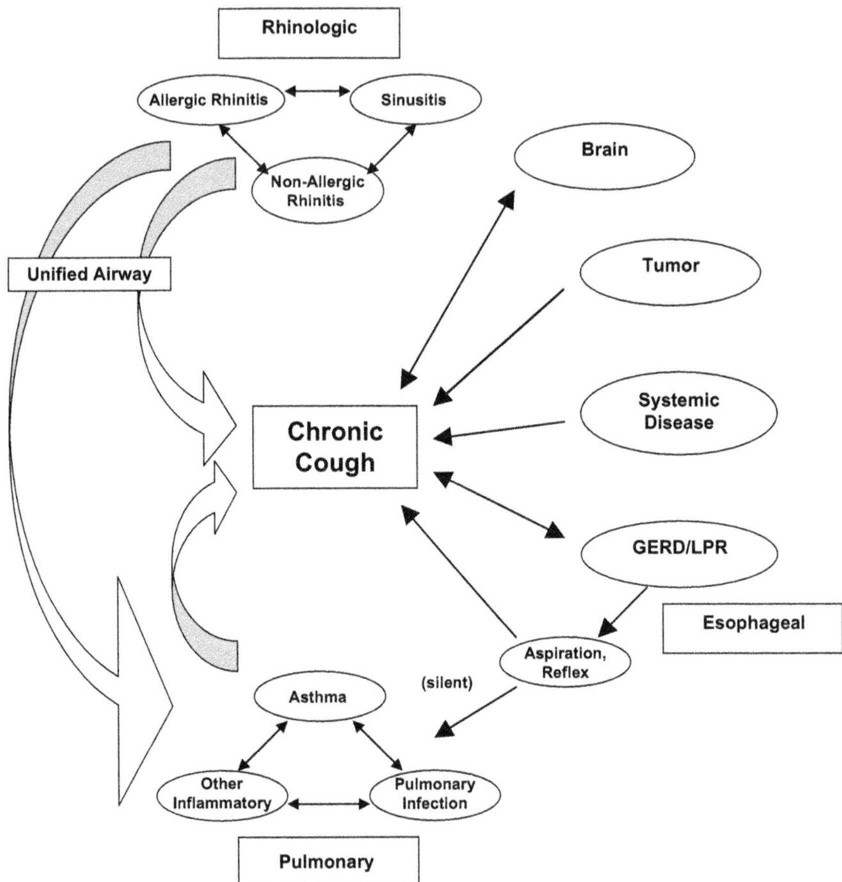

Fig. 1. Inter-relatedness of clinical disease relating to cough. Multiple mechanisms exist at both the local and systemic levels to account for synergy in exacerbation of disease processes. Note: systemic disease includes congestive heart failure (CHF), hypertension treated with angiotensin converting enzyme inhibitors (ACEi), and cystic fibrosis (CF). Tumor may have a direct effect on nerves triggering cough, particularly all branches of the vagus. It may also result in an indirect cause of cough through a post-obstructive inflammatory/infectious process in the lung or paranasal sinuses. There are a number of mechanisms by which gastroesophageal reflux disease (GERD) may trigger cough, both directly related to gross or microspiration, as well as through neurologic reflex (see text). Aspiration may also occur independent of GERD.

The role of gastroesophageal reflux disease (GERD) or laryngopharyngeal reflux (LPR) in inducing cough as a protective mechanism of aspiration is increasingly recognized, even if the gastric chyme extends only to the distal esophagus. The presence of vagal-mediated neural reflexes that produces cough in response to distal esophageal reflux may also produce an indirect effect on the lung through the esophageal-bronchial reflex. Silent, or "microaspiration" of food contents, saliva or refluxed contents may not initially trigger a cough, but produce a chronic inflammatory condition in the lung that does result in cough. We also know that diaphragmatic movements as a result of cough may precipitate GERD or LPR. Cough sensitivity is further modulated by the interplay of these disease states, the potential additive effects of chronic disease versus acute exacerbation, baseline neurologic disease, certain medications and the presence of microaspiration. And lack of a cough when needed, may result in the devastating effects from aspiration or impaired pulmonary toilet.

The brain and its relationship with cough is seen as a "two-sided arrow" in **Fig. 1**. Clearly the cortex of the brain may initiate a cough voluntarily, as well as attempt to suppress it. From the other side of the nervous pathway, sensory afferent fibers stimulate brainstem nuclei to trigger the cough reflex. In the brainstem, there is also considerable overlap between cough and respiratory nuclei. This convergence between higher cortical influence, and primitive brainstem reflexes may result in the clinical presentation of laryngeal spasm, paradoxical vocal fold motion, and other forms of disordered breathing.

When one studies the triggers of cough, it becomes straightforward to recognize that there is an intense interplay of physiologic mechanisms. These are described in **Fig. 2**, and includes the roles of:

- Sensory receptors – chemical and mechanical (temperature and pH-sensitive).
- Transient receptor potential (TRP) family of ion channels and especially overexpression of TRPV1 (the capsaicin receptor) may explain the overly sensitive cough reflex in unexplained cough.
- Peripheral nerve afferent vagal fibers - rapidly adapting stretch receptors (RAR) associated with small diameter myelinated fibers, cough receptors, and the pulmonary and bronchial C-fiber receptors. There are also likely vagal-mediated reflexes triggering cough from sources outside the lung.
- Airway mucus – viscosity and the presence of cellular and secreted inflammatory mediators. It may be postulated that reflexive vascular dilation leads to transudate of fluid that affects mucus viscosity, and also leads to increased blood flow of the submucosal seromucinous glands to increase or change the nature of seromucinous secretions.
- Neurogenic mediators – tachykinins such as substance P and other sub-epithelial chemicals that mediate the afferent neural response to sensory triggers. (While these mediators have been shown to play a role in cough in animal models, evidence to support this in humans has yet to be demonstrated).
- Systemic inflammation – both cellular and humoral, and
- Central neurologic integration – including brainstem overlap between nuclei responsible for cough and respiration.

While precise mechanisms involving these triggers are still being explored, one may envision a seamless systemic communication between each of these factors, and the upper and lower respiratory, gastrointestinal, and neuromuscular systems.

This recent comprehensive understanding that "cough" as a reflection of underlying disease pays tribute to the multifactorial contributions. It also enhances recognition of the respiratory and upper digestive tracts as a "physiologic unit," with the larynx at the epicenter.

The three main goals of this edition are to:

1) Highlight the advances that have been made in understanding and managing cough in a clinically-relevant forum
2) Bring evidence-based clinical guidelines pioneered by the American College of Chest Physicians (ACCP) to the otolaryngology community in a concise presentation
3) Build-out issues with special interest to general otolaryngologists and laryngologists. Because the evaluation and management of cough is an interdisciplinary

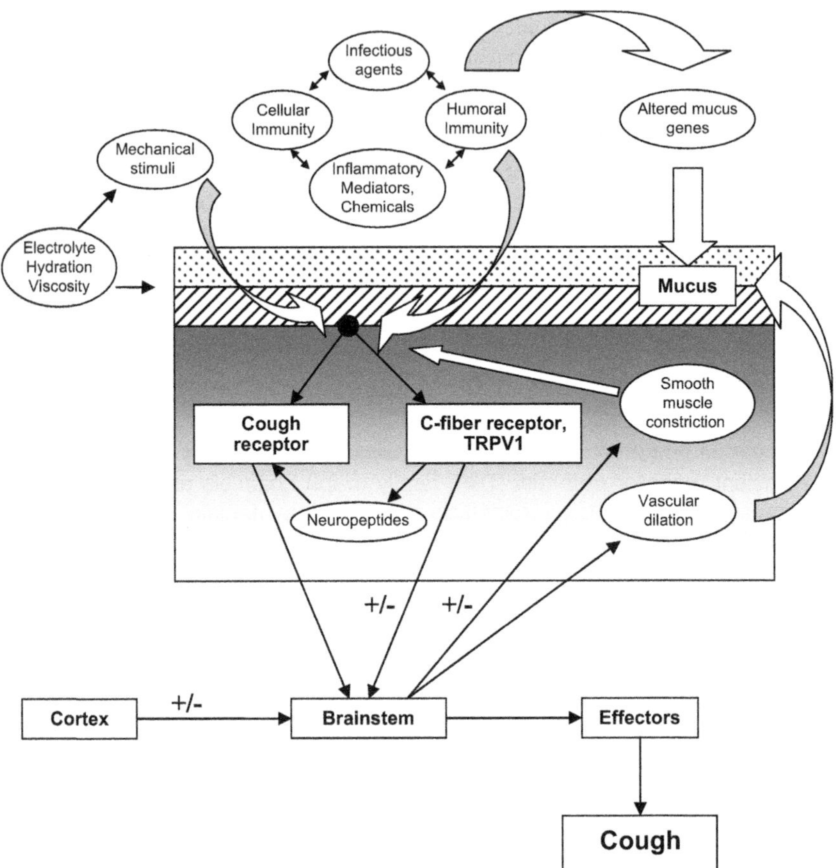

Fig. 2. Inter-relatedness of mechanisms inducing cough. Note: "•" denotes sensory receptor. Sensory receptors may include both cough receptors, as well as c-fiber receptors in the lung. Although the latter communicates with slower conducting fibers to the brainstem, strong stimuli may result in an inhibitory effect. The transient receptor potential (TRP) family of ion channels and especially over-expression of TRPV1 (the capsaicin receptor) may also play a critical role on sensory triggers for cough. Also note that the cortex may have voluntary initiation of cough, as well as intended cough suppression.

problem, it is important that all clinicians who manage this problem are reading from the same script. We also expect that general medicine practitioners would appreciate this information as a focused compendium of current knowledge regarding the evaluation, diagnosis and treatment of patients with chronic cough.

As we move to more value-based medical care, it is important to respect clinical guidelines, but also to construct a means to improve the present standard of care. The interdisciplinary problem of cough is ideally suited to a multispecialty clinic in order to 1) integrate communication among professionals versed in the interplay of this complex disease, 2) improve efficiency and outcomes, and 3) avoid sequential care that results in redundant testing and ultimately delays diagnoses.

While the ACCP guidelines are driven by evidence, medicine is an evolving science and anecdotal observation may yet need to be explained. We expect the following chapters will draw the reader into the subject, and we look forward to expanding the dialogue regarding chronic cough. In many ways, we see this collaboration as symbolic of the interdisciplinary nature of disease, and would emphasize our shared efforts in maximizing the care of these patients.

Kenneth W. Altman, MD, PhD
Department of Otolaryngology-Head and Neck Surgery
Mount Sinai School of Medicine
Annenberg 10th Floor, One Gustave Levy Place
Box 1189
New York, NY 10029, USA

Richard S. Irwin, MD
Division of Pulmonary Allergy
and Critical Care Medicine
University of Massachusetts Medical School
55 Lake Avenue North
Worcester, MA 01655, USA

E-mail addresses:
Kenneth.Altman@mountsinai.org (K.W. Altman)
Richard.Irwin@umassmemorial.org (R.S. Irwin)

REFERENCES

1. Schappert SM, Burt CW. Ambulatory care visits to physicians offices, hospital outpatient departments, and emergency departments: United States, 2001–2002. National Center of Health Statistics. Vital Health Stat 2006;13:1–66.
2. ACNielsen Strategic Planner. The Nielsen Company; 2007. p. 1.

Cough: A Worldwide Problem

J. Mark Madison, MD*, Richard S. Irwin, MD

KEYWORDS

- Cough • Complications • Differential diagnosis
- Asthma • Gastroesophageal reflux disease
- Upper airway cough syndrome

The diagnostic evaluation of cough can be challenging for physicians because it is a nonspecific symptom of respiratory disease with a broad differential diagnosis. An organized approach that first determines the duration of the symptom is highly effective for patient evaluation and management.[1–7] This approach is important because ineffective or inefficient strategies in evaluating cough may themselves negatively impact patient satisfaction, worsen a patient's sense of helplessness, and lower the quality of life.[8] This article focuses on diagnostic evaluation and emphasizes that guidelines from around the world share common features that have served physicians well in various clinical settings.[1,9–12] Although this article concentrates on the differential diagnosis of cough in immunocompetent adult patients, evaluations of cough in immunocompromised or pediatric patients also share many common features.[2]

EPIDEMIOLOGY

Cough is the single most common symptom for which patients worldwide seek medical attention.[13–15] Cough is an important respiratory symptom because it can not only sometimes suggest serious underlying medical conditions but also cause serious complications and significantly affect a patient's lifestyle and sense of well-being.[16]

Questionnaire surveys have estimated the prevalence of cough to be as high as 9% to 33% of the population.[17,18] With prevalence this high and the seriousness with which it is regarded by patients, it is not surprising that cough was the most frequent symptom for ambulatory care visits in 2001 to 2002 in the United States, accounting for 3.1% of visits.[13] In the United States alone, 2006 sales for over-the-counter cough and cold remedies exceeded $3.6 billion.[19] Guidelines to help health care providers diagnose and manage cough have been published in North America,[1] Europe,[9,10] South America,[12] and Asia.[11] reflecting its magnitude and importance to medical

Division of Pulmonary, Allergy and Critical Care Medicine, University of Massachusetts Medical School, 55 Lake Avenue, North, Worcester, MA 01655, USA
* Corresponding author.
E-mail address: Mark.madison@umassmed.edu (J.M. Madison).

Otolaryngol Clin N Am 43 (2010) 1–13
doi:10.1016/j.otc.2009.11.001
oto.theclinics.com
0030-6665/10/$ – see front matter

care around the world. To help even more patients with this common symptom, efforts have been made to develop an online service for diagnosing and advising patients experiencing cough.[20]

COMPLICATIONS OF COUGH

Cough is a respiratory reflex mediated by sensory afferents of the vagus nerve.[17,21] It is an important respiratory clearance mechanism that is stimulated by inflammatory and mechanical irritation of the airways and is especially important when normal mucociliary transport mechanisms are overwhelmed or inadequate. Atelectasis, pneumonia, lung abscess, bronchiectasis, and pulmonary fibrosis may occur when cough is ineffective in its protective role.

An individual cough typically has three main phases: a brief inspiratory phase; a compressive phase, in which the glottis closes and intrathoracic pressure builds as a result of expiratory muscle contraction; and, finally, an expiratory phase, which involves opening of the glottis and a sudden release of air at high velocity.[22] Cough effectiveness depends primarily on achieving a high expiratory air flow and a high linear velocity of the air column. The high intrathoracic pressures (up to 300 mm Hg) achieved during the expiration phase and high velocities of airflow (up to 500 miles per hour) during vigorous coughing can cause various cardiovascular, central nervous system, gastrointestinal, musculoskeletal, respiratory, and miscellaneous complications, many of which can be serious, including syncope, rib fractures, and pneumothoraces (**Box 1**).[23]

One important and common complication of chronic cough is a significant decrease in quality of life stemming from both psychological and physical adverse occurrences such as fear of serious illness, self-consciousness in social situations, urinary incontinence, and other functional impairments.[16] The marked decrease in health-related quality of life is likely responsible for cough being the most common symptom bringing patients to medical attention.

CLASSIFYING COUGH ACCORDING TO DURATION

Classifying cough based on its duration helps narrow diagnostic possibilities, is a widely accepted approach to differential diagnosis, and is the foundation of strategies described in consensus guidelines around the world.[1,9–11] Cough is categorized as either acute (ie, lasting <3 weeks); subacute (ie, lasting 3–8 weeks); or chronic (ie, lasting >8 weeks).[1,3] Acute cough is usually transient, of minor consequence, and most commonly caused by the common cold, although it can occasionally be associated with life-threatening conditions, such as pulmonary thromboembolism, congestive heart failure, and pneumonia.

The category of subacute cough is most commonly a postinfectious phenomenon in which cough develops during a respiratory infection that is more severe than an uncomplicated common cold (eg, pertussis) and then resolves spontaneously within 8 weeks. When cough persists beyond 3 weeks without any obvious respiratory infection, guidelines recommend beginning the workup for chronic cough even before 8 weeks, because it probably will not resolve on its own.[1]

DIFFERENTIAL DIAGNOSIS FOR ACUTE COUGH

Upper respiratory tract infections, especially the common cold, are the most common causes of acute cough (**Table 1**). The prevalence of cough in patients who have untreated common colds ranges from 83% during the first 48 hours to 26% at day

Box 1
Complications of cough

Respiratory

- Pneumothorax
- Pneumomediastinum
- Pneumoperitoneum
- Pneumoretroperitoneum
- Subcutaneous emphysema
- Laryngeal trauma
- Tracheobronchial rupture
- Tracheobronchial inflammation
- Exacerbation of asthma
- Lung herniation

Cardiovascular

- Systemic hypotension
- Syncope
- Subconjunctival hemorrhage
- Arrhythmias

Gastrointestinal

- Cough-induced gastroesophageal reflux
- Splenic rupture
- Inguinal herniation

Genitourinary

- Urinary incontinence
- Bladder inversion

Musculoskeletal

- Rupture of rectus abdominis muscles
- Rib fractures

Neurologic

- Cough syncope
- Headache
- Air embolism
- Cerebrospinal fluid rhinorrhea
- Cervical radiculopathy
- Malfunctioning ventriculoatrial shunts
- Seizures
- Vertebral artery dissection

Miscellaneous

- Petechiae and purpura
- Wound dehiscence
- Constitutional symptoms
- Lifestyle changes

Table 1
Common causes of cough

Cough Classification	Most Common Causes
Acute cough	Viral upper respiratory tract infection (eg, common cold) Exacerbation of underlying lung disorder (eg, asthma) Acute environmental exposure Acute cardiopulmonary disease (eg, pneumonia, pulmonary embolism, congestive heart failure)
Subacute cough	Postinfectious cough (eg, viral upper respiratory tract infection, pertussis infection, exacerbation of underlying lung disorder) Non-postinfectious cough (chronic cough)
Chronic cough	Active cigarette smoking or other chronic irritant Angiotensin converting enzyme inhibitor use Radiographically apparent disease processes of the lung If normal chest radiograph, most common causes are: • upper airway cough syndrome • asthma • nonasthmatic eosinophilic bronchitis • gastroesophageal reflux disease

14.[24] During that 14-day period, the prevalence of cough as a symptom progressively decreases, similar to that of other symptoms associated with the common cold, such as sensation of postnasal drip, throat clearing, nasal obstruction, and nasal discharge.

The diagnosis of the common cold is usually straightforward when immunocompetent patients present with an acute upper respiratory illness characterized by symptoms and signs referable predominantly to the nasal passages (eg, rhinorrhea, sneezing, nasal obstruction, postnasal drip). Patients may or may not have fever, lacrimation, and throat irritation, and physical examination of the chest is normal. In this setting, diagnostic testing has a low yield, with chest roentgenograms being normal in greater than 97% of cases.[25] However, with acute cough in immunocompromised patients, especially those who have AIDS or are at risk for developing AIDS, the clinician should address pneumonia secondary to *Pneumocystis jiroveci* and *Mycobacterium tuberculosis* early in the evaluation, even if the physical examination and chest roentgenogram are normal.[26]

Acute cough is also commonly caused by allergic rhinitis, acute bacterial sinusitis, acute exacerbation of asthma or chronic obstructive pulmonary disease, and the initial catarrhal stage of *Bordetella pertussis* infection. Acute cough also can be the presenting manifestation of pneumonia, congestive heart failure, pulmonary thromboembolism, or conditions that predispose to aspiration. Approximately 50% of patients who have documented pulmonary thromboembolism complain of cough, and cough is occasionally the predominant complaint.[27] In evaluating patients who have acute cough, clinicians must decide whether the patient has a life-threatening condition (eg, pneumonia or pulmonary thromboembolism) or not (eg, common cold) and conduct further evaluation and management accordingly.

DIFFERENTIAL DIAGNOSIS FOR SUBACUTE COUGH

The main diagnostic distinction to make when evaluating subacute cough is whether the cough is postinfectious (see **Table 1**).[28,29] Postinfectious cough begins during an acute respiratory tract infection that is not complicated by pneumonia and that ultimately resolves without treatment.[28] The most common causes are viral infections,

B pertussis infection, bacterial sinusitis, and exacerbations of preexisting diseases, such as asthma, chronic bronchitis, or bronchiectasis. For a cough that has persisted for 3 to 8 weeks but did not begin during an obvious upper respiratory tract infection, the most common causes are the same as for chronic cough (see below).

Infection with *B pertussis* is one cause of postinfectious cough and is a diagnosis suggested by recent *B pertussis* infections in the community, a patient's history of contact with a known case, a cough with a biphasic course (ie, worsening after initial improvement), or a characteristic "whoop" or cough–vomit syndrome.[28] Of course, a biphasic course for cough should lead physicians to consider other causes of cough, such as flares in asthma, chronic bronchitis, and bronchiectasis, but classically *B pertussis* infection should always be considered when cough follows a biphasic course.

After a 1- to 3-week incubation period, a catarrhal phase occurs consisting of conjunctivitis, rhinorrhea, fever, malaise, and cough, followed by a paroxysmal phase featuring worsening of the cough. Cough from pertussis usually lasts 4 to 6 weeks, but may persist for months. Laboratory confirmation of *B pertussis* in a clinical setting can be difficult to establish because a delay usually occurs between onset of cough and suspicion of the disease. No reliable serologic test for *B pertussis* is readily available. Cultures of nasopharyngeal secretions are usually negative beyond 2 weeks of infection, and confirmatory serologic testing requires paired acute and convalescent sera samples. Polymerase chain reaction tests for *B pertussis* have not yet been standardized. The U.S. Advisory Committee on Immunization Practices has recommended dTap vaccine for adolescents and adults up to 65 years of age,[28] reflecting the frequency and importance of this highly transmittable disease.

Acute bronchitis can result in subacute cough, but the diagnosis should only be made when the clinician has excluded pneumonia, the common cold, acute asthma, and, in smokers, an exacerbation of chronic bronchitis.[30] Viral cultures, serologic assays, and sputum analysis should not be performed routinely for acute bronchitis.

DIFFERENTIAL DIAGNOSIS FOR CHRONIC COUGH

Because most respiratory illnesses may cause cough sometime during the course of the illness, and because the frequencies of many respiratory illnesses vary worldwide, the differential diagnosis of cough and the more likely causes in a given patient can vary among different countries and regions of the world. Fortunately, however, for physicians evaluating chronic cough in patients, relatively few conditions account for most cases, which is true in Asia,[11] North America,[1] South America,[12] and Europe[9,10] alike (see **Table 1**). When considering the differential diagnosis for chronic cough, clinicians should recognize multiple, simultaneous causes may be contributing to the cough in at least 25% of cases.[2] In a small percentage of patients, as many as five concomitant causes contributing to cough have been reported.

When evaluating a patient for chronic cough, chest radiograph is an important first step. Any abnormality apparent on the chest radiograph should be pursued first as a potential contributing cause.[1,3] For example, chronic cough can be a symptom of many respiratory disorders that may be evident on chest radiograph, such as bronchogenic carcinoma, interstitial lung disease, and bronchiectasis.[31–34] However, even when a seemingly obvious cause of cough has been identified with chest radiograph, clinicians should not conclude that the cause of cough is established until specific treatment has eliminated the cough entirely. If the cough is not completely relieved with specific treatment, then physicians should consider that other, more common causes of chronic cough may be contributing simultaneously.

The nuances of integrating the diagnosis of chronic cough with empiric trials of treatment for upper airway cough syndrome (UACS), gastroesophageal reflux disease (GERD), and asthma are described in-depth in the most recent American College of Chest Physicians (ACCP) guidelines.[1]

CHRONIC BRONCHITIS

In early prospective studies of adult patients who have normal, or near-normal chest radiographs, chronic bronchitis was among the most common causes of cough.[2,35] Because of the high prevalence of smoking in society and the high frequency of cough among cigarette smokers, it is not surprising that chronic bronchitis is such a common cause of chronic cough.[36] Therefore, if a patient who has chronic cough is a cigarette smoker or is chronically exposed to other environmental irritants that cause chronic bronchitis, that irritant exposure should be eliminated before initiating extensive diagnostic testing. When chronic cough is caused by chronic bronchitis secondary to cigarette smoking, cough improves in up to 94% of cases after abstinence from cigarettes for at least 4 weeks. In the absence of smoking or environmental irritants, patients who have a chronic cough–phlegm syndrome should not be diagnosed as having chronic bronchitis because it does not meet definitions (see British Medical Research Council definition; Lancet, 1965[37]) and can be caused by UACS, GERD, bronchiectasis, and asthma instead.

ANGIOTENSIN-CONVERTING ENZYME INHIBITORS

Angiotensin-converting enzyme (ACE) inhibitor medications are another common cause of chronic cough.[38,39] Although the reported frequency of cough associated with ACE inhibitors has varied widely, from 0.2% to 33%, prospective studies have shown that ACE inhibitors account for 2% of chronic cough.[2] Cough has been reported to occur within a few hours of taking a first dose in many patients, but may not become apparent for weeks, months, or even longer.

If clinically feasible, ACE inhibitor medications should be discontinued before extensive diagnostic testing is performed for chronic cough. The diagnosis of cough caused by an ACE inhibitor medication can only be established when cough disappears on elimination of the drug. Assuming that cough will always disappear within 2 weeks is a pitfall in management, because the median time to resolution has been shown to be 26 days.[40] Because cough caused by ACE inhibitors is a class effect and not dose-related, substituting one ACE inhibitor for another will not likely improve the cough.[1] However, when clinically feasible and appropriate, substituting an angiotensin II receptor antagonist for the ACE inhibitor should eliminate cough caused by ACE inhibitor medications.[40]

COMMON CLINICAL PROFILE

Often clinicians have the challenge of identifying the cause of chronic cough when the chest radiograph is normal, or near-normal, and the patient is a nonsmoker who does not take ACE inhibitor medications. Fortunately, for patients having this common clinical profile, few conditions account for most instances of chronic cough, including asthma, UACS from rhinosinus conditions, and GERD. In nonsmokers, chronic cough is almost uniformly caused by these conditions, alone or in combination.[4]

Another common cause of chronic cough is nonasthmatic eosinophilic bronchitis (NAEB), an eosinophilic inflammatory disorder of the airways distinct from asthma.[41–44] Although NAEB has been more commonly reported outside of the United

States, this disorder may be responsible for as many as 10% to 30% of chronic cough cases.

Upper Airway Cough Syndrome

UACS is the result of rhinosinus conditions that may cause cough through direct mechanical stimulation or causing irritation and inflammation of tissues in the pharynx and larynx.[45,46] Why chronic cough develops in only a minority of patients who have rhinosinus disease is unknown. Typically, patients who have UACS describe the sensation of fluid dripping down into their throats, nasal discharge, or the need to frequently clear their throats, and physical examination of the nasopharynx and oropharynx shows mucoid or mucopurulent secretions or a cobblestoned appearance of the mucosa. Unfortunately, none of these criteria alone is very sensitive or specific.

Moreover, in some patients, chronic cough may be the only symptom of UACS (so-called silent UACS), primarily because they do not sense the drip as an irritation or appreciate that they are frequently clearing their throats when it is obvious to others. Therefore, UACS is often diagnosed based on response to empiric therapeutic trials.[1] Because postnasal drip and throat clearing are common complaints in the general population and in patients who have chronic cough from other conditions, cough can be definitively ascribed to UACS only when it responds to specific therapy for UACS.

Asthma

Asthma should be suspected as the cause of chronic cough when patients complain of episodic wheezing and shortness of breath and cough and wheezing is heard on chest examination; when pulmonary function testing shows reversible airflow obstruction even in the absence of wheezing; or when methacholine inhalation challenge testing is positive in a patient who has normal or near-normal results on routine spirometry. However, chronic cough can be the sole presenting manifestation of asthma (ie, cough-variant asthma).[47,48] In a prospective study of chronic cough, cough was the only symptom of asthma in 28% of asthmatics.[2] Cough-variant asthma is important to recognize because treatment can relieve the cough and decrease the airway remodeling that occurs with asthma.[49]

Nonspecific pharmacologic bronchoprovocation challenge testing is extremely helpful in ruling out asthma as a possible cause of chronic cough. Although it has a positive predictive value of only 60% to 80%, it has a negative predictive value that approaches 100%.[2] Therefore, a negative methacholine challenge essentially rules out asthma as a cause of chronic cough. An exception would be patients who have occupational asthma in its earliest stage.[50] In these cases, however, the methacholine challenge should become positive as the workplace exposure continues. False-positive results on methacholine challenge testing have been reported to occur in 22% of patients undergoing evaluation for chronic cough.[2] Therefore, a positive test alone is not diagnostic of asthma as the cause of chronic cough.

Furthermore, asthma should not be diagnosed solely based on the clinical examination because this has been shown to be unreliable. Because not all wheezes are from asthma and the presence of bronchial hyperresponsiveness does not necessarily mean that asthma is the cause of cough, diagnosing asthma as the cause of chronic cough requires that the cough respond to specific therapy for asthma and that the patient's subsequent clinical course be consistent with asthma.

Nonasthmatic Eosinophilic Bronchitis

NAEB should be suspected as a cause of chronic cough when patients have sputum eosinophilia but no evidence of bronchial hyperresponsiveness or variable airflow obstruction.[41–44] The pathogenesis is unknown and the natural history of this condition is not well established. Although NAEB may be transient or episodic, one study suggested that without treatment, NAEB is persistent in most patients for at least 1 year and possibly longer.[44]

Although NAEB has been associated with occupational sensitizers and inhaled allergens,[51] it also may occur spontaneously. NAEB differs histopathologically from asthma in that the principal site of mast cell infiltration is mucosa rather than smooth muscle and mucosa.[52] NAEB and its treatment are discussed elsewhere in this issue.

Gastroesophageal Reflux Disease

The mechanism through which GERD causes chronic cough is not known. Although GERD can stimulate cough by irritating the upper respiratory tract without aspiration, or the lower respiratory tract with aspiration, GERD may often cause chronic cough by stimulating an esophageal–bronchial reflex in the mucosa of the distal esophagus.[53,54] How refluxed gastric contents stimulate afferent nerves of the esophagus to cause cough is unknown, but most data suggest that gastric acid per se is not the sole trigger of cough in most patients.[53,55] That is, increasing evidence indicates that chronic cough can be caused by nonacid reflux and acid reflux. Therefore, the term *acid reflux* can be misleading when describing chronic cough caused by GERD.

GERD should be suspected as the cause of chronic cough whenever a patient who has cough complains of daily heartburn and regurgitation.[53] Failure to obtain a history of nocturnal coughing does not exclude GERD as a cause of cough. When the chest radiograph is normal, cough from GERD most commonly occurs while the patient is awake and upright and usually does not occur or is not noted at all during sleep. However, chronic cough may be the only symptom of GERD in 43% to 75% of cases.[2,55] In the absence of gastrointestinal symptoms, 92% of patients who have chronic cough caused by GERD have the following clinical profile: nonsmoker, no ACE inhibitor, normal or nearly normal chest radiograph, and asthma, UACS, and NAEB all have been ruled out.

Combining 24-hour esophageal pH monitoring with a symptom diary can help confirm that GERD is causing a patient's chronic cough.[2,53,55] The pH monitoring findings can be considered consistent with GERD as the cause of chronic cough when reflux events (acid or alkaline) are associated with cough recorded in the diary, or when any reflux parameter falls outside of the normal range.[53] However, the conventional diagnostic indices of GERD (eg, percentage of time that pH is less than 4.0) that gastroenterologists use to diagnose reflux esophagitis can be misleadingly normal in patients who have cough from GERD. The test should be interpreted as normal only when conventional indices for acid reflux are within the normal range and no reflux-induced coughs are identified during the 24-hour pH monitoring study.[55]

Confirmation of GERD as the cause of cough requires that the cough disappear when the patient is treated with antireflux therapy. The recent development of simultaneous 24-hour monitoring of esophageal impedance and pH will likely expand understanding of cough from GERD because acid, alkaline, and neutral reflux events will be detectable and better-correlated with instances of cough. Because no uniform agreement exists on how to interpret these tests, the ACCP Cough Guideline committee recommends empiric therapy initially rather than esophageal monitoring.

Miscellaneous Conditions

Conditions other than cigarette smoking, ACE inhibitor use, UACS, asthma, NAEB, and GERD have usually made up no more than 6% of the causes of chronic cough in prospective studies.[2,56] Although these other causes of cough include virtually any condition that may affect the afferent limb of the cough reflex, the more frequently described miscellaneous causes are listed in **Box 2**.[57]

Chronic cough from bronchiectasis most likely results from the accumulation of excessive secretions because of excessive production, inadequate clearance, or both. Although bronchiectasis should be suspected when cough is associated with expectoration of greater than 30 mL of purulent sputum in 24 hours, bronchorrhea is not specific for bronchiectasis. In 40% of cases, chronic cough with bronchorrhea is caused by UACS, not bronchiectasis.[34] Plain chest radiographs often suggest bronchiectasis when they show increased lung markings and size and loss of definition of segmental markings. When bronchiectasis is not apparent on a plain chest roentgenogram, but suspicion for this diagnosis remains high, high-resolution chest CT is the optimal method for further evaluation.[34]

Difficulty swallowing from any cause may result in chronic cough because of recurrent aspiration of material into the airway.[58] Recurrent aspiration is the cause of cough in approximately 1% of patients presenting to a chronic cough clinic.[2] However, recurrent aspiration does not necessarily cause chronic cough, perhaps because mechanical cough receptors become desensitized with prolonged or frequent stimulation. When pharyngeal dysfunction or aspiration is suspected, referral to a speech and swallowing specialist for videofluoroscopic swallow evaluation or flexible endoscopic evaluation of swallowing is appropriate.

Although bronchogenic carcinoma is not a common cause of chronic cough, it should be considered when the chest radiograph is abnormal, especially when the film shows centrally located lesions.[2,59] Cough is a presenting symptom in 21% to 87% of patients who have bronchogenic carcinoma, but occurs in 70% to 90% of patients during the course of the disease.[31] In long-term cigarette smokers, the new development of a chronic cough or a change in the character of cough should suggest bronchogenic carcinoma.[60]

Chronic cough, along with the symptom of shortness of breath, is a frequent presenting symptom in interstitial lung disease.[33,61,62] However, in patients who have interstitial lung disease presenting with chronic cough, the interstitial lung disease, even if prominent radiographically, is not necessarily causing the cough.[32] One prospective study in patients who had known interstitial lung disease found that 18

Box 2
Miscellaneous causes of chronic cough

Bronchogenic carcinoma

Metastatic carcinoma

Sarcoidosis

Left ventricular failure

Aspiration from a Zenker diverticulum or difficulty in swallowing

Benign and malignant laryngeal lesions

Psychogenic

Tuberculosis (the latter especially in underdeveloped countries and high-risk groups)

of 30 episodes of chronic cough were the result of other conditions, including UACS, asthma, GERD, bronchiectasis, and exacerbation of chronic obstructive pulmonary disease.[32]

Psychogenic cough is uncommon and should never be diagnosed until all other causes, both common and uncommon, are ruled out.[2,63] Experts have suggested that patients who have psychogenic cough typically do not cough at night and have barking or honking coughs, but these characteristics are not diagnostically helpful. For instance, cough from any variety of diseases is unlikely to occur once patients fall asleep and may well be barking or honking without any diagnostic implication. Other uncommon causes of chronic cough, such as irritating lesions in the external auditory canal, have been summarized and these, along with the more common causes of cough described earlier, must all be excluded before psychogenic cough is diagnosed.[55,63] Please see the chapter on unexplained cough for further discussion of psychogenic cough in this issue.

SUMMARY

Evaluating cough is challenging for primary care physicians, pulmonologists, allergists, and otolaryngologists worldwide. However, an organized approach that starts with classifying cough according to the duration of the symptom has been effective in clinical settings in Asia,[11] North America,[1] South America,[12] and Europe.[9,10] Acute cough lasts less than 3 weeks and is most commonly caused by the common cold. Subacute cough lasts 3 to 8 weeks and is commonly postinfectious in origin. Chronic cough lasts more than 8 weeks. Once cigarette smoking, ACE inhibitor use, and an abnormal chest radiograph have been excluded, chronic cough is most commonly caused by UACS, asthma, NAEB, or GERD.

REFERENCES

1. Irwin RS, Baumann MH, Bolser DC, et al. Diagnosis and management of cough executive summary: ACCP evidence-based clinical practice guidelines. Chest 2006;129:1S–23S.
2. Irwin RS, Curley FJ, French CL. Chronic cough: the spectrum and frequency of causes, key components of the diagnostic evaluation, and outcome of specific therapy. Am Rev Respir Dis 1990;141:640–7.
3. Irwin RS, Madison JM. The diagnosis and treatment of cough. N Engl J Med 2000;343:1715–21.
4. Irwin RS, Madison JM. The persistently troublesome cough. Am J Respir Crit Care Med 2002;165:1469–74.
5. Madison JM, Irwin RS. Diagnosis and treatment of cough. Respiratory medicine. In: Dale DC, Federman DD, editors. ACP medicine. New York: WebMD Inc; 2007. p. 1–10.
6. Madison JM, Irwin RS. Chronic cough with a normal CXR. In: Brown K, Lee-Chiong T, editors. Oxford American handbook of pulmonary medicine. New York: Oxford University Press, Inc; 2009. p. 523–38.
7. Madison JM, Irwin RS. Diagnosis and treatment of acute, subacute and chronic cough in adults. Available at: http://www.antimicrobe.org. Accessed November 16, 2009.
8. Kuzniar TJ, Morgenthaler TI, Afessa B, et al. Chronic cough from the patient's perspective. Mayo Clin Proc 2007;82:56–60.
9. Morice AH, McGarvey L, Pavord I. Recommendations for the management of cough in adults. Thorax 2006;61:i1–24.

10. Morice. AH and committee members. The diagnosis and management of chronic cough. Eur Respir J 2004;24:481–92.
11. Kohno S, Ishida T, Uchida Y, et al. The Japanese respiratory society guidelines for the management of cough. Respirology 2006;11:S135–86.
12. II Brazilian guidelines for the management of chronic cough. J Bras Pneumol 2006;32:S403–46.
13. Schappert SM, Burt CW. Ambulatory care visits to physicians offices, hospital outpatient departments, and emergency departments: United States, 2001–2002. National Center of Health Statistics. Vital Health Stat 20 2006;13:1–66.
14. Office of Population Censuses and Surveys. Morbidity statistics from general practice: 4th national study 1991–1992. London: Her Majesty's Stationery Office; 1995. MB5 no. 3.
15. Morice AH, Fontana GA, Belvisi MG, et al. ERS guidelines on the assessment of cough. Eur Respir J 2007;29:1256–76.
16. French C, Irwin RS, Curley FJ, et al. Impact of chronic cough on quality of life. Arch Intern Med 1998;158:1657–61.
17. Chung KF, Pavord ID. Chronic cough 1. Prevalence, pathogenesis, and causes of chronic cough. Lancet 2008;371:1364–74.
18. Morice AH. Review series: chronic cough: epidemiology. Chron Respir Dis 2008; 5:43–7.
19. ACNielsen Strategic Planner. The Nielsen Company; 2007. p. 1.
20. Dettmar PW, Strugala V, Fathi H, et al. The online Cough Clinic: developing guideline-based diagnosis and advice. Eur Respir J 2009;34:819–24.
21. McCool FD. Global physiology and pathophysiology of cough: ACCP evidence-based clinical practice guidelines. Chest 2006;129(Suppl 1):48S–53S.
22. Bianco S, Robuschi M. Mechanics of cough. In: Braga PC, Alegra L, editors. Cough. New York: Raven Press; 1989. p. 29–36.
23. Irwin RS. Cough. In: Irwin RS, Curley FJ, Grossman RF, editors. Diagnosis and treatment of symptoms of the respiratory tract. Armonk (NY): Futura Publishing Company; 1997. p. 1–54.
24. Curley FJ, Irwin RS, Pratter MR, et al. Cough and the common cold. Am Rev Respir Dis 1988;138:305–11.
25. Diehr P, Wood RW, Bushyhead JB, et al. Prediction of pneumonia in outpatients with acute cough. J Chronic Dis 1984;37:215–25.
26. Rosen MJ. Cough in the immunocompromised host: ACCP evidence-based clinical practice guidelines. Chest 2006;129(Suppl 1):204S–5S.
27. Moser KM. Pulmonary embolism. Am Rev Respir Dis 1977;115:829–52.
28. Braman SS. Postinfectious cough: ACCP evidence-based clinical practice guidelines. Chest 2006;129(Suppl 1):138S–46S.
29. Kwon NH, Oh MJ, Min TH, et al. Causes and clinical features of subacute cough. Chest 2006;129:1142–7.
30. Braman SS. Chronic cough due to acute bronchitis: ACCP evidence-based clinical practice guidelines. Chest 2006;129(Suppl 1):95S–103S.
31. Kvale PA. Chronic cough due to lung tumors: ACCP evidence-based clinical practice guidelines. Chest 2006;129(Suppl 1):147S–53S.
32. Madison JM, Irwin RS. Chronic cough in adults with interstitial lung disease. Curr Opin Pulm Med 2005;11:412–6.
33. Brown KK. Chronic cough due to chronic interstitial pulmonary diseases: ACCP evidence-based clinical practice guidelines. Chest 2006;129(Suppl 1):180S–5S.
34. Rosen MJ. Chronic cough due to bronchiectasis: ACCP evidence-based clinical practice guidelines. Chest 2006;129(Suppl 1):122S–31S.

35. Irwin RS, Corrao WM, Pratter MR. Chronic persistent cough in the adult: the spectrum and frequency of causes and successful outcome of specific therapy. Am Rev Respir Dis 1981;123:413–7.
36. Pavord ID, Chung KF. Chronic cough 2, Management of chronic cough. Lancet 2008;371:1375–84.
37. Medical Research Council. Committee report on the aetiology of chronic bronchitis: definition and classification of chronic bronchitis for clinical and epidemiologic purposes. Lancet 1965;1:775–8.
38. Israili ZH, Hall WD. Cough and angioneurotic edema associated with angiotensin-converting enzyme inhibitor therapy: a review of the literature and pathophysiology. Ann Intern Med 1992;117:234–42.
39. Dicpinigaitis PV. Angiotensin-converting enzyme inhibitor–induced cough: ACCP evidence-based clinical practice guidelines. Chest 2006;129(Suppl 1): 169S–73S.
40. Lacourciere Y, Brunner H, Irwin R, et al. Effects of modulators of the renin-angiotensin-aldosterone system on cough. J Hypertens 1994;12:1387–93.
41. Gibson PG, Dolovich J, Denburg J, et al. Chronic cough: eosinophilic bronchitis without asthma. Lancet 1989;1:1346–8.
42. Brightling CE. Chronic cough due to nonasthmatic eosinophilic bronchitis: ACCP evidence-based clinical practice guidelines. Chest 2006;129(Suppl 1): 116S–21S.
43. Ayik SO, Basoglu OK, Erdine M, et al. Eosinophilic bronchitis as a cause of chronic cough. Respir Med 2003;97:695–701.
44. Berry MA, Brightling CE, Hargadon B, et al. Observational study of the natural history of eosinophilic bronchitis. Clin Exp Allergy 2005;35:598–601.
45. Pratter MR. Chronic upper airway cough syndrome secondary to rhinosinus diseases (previously referred to as postnasal drip syndrome): ACCP evidence-based clinical practice guidelines. Chest 2006;129(Suppl 1):63S–71S.
46. Sanu A, Eccles R. Postnasal drip syndrome. Two hundred years of controversy between UK and USA. Rhinology 2008;46:86–91.
47. Dicpinigaitis PV. Chronic cough due to asthma: ACCP evidence-based clinical practice guidelines. Chest 2006;129(Suppl 1):75S–9S.
48. Corrao WM, Braman SS, Irwin RS. Chronic cough as the sole presenting manifestation of bronchial asthma. N Engl J Med 1979;300:633–7.
49. Niimi A, Matsumoto H, Minakuchi M, et al. Airway remodeling in cough-variant asthma. Lancet 2000;356:564–5.
50. Hargreave FE, Ramsdale EH, Pugsley SO. Occupational asthma without bronchial hyper-responsiveness. Am Rev Respir Dis 1984;130:513–5.
51. Lemiere C, Efthimiadis A, Hargreave FE. Occupational eosinophilic bronchitis without asthma: an unknown occupational airway disease. J Allergy Clin Immunol 1997;100:852–3.
52. Brightling CE, Bradding P, Symon FA, et al. Mast-cell infiltration of airway smooth muscle in asthma. N Engl J Med 2002;346:1699–705.
53. Irwin RS, French CL, Curley FJ, et al. Chronic cough due to gastroesophageal reflux: clinical, diagnostic, and pathogenetic aspects. Chest 1993;104:1511–7.
54. Ing AJ, Ngu MC, Breslin AB. Pathogenesis of chronic persistent cough associated with gastroesophageal reflux. Am J Respir Crit Care Med 1994;149: 160–7.
55. Irwin RS. Chronic cough due to gastroesophageal reflux disease: ACCP evidence-based clinical practice guidelines. Chest 2006;129(Suppl 1): 80S–94S.

56. Prakash UB. Uncommon causes of cough. Chest 2006;129(Suppl 1):206S–19S.
57. Rosen MJ. Chronic cough due to tuberculosis and other infections. Chest 2006; 129(Suppl 1):197S–201S.
58. Smith Hammond CA, Goldstein LB. Cough and aspiration of food and liquids due to oral-pharyngeal dysphagia: ACCP evidence-based clinical practice guidelines. Chest 2006;129(Suppl 1):154S–68S.
59. Hyde L, Hyde CI. Clinical manifestations of lung cancer. Chest 1974;65:299–306.
60. Hoffstein V. Persistent cough in nonsmokers. Can Respir J 1994;1:40–7.
61. Guerry-Force ML, Muller NL, Wright JL, et al. A comparison of bronchiolitis obliterans with organizing pneumonia, usual interstitial pneumonia and small airways disease. Am Rev Respir Dis 1987;135:705–12.
62. Hope-Gill BD, Hilldrup S, Davies C, et al. A study of the cough reflex in idiopathic pulmonary fibrosis. Am J Respir Crit Care Med 2003;168:995–1002.
63. Irwin RS, Glomb WB, Chang AB. Habit cough, tic cough, and psychogenic cough in adult and pediatric populations: ACCP evidence-based clinical practice guidelines. Chest 2006;129(Suppl 1):174S–9S.

Afferent Nerves Regulating the Cough Reflex: Mechanisms and Mediators of Cough in Disease

Brendan J. Canning, PhD

KEYWORDS

• Capsaicin • Vagal • Bradykinin • N-Methyl-D-Aspartate

The cough reflex protects the airways and lungs from aspiration, inhaled irritants, particulates, and pathogens and clears the air spaces of accumulated secretions. Studies in animals provide conclusive evidence that cough is initiated by activation of vagal afferent nerves. Precisely which afferent nerve subtypes regulate cough has been debated and reviewed elsewhere.[1] In this review, the author describes the stimuli that initiate cough and the mechanisms by which these stimuli activate airway sensory nerves. These data are related to the known physiologic properties of bronchopulmonary afferent nerve subtypes. The review concludes with a discussion of the potential interactions between afferent nerve subtypes and the possible mechanisms of altered cough reflexes in disease.

CHEMICAL AND MECHANICAL STIMULI THAT INITIATE COUGHING

Multiple chemical and mechanical stimuli initiate coughing in humans and in animals.[1–4] Several of these stimuli, including capsaicin, citric acid, hypertonic saline, and low chloride buffers/solutions are often used to evoke cough experimentally. Other stimuli known to initiate coughing in animals and humans include particulate/dust; mechanical/vibratory stimulation of the airway mucosa larynx or chest wall; chemical irritants, such as resiniferatoxin, cinnamaldehyde, and allyl isothiocyanate (AITC); and the

Funding for the authors research is provided by a grant from the National Institutes of Health (HL083192).
Financial disclosure: The author's research is funded by grants from the National Institutes of Health and by grants from Eisai, Glaxo-Smithkline, Merck, and Sanofi-Aventis. The author has no other financial interests relevant to the contents of this article.
Department of Medicine, Division of Allergy and Clinical Immunology, Johns Hopkins Asthma and Allergy Center, 5501 Hopkins Bayview Circle, Baltimore, MD 21224, USA
E-mail address: bjc@jhmi.edu

Otolaryngol Clin N Am 43 (2010) 15–25
doi:10.1016/j.otc.2009.11.012 oto.theclinics.com

autacoids bradykinin, anandamide, and prostaglandin E2 (PGE2). Although seemingly varied in origin and chemical composition, many of these stimuli share common modes of action. For example, acids/protons, capsaicin, resiniferatoxin, and anandamide all act in part or entirely by activation of the ion channel/receptor transient receptor potential vanilloid 1(TRPV1).[3,5–12] Bradykinin and PGE2 may also act in part through TRPV1 activation.[13–16] Cinnamaldehyde, AITC, and several other known respiratory irritants (eg, cigarette smoke, toluene diisocyanate) activate the ion channel transient receptor potential ankyrin (TRPA1).[17–19] Knowing the specific ion channels and receptors for the stimuli that initiate cough is important, as this information can be used to identify which afferent nerves express these ion channels and receptors. This information can then be used to identify possible mechanisms for coughing in disease, but may also suggest therapeutic approaches to restore normal cough function and sensitivity (**Table 1**).

The stimuli that do not initiate coughing are equally helpful when attempting to identify the specific vagal afferent nerve subtypes that regulate this reflex (**Table 2**). These stimuli may also suggest a great complexity underlying the cough associated with disease. Consider, for example, three of the most common causes of chronic cough: asthma, gastroesophageal reflux disease (GERD), and upper airway inflammatory diseases (eg, allergic rhinitis, sinusitis).

These conditions are often found simultaneously in patients who have chronic cough.[20,21] Although none of these disorders are adequately described by a single presenting symptom, it is generally agreed that reversible airways obstruction, acidic refluxate in the esophagus, and inflammation of the upper airways are characteristics of asthma, GERD, and upper airway diseases, respectively. Remarkably, however, bronchospasm, acid in the esophagus and upper airway challenges with a variety of inflammatory mediators are consistently ineffective at initiating cough in animals or human subjects.[1,22–24] The inability of these stimuli to initiate cough is not because they fail to activate sensory nerves. Histamine, capsaicin, allergen, and bradykinin all initiate sneezing and reflex-dependent mucus secretion when delivered selectively to the upper airways; whereas the bronchoconstrictors histamine, substance P, and even methacholine evoke reflex-dependent changes in autonomic tone in the airways; changes in breathing pattern; and respiratory sensations, such as chest tightness and dyspnea.[1,22,25,26] Esophageal acidification is known to evoke reflex bronchospasm in animals and in human subjects but has rarely if ever been reported to initiate coughing.[24,26–30] Observations such as these argue against the afferent nerves responding to these stimuli as the primary initiators of cough in disease, which implies the involvement of other afferent nerves and afferent-nerve subtype interactions in disease. Defining precisely how these afferent nerves interact to produce the coughing

Table 1
Stimuli initiating cough: mode of action and afferent nerve targets

Stimulus	Mode of Action	Afferent Nerves Targeted
Capsaicin	TRPV1	C fibers
Bradykinin	Bradykinin B2 receptors	C fibers
Acid	TRPV1, acid-sensing ion channels	C fibers, cough receptors
Particulates	Unknown	Cough receptors, C fibers
TRPA1 agonists	TRPA1	C fibers
Prostaglandin E2	Prostaglandin EP3 receptors	C fibers
Nicotine	Nicotinic receptors	C fibers

Table 2
Stimuli that do not initiate cough: reflexes evoked, afferent nerves activated

Stimulus	Reflexes Evoked	Afferent Nerves Targeted
Bronchoconstriction[a]	Mucus secretion, tachypnea	RARs
Esophageal acid	Bronchospasm, mucus secretion	Esophageal nociceptors
Upper airway stimulation	Sneeze, mucus secretion	Trigeminal afferent nerves
Inc. airway luminal pressure	Respiratory slowing	SARs
Dec. airway luminal pressure	Tachypnea	RARs
Adenosine	Tachypnea, dyspnea	RARs, C fibers
Pulmonary embolism	Tachypnea, dyspnea	RARs, C fibers

Abbreviations: Dec, decrease; Inc, increase; RARs, rapidly adapting receptors; SARs, slowly adapting receptors.

[a] Bronchoconstrictors including histamine, methacholine, leukotriene D4, thromboxane A2, and neurokinin. Failure to reliably evoke coughing in humans or in animals despite initiating reflex bronchospasm and mucus secretion, an increase in respiratory rate and dyspnea.

observed in diseases, such as asthma and GERD, are likely be critical to the development of better therapeutic strategies for the treatment of chronic cough.

AFFERENT NERVES REGULATING THE COUGH REFLEX

Coughing can be partitioned into at least four phases. The initial phase comprises the encoding of action potentials by the afferent nerves directly responding to the tussive stimulus and the subsequent reconfiguration of the respiratory motor drive within the brainstem. This initial phase immediately precedes any change in respiratory muscle activity. The second phase is the enhanced inspiratory effort that accompanies cough. The expiratory phase of cough has two components: (1) an initial compressive phase when expiration is initiated against a restricted or occluded upper airway; and (2) the expulsive phase, when the upper airways are dilated, allowing forceful expiration and the high airflow velocities that facilitate airway clearance.

Depending on the stimulus and social situation, the number and forcefulness of the resulting coughs can vary substantially. Given this complexity and the multiple elements involved (lower and upper airways, respiratory muscles, brain stem), it is apparent that multiple afferent nerve subtypes act in concert to regulate the sensitivity, forcefulness, and repetitions of coughs in response to all tussive stimuli. The following discussion focuses only on those afferents involved in the initial encoding phase of cough (**Fig. 1**).

C Fibers

Bronchopulmonary C fibers are identified physiologically by their action potential conduction velocity, which falls in the *C* range ($\leq$1 m/s) of the compound action potential. C fibers comprise the majority of afferent nerves innervating the airways and lungs, terminating in the mucosa and submucosa of the nose, pharynx, larynx, trachea, bronchi, and throughout the lungs. C fibers project to the airways from the jugular and nodose ganglia of the vagus nerves, and from thoracic dorsal root ganglia.[1,31–33]

Bronchopulmonary C fibers are activated by capsaicin, bradykinin (**Fig. 2**), protons, nicotine, and the TRPA1 agonists cinnamaldehyde and AITC. C fibers are selectively desensitized by high-dose capsaicin treatment that also prevents coughing evoked by

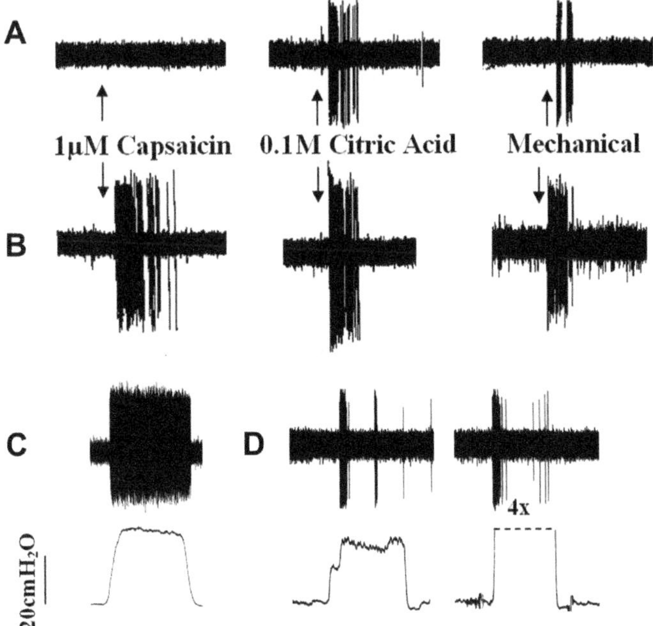

Fig. 1. Representative extracellular recordings from the vagal afferent nerve subtypes innervating the airways and lungs. (*Reproduced from* Canning BJ, Mazzone SB, Meeker SN, et al. Identification of the tracheal and laryngeal afferent neurones mediating cough in anaesthetized guinea-pigs. J Physiol 2004;557:543–58; with permission.)

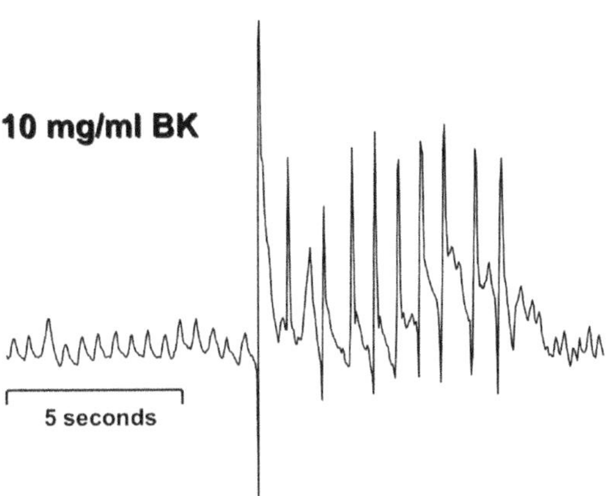

Fig. 2. A representative trace of coughing recorded from a guinea pig following exposure to an aerosol of bradykinin (BK) is shown. Many animal species cough in response to the same stimuli that initiate coughing in human subjects, which permits more mechanistic studies of the cough reflex and has led to the development of novel therapeutic strategies for the treatment of cough. (*Reproduced from* Canning BJ, Mazzone SB, Meeker SN, et al. Identification of the tracheal and laryngeal afferent neurones mediating cough in anaesthetized guinea-pigs. J Physiol 2004;557:543–58; with permission.)

citric acid.[34] In guinea pigs, C fibers use the peptide neurotransmitters substance P and neurokinin A that act primarily by way of neurokinin$_1$ (NK_1), NK_2, and NK_3 receptors. Neurokinin-receptor antagonists prevent coughing evoked in guinea pigs by capsaicin and citric acid.[35–38] These results and observations provide conclusive evidence that C-fiber activation initiates coughing.

Despite the overwhelming evidence that C-fiber activation can initiate coughing, the role of C fibers in cough remains controversial. Much of the controversy arises from the inability of C-fiber selective stimuli to initiate coughing in anesthetized animals.[1,22,26,39,40] It seems likely that anesthesia selectively inhibits C-fiber–dependent coughing. But anesthesia does not readily explain the observation that C-fiber activation not only fails to initiate coughing in anesthetized animals but also actively inhibits coughing evoked by activation of other afferent nerves subtypes.[39,40] The author speculated that these opposing effects of C fibers on cough might be attributable to the opposing actions of C-fiber subtypes. Studies performed in guinea pigs using stimuli that are selective for vagal C-fiber subtypes suggest that C fibers arising from the nodose ganglia can acutely inhibit coughing, whereas activation of C fibers arising from the jugular ganglia sensitize or initiate coughing.[41,42] Circumstantial evidence suggests that C-fiber subtypes in humans play similar opposing roles.[2,43–45]

RAPIDLY ADAPTING RECEPTORS

Rapidly adapting receptors (RAR) are mechanoreceptors that respond to the dynamic physical forces associated with lung inflation and deflation. RARs are also activated by punctate mechanical stimuli and airway smooth muscle contraction.[31,46–48] The seminal work of Widdicombe has been interpreted as evidence that RARs play an essential role in the initiation of cough.[46,49] A critical reassessment of Widdicombe's studies suggests otherwise.[41]

Central to the thesis that RARs play a role in the initiation of cough in anesthetized animals has been the inability of C-fiber–selective stimuli to initiate cough, and the sensitivity of the cough reflex to vagal cooling temperatures that target myelinated afferent nerves, such as RARs.[40,46,49] Slowly adapting receptors (SAR), the stretch receptors that regulate the Hering-Breuer reflex, are not implicated in the initiation of cough,[1,41,46,49] and with C-fiber–selective stimuli failing to evoke cough and nearly all airway sensory nerve classification schemes limited to three types (C fibers, RARs, and SARs), RARs have been implicated largely by default.[1,31,41,47–49] But there is overwhelming evidence against a role for RARs in cough. Hyperventilation and maximal inspiratory efforts against a closed glottis, for example, are effective at activating RARs and consistently ineffective at initiating cough.[1,41] Bronchoconstrictors, such as histamine, neurokinin A, the cysteinyl leukotrienes, and even methacholine, are also effective stimulants of RARs but rarely if ever initiate coughing.[1,22,41,48,50]

The imprecise semantics often used in describing airway afferent nerve subtypes likely contributes to the misconception that RARs regulate coughing. The term RAR is used to describe a variety of afferent nerve subtypes that differ substantially in peripheral termination sites, sensitivity to mechanical stimuli, and in the reflexes initiated upon their activation. The term *rapidly adapting*, when used as a means of differentiating airway afferent nerve subtypes, should refer only to the response of afferent nerves to sustained lung inflation. Indeed, RARs adapt only modestly to smooth muscle contraction/bronchoconstriction or lung deflation.[1,41] By contrast, most bronchopulmonary afferent nerves adapt rapidly to punctate mechanical stimuli. Studies in guinea pigs and a reappraisal of Widdicombe's work performed in cats suggests that vagal afferent nerves that are distinct from RARs but possessing RAR like characteristics likely regulate the coughing studied in anesthetized animals.[41,48]

COUGH RECEPTORS

Coughing can be initiated in anesthetized animals by mechanically probing the laryngeal, tracheal, or bronchial mucosa or by acid applied topically to the mucosa of these airways.[22,35,41,48–50] C-fiber selective stimuli (eg, capsaicin and bradykinin) consistently fail to initiate coughing, as does sustained lung inflation (which activates SARs), or the bronchoconstrictors histamines, neurokinin A and methacholine. Sustained or dynamic increases or decreases in intraluminal pressure in an isolated segment of the extrathoracic trachea also fails to initiate coughing, whereas acid applied topically to this tracheal segment readily initiates cough. Electrophysiological analyses combined with these physiologic studies of cough suggest that a vagal afferent nerve subtype distinct from RARs, SARs, and C fibers plays an essential role in the initiation of cough.[22,26,41,48]

The cough receptors are myelinated as evidenced by their action potential conduction velocity (~5 m/s) and terminate almost exclusively in the larynx, trachea, and extrapulmonary bronchi. These afferents are insensitive to airway smooth muscle contraction or changes in intraluminal pressure, but are exquisitely sensitive to punctate mechanical stimuli. The cough receptors are also activated by acid and by the voltage-gated K+ channel blocker 4-aminopyridine.[22,48]

Cough receptors terminate peripherally in the submucosa of the laryngeal, tracheal, and bronchial mucosa.[22,48,51,52] The termination of these afferent nerves branch extensively in a circumferential arbor, adhered to the subepithelial matrix and largely uncoupled to the underlying smooth muscle. Their structure and sites of termination give the appearance of a spider adhered to its web, sensing mechanical stimuli transduced through the intricate structure of the extracellular matrix. Their sites of termination and sensitivity to acid and to punctate mechanical stimuli render the cough receptors ideally suited to protect the airways from aspiration and to facilitate clearance of accumulated secretions.

Physiologic and pharmacologic studies have identified several mechanisms regulating cough-receptor excitability.[22,48,52,53] The cough receptors are insensitive to capsaicin and bradykinin, and therefore do not express the capsaicin receptor TRPV1. Acid activates the cough receptors, perhaps through gating of acid-sensing ion channels. Other regulatory mechanisms identified on the peripheral terminals of the cough receptors include unique isozymes of Na+-K+-ATPase and the Na+-K+-2Cl- transporter and voltage-gated sodium and chloride channels. Centrally, the cough receptors use glutamate acting by way of N-Methyl-D-Aspartate (NMDA) and non-NMDA receptors to initiate coughing.[1,54]

AFFERENT NERVE INTERACTIONS IN COUGH AND MECHANISMS OF COUGH IN DISEASE

There is considerable evidence for vagal afferent nerve convergence onto subpopulations of relay neurons in the nucleus of the solitary tract. Such convergence may account for the imprecise nature of visceral reflexes, whereby vagal afferent nerve activation in one organ reflexively initiates changes in autonomic outflow to other organs.[42,55,56] Similar interactions likely regulate the cough reflex and may explain the extrapulmonary origins of cough in some patients.

Studies performed in guinea pigs suggest that bronchopulmonary C fibers and cough receptors may act synergistically to regulate coughing.[42] As discussed

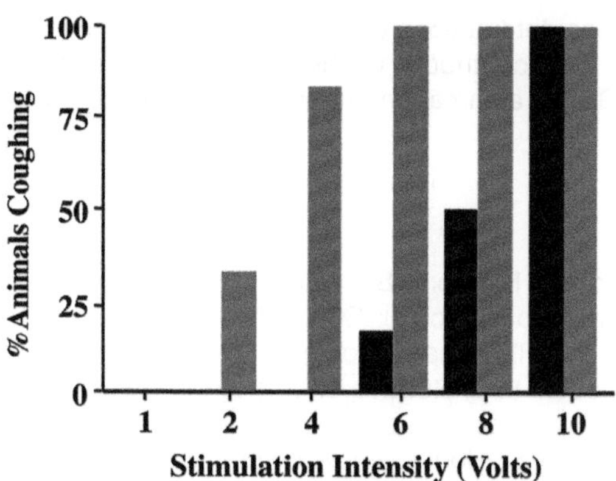

Fig. 3. Cough reflex sensitivity can be enhanced by coincident activation of airway afferent nerve subtypes. Coughing was evoked electrically from the tracheal mucosa of anesthetized guinea pigs. Optimal stimulation frequencies (16 Hz) and pulse duration were maintained during 10-second stimuli delivered at varying stimulation voltages. The percentage of animals coughing at various voltages was determined in animals inhaling saline (*black bars*) or the C-fiber stimulant bradykinin (1mg/mL; *gray bars*). (*Reproduced from* Mazzone SB, Mori N, Canning BJ. Synergistic interactions between airway afferent nerve subtypes regulating the cough reflex in guinea-pigs. J Physiol 2005;569:559–73; with permission.)

previously, C-fiber activation is consistently ineffective at initiating cough in anesthetized animals. But C-fiber activation coincident with cough-receptor stimulation produces a heightened sensitivity to tussive challenge (**Fig. 3**). This sensitizing effect of C-fiber activation is similar to the central sensitization attributed to somatic C fibers in models of pain.[57] Like central sensitization in somatic tissues, neurokinin-receptor antagonists prevent the sensitizing effects of bronchopulmonary C-fiber activation in cough.

Vagal afferent nerve interactions may account for the coughing attributed to gastroesophageal reflux disease. Refluxate or acid in the esophagus are very ineffective at initiating cough in animals or in humans and refluxate rarely reaches the airways or even the pharynx. But acid or capsaicin infusion into the esophageal lumen markedly enhances airway sensitivity to tussive stimuli.[58,59] This sensitizing effect of acid or capsaicin in the esophagus on subsequently evoked cough suggests that in patients presenting with GERD cough, in addition to the sensitizing refluxate in the esophagus, some tussive stimuli or condition within the airways ultimately initiates coughing. Evidence for airway inflammation in GERD has been presented.[60–63] A similar sensitizing effect on cough may also account for the coughing associated with upper airways diseases.[64]

SUMMARY

The cough reflex is initiated by activation of bronchopulmonary C fibers and the mechanically-sensitive cough receptors. Stimuli initiating cough through activation of one or both of these vagal afferent nerves include capsaicin, acid, bradykinin, cinnamaldehyde, cigarette smoke, and non-isotonic aerosols. Multiple ion channels and cell surface receptors regulating the response to these tussive stimuli have been identified. The cough receptors and C fibers may interact centrally to produce a heightened sensitivity to challenge. Interactions of afferent pathways innervating the esophagus and upper airways may contribute to the heightened cough sensitivity in chronic diseases, such as GERD, asthma, and upper airways disorders.

REFERENCES

1. Canning BJ, Mori N, Mazzone SB. Vagal afferent nerves regulating the cough reflex. Respir Physiolo Neurobiol 2006;152(3):223–42.
2. Karlsson JA, Fuller RW. Pharmacological regulation of the cough reflex–from experimental models to antitussive effects in Man. Pulm Pharmacol Ther 1999; 12:215–28.
3. Laude EA, Higgins KS, Morice AH. A comparative study of the effects of citric acid, capsaicin and resiniferatoxin on the cough challenge in guinea-pig and man. Pulm Pharmacol 1993;6:171–5.
4. Maher SA, Belvisi MG. Prostanoids and the cough reflex. Lung 2009. [Epub ahead of print].
5. Bolser DC, Aziz SM, Chapman RW. Ruthenium red decreases capsaicin and citric acid-induced cough in guinea pigs. Neurosci Lett 1991;126:131–3.
6. Jia Y, McLeod RL, Wang X, et al. Anandamide induces cough in conscious guinea-pigs through VR1 receptors. Br J Pharmacol 2002;137:831–6.
7. Gu Q, Lee LY. Characterization of acid signaling in rat vagal pulmonary sensory neurons. Am J Physiol Regul Integr Comp Physiol 2006;291(1):L58–65.
8. Kollarik M, Undem BJ. Mechanisms of acid-induced activation of airway afferent nerve fibres in guinea-pig. J Physiol 2002;543:591–600.
9. Lalloo UG, Fox AJ, Belvisi MG, et al. Capsazepine inhibits cough induced by capsaicin and citric acid but not by hypertonic saline in guinea pigs. J Appl Phys 1995;79:1082–7.
10. Leung SY, Niimi A, Williams AS, et al. Inhibition of citric acid- and capsaicin-induced cough by novel TRPV-1 antagonist, V112220, in guinea-pig. Cough 2007;3:10.
11. Lin YS, Lee LY. Stimulation of pulmonary vagal C-fibres by anandamide in anaesthetized rats: role of vanilloid type 1 receptors. J Physiol 2002;539(Pt 3): 947–55.
12. Trevisani M, Milan A, Gatti R, et al. Antitussive activity of iodo-resiniferatoxin in guinea pigs. Thorax 2004;59:769–72.
13. Carr MJ, Kollarik M, Meeker SN, et al. A role for TRPV1 in bradykinin-induced excitation of vagal airway afferent nerve terminals. J Pharmacol Exp Ther 2003; 304(3):1275–9.
14. Kollarik M, Undem BJ. Activation of bronchopulmonary vagal afferent nerves with bradykinin, acid and vanilloid receptor agonists in wild-type and TRPV1-/- mice. J Physiol 2004;555(Pt 1):115–23.
15. Schnizler K, Shutov LP, Van Kanegan MJ, et al. Protein kinase A anchoring via AKAP150 is essential for TRPV1 modulation by forskolin and prostaglandin E2 in mouse sensory neurons. J Neurosci 2008;28(19):4904–17.
16. Ho CY, Gu Q, Hong JL, et al. Prostaglandin E(2) enhances chemical and mechanical sensitivities of pulmonary C fibers in the rat. Am J Respir Crit Care Med 2000; 162(2 Pt 1):528–33.
17. Andrè E, Gatti R, Trevisani M, et al. Transient receptor potential ankyrin receptor 1 is a novel target for pro-tussive agents. Br J Pharmacol 2009; 158(6):1621–8.

18. Birrell MA, Belvisi MG, Grace M, et al. TRPA1 agonists evoke coughing in guinea-pig and human volunteers. Am J Respir Crit Care Med 2009;180(11):1042–7.
19. Taylor-Clark TE, Nassenstein C, McAlexander MA, et al. TRPA1: a potential target for anti-tussive therapy. Pulm Pharmacol Ther 2009;22(2):71–4.
20. Irwin RS, Baumann MH, Bolser DC, et al. Diagnosis and management of cough executive summary: ACCP evidence-based clinical practice guidelines. Chest 2006;129(Suppl 1):1S–23S.
21. Morice AH, Fontana GA, Sovijarvi AR, et al. ERS task force. The diagnosis and management of chronic cough. Eur Respir J 2004;24(3):481–92.
22. Canning BJ, Farmer DG, Mori N. Mechanistic studies of acid-evoked coughing in anesthetized guinea pigs. Am J Physiol Regul Integr Comp Physiol 2006;291: R454–63.
23. Ing AJ, Ngu MC, Breslin AB. Pathogenesis of chronic persistent cough associated with gastroesophageal reflux. Am J Respir Crit Care Med 1994;149(1):160–7.
24. Irwin RS, French CL, Curley FJ, et al. Chronic cough due to gastroesophageal reflux. Clinical, diagnostic, and pathogenetic aspects. Chest 1993;104(5):1511–7.
25. Canning BJ. Reflex regulation of airway smooth muscle tone. J Appl Phys 2006; 101(3):971–85.
26. Chou YL, Scarupa MD, Mori N, et al. Differential effects of airway afferent nerve subtypes on cough and respiration in anesthetized guinea pigs. Am J Physiol Regul Integr Comp Physiol 2008;295(5):R1572–84.
27. Mansfield LE, Stein MR. Gastroesophageal reflux and asthma: a possible reflex mechanism. Ann Allergy 1978;41(4):224–6.
28. Schan CA, Harding SM, Haile JM, et al. Gastroesophageal reflux-induced bronchoconstriction. An intraesophageal acid infusion study using state-of-the-art technology. Chest 1994;106(3):731–7.
29. Mazzone SB, Canning BJ. Evidence for differential reflex regulation of cholinergic and noncholinergic parasympathetic nerves innervating the airways. Am J Respir Crit Care Med 2002;165(8):1076–83.
30. Spaulding HS Jr, Mansfield LE, Stein MR, et al. Further investigation of the association between gastroesophageal reflux and bronchoconstriction. J Allergy Clin Immunol 1982;69(6):516–21.
31. Coleridge JC, Coleridge HM. Afferent vagal C fibre innervation of the lungs and airways and its functional significance. Rev Physiol Biochem Pharmacol 1984;99: 1–110.
32. Kollarik M, Dinh QT, Fischer A, et al. Capsaicin-sensitive and -insensitive vagal bronchopulmonary C-fibres in the mouse. J Physiol 2003;551:869–79.
33. Undem BJ, Chuaychoo B, Lee MG, et al. Subtypes of vagal afferent C-fibres in guinea-pig lungs. J Physiol 2004;556:905–17.
34. Forsberg K, Karlsson JA, Theodorsson E, et al. Cough and bronchoconstriction mediated by capsaicin-sensitive sensory neurons in the guinea-pig. Pulm Pharmacol 1988;1:33–9.
35. Bolser DC, DeGennaro FC, O'Reilly S, et al. Central antitussive activity of the NK1 and NK2 tachykinin receptor antagonists, CP-99,994 and SR 48968, in the guinea-pig and cat. Br J Pharmacol 1997;121:165–70.
36. Daoui S, Cognon C, Naline E, et al. Involvement of tachykinin NK3 receptors in citric acid-induced cough and bronchial responses in guinea pigs. Am J Respir Crit Care Med 1998;158:42–8.
37. Girard V, Naline E, Vilain P, et al. Effect of the two tachykinin antagonists, SR 48968 and SR 140333, on cough induced by citric acid in the unanaesthetized guinea pig. Eur Respir J 1995;8:1110–4.

38. Ujiie Y, Sekizawa K, Aikawa T, et al. Evidence for substance P as an endogenous substance causing cough in guinea pigs. Am Rev Respir Dis 1993;148(6 Pt 1): 1628–32.
39. Tatar M, Webber SE, Widdicombe JG. Lung C-fibre receptor activation and defensive reflexes in anaesthetized cats. J Physiol 1988;402:411–20.
40. Tatar M, Sant'Ambrogio G, Sant'Ambrogio FB. Laryngeal and tracheobronchial cough in anesthetized dogs. J Appl Phys 1994;76:2672–9.
41. Canning BJ, Chou YL. Cough sensors. I. Physiological and pharmacological properties of the afferent nerves regulating cough. Handb Exp Pharmacol 2009;187:23–47.
42. Mazzone SB, Mori N, Canning BJ. Synergistic interactions between airway afferent nerve subtypes regulating the cough reflex in guinea-pigs. J Physiol 2005;569:559–73.
43. Stone RA, Worsdell YM, Fuller RW, et al. Effects of 5-hydroxytryptamine and 5-hydroxytryptophan infusion on the human cough reflex. J Appl Phys 1993;74: 396–401.
44. Winning AJ, Hamilton RD, Shea SA, et al. Respiratory and cardiovascular effects of central and peripheral intravenous injections of capsaicin in man: evidence for pulmonary chemosensitivity. Clin Sci (Lond) 1986;71(5):519–26.
45. Burki NK, Dale WJ, Lee LY. Intravenous adenosine and dyspnea in humans. J Appl Phys 2005;98:180–5.
46. Widdicombe JG. Receptors in the trachea and bronchi of the cat. J Physiol 1954; 123:71–104.
47. Ho CY, Gu Q, Lin YS, et al. Sensitivity of vagal afferent endings to chemical irritants in the rat lung. Respir Physiol 2001;127:113–24.
48. Canning BJ, Mazzone SB, Meeker SN, et al. Identification of the tracheal and laryngeal afferent neurones mediating cough in anaesthetized guinea-pigs. J Physiol 2004;557:543–58.
49. Widdicombe JG. Respiratory reflexes from the trachea and bronchi of the cat. J Physiol 1954;123:55–70.
50. House A, Celly C, Skeans S, et al. Cough reflex in allergic dogs. Eur J Pharmacol 2004;492:251–8.
51. Hunter DD, Undem BJ. Identification and substance P content of vagal afferent neurons innervating the epithelium of the guinea pig trachea. Am J Respir Crit Care Med 1999;159:1943–8.
52. Mazzone SB, Reynolds SR, Mori N, et al. Selective expression of a sodium pump isozyme by cough receptors and evidence for its essential role in regulating cough. J Neurosci 2009;29(43):13662–71.
53. Mazzone SB, McGovern AE. Na+-K+-2Cl- cotransporters and Cl- channels regulate citric acid cough in guinea pigs. J Appl Phys 2006;101(2):635–43.
54. Canning BJ. Central regulation of the cough reflex: therapeutic implications. Pulm Pharmacol Ther 2009;22(2):75–81.
55. Paton JF. Pattern of cardiorespiratory afferent convergence to solitary tract neurons driven by pulmonary vagal C-fiber stimulation in the mouse. J Neurophysiol 1998;79(5):2365–73.
56. Silva-Carvalho L, Paton JF, Rocha I, et al. Convergence properties of solitary tract neurons responsive to cardiac receptor stimulation in the anesthetized cat. J Neurophysiol 1998;79(5):2374–82.
57. Latremoliere A, Woolf CJ. Central sensitization: a generator of pain hypersensitivity by central neural plasticity. J Pain 2009;10(9):895–926.

58. Javorkova N, Varechova S, Pecova R, et al. Acidification of the oesophagus acutely increases the cough sensitivity in patients with gastro-oesophageal reflux and chronic cough. Neurogastroenterol Motil 2008;20(2):119–24.
59. Wu DN, Yamauchi K, Kobayashi H, et al. Effects of esophageal acid perfusion on cough responsiveness in patients with bronchial asthma. Chest 2002;122(2):505–9.
60. Patterson RN, Johnston BT, Ardill JE, et al. Increased tachykinin levels in induced sputum from asthmatic and cough patients with acid reflux. Thorax 2007;62(6): 491–5.
61. Sacco O, Silvestri M, Sabatini F, et al. IL-8 and airway neutrophilia in children with gastroesophageal reflux and asthma-like symptoms. Respir Med 2006;100(2): 307–15.
62. Chang AB, Gibson PG, Ardill J, et al. Calcitonin gene-related peptide relates to cough sensitivity in children with chronic cough. Eur Respir J 2007;30(1):66–72.
63. Groneberg DA, Niimi A, Dinh QT, et al. Increased expression of transient receptor potential vanilloid-1 in airway nerves of chronic cough. Am J Respir Crit Care Med 2004;170(12):1276–80.
64. Plevkova J, Kollarik M, Brozmanova M, et al. Modulation of experimentally-induced cough by stimulation of nasal mucosa in cats and guinea pigs. Respir Physiolo Neurobiol 2004;142(2–3):225–35.

Mucus and Mucins

Bruce K. Rubin, MEngr, MD, MBA, FRCPC

KEYWORDS

- Sputum • Mucus • Mucins • Phlegm • Cough
- Rheology • Tenacity

Normal airway mucus lines epithelial surfaces that are potentially exposed to the outside environment. Mucins and mucus can detoxify noxious or reactive aerosols, decrease ambient water loss for the epithelia, and capture and clear inhaled pathogens and particles. The normal mucin network may also inhibit bacterial biofilm formation. The major macromolecular constituents of normal mucus are the secreted gel-forming mucin glycoproteins. Phlegm production is a hallmark of chronic inflammatory airway diseases such as bronchiectasis, chronic bronchitis, and cystic fibrosis. When expectorated, phlegm is called sputum. Sputum has altered macromolecular and polymer composition and biophysical properties, which vary with disease. Mucin glycoprotein overproduction and hypersecretion are common features of chronic inflammatory airway disease. However, in some pathologic conditions such as cystic fibrosis, airway sputum contains little intact mucin and has increased content of DNA, filamentous actin, and lipids. Cough clearance is a secondary airway defense when mucociliary clearance is impaired. The effectiveness of cough depends on volume and flow of exhaled air and the biophysical properties of airway phlegm.

Mucus secretion and clearance is the primary physical defense of the airway epithelium. The energy intensive process of mucin synthesis, oligomerization, granule storage, and, finally, exocytosis serves as protection for epithelial surfaces exposed to an external environment. Mucus secretion defends the eyes, nose, middle ear, airways, and urogenital tract from microbial invasion. Mucin polymers, or mucus, prevent water loss and dehydration of these epithelia, and mucus production and clearance by cilia are an important means of airway hygiene.

While mucus plays a defensive role, mucus overproduction can overwhelm mucociliary clearance, producing airflow obstruction. Infection and inflammation in the airway leads to poor mucus clearance, stimulates mucus secretion and production,[1] and can cause ciliary dysfunction.[2] Retained secretion containing mucus and inflammatory products with DNA and filamentous (F)-actin copolymers (**Fig. 1**) is called phlegm from the Greek word for inflammation.[3] Excessive phlegm is cleared by cough, which can be an effective secondary defense of the airway. When phlegm is expectorated, it is then called sputum.

Department of Pediatrics, Virginia Commonwealth University School of Medicine, 1001 East Marshall Street, P.O. Box 980646, Richmond, VA 23298, USA
E-mail address: brubin@vcu.edu

Otolaryngol Clin N Am 43 (2010) 27–34
doi:10.1016/j.otc.2009.11.002
0030-6665/10/$ – see front matter

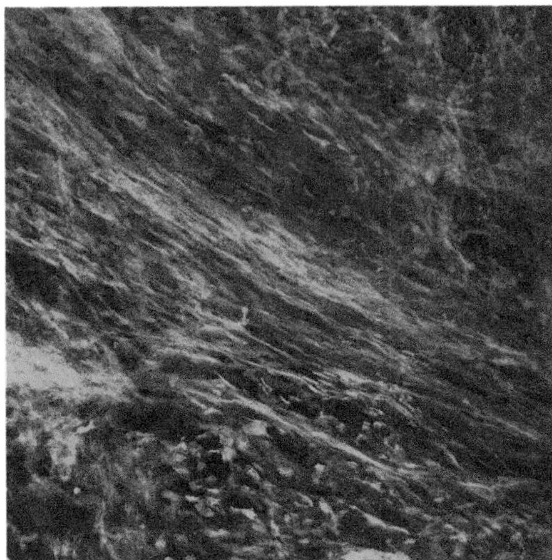

Fig. 1. Confocal micrograph of cystic fibrosis sputum showing prominent copolymers of DNA and F-actin, in green, but no significant amount of mucin.

COMPOSITION OF MUCUS AND PHLEGM

Mucus is the normal secretory product lining the epithelium. It is more than 90% water with the principal polymeric component being the gel-forming mucins MUC5B and MUC5AC. The former is a primary secretory polymeric protein from submucosal glands and the latter is the main gel-forming mucin from surface mucous or goblet cells.[4] There are small amounts of MUC2 in the airways of persons with chronic infection and inflammation such as in bronchiectasis or cystic fibrosis (CF). MUC7 is expressed in serous cells of the submucosal glands but gene expression levels are not altered in chronic airway diseases such as CF.[5] In health, these gel-forming mucins form long, linearly linked oligomers joined by disulfide bonds. In normal mucus, there is minimal intramolecular cross-linking and the polymeric nature comes from the length of the oligomers and their entanglement, producing what has been called a "tangled network."[4] The abnormal sputum structure seen in conditions like plastic bronchitis or fatal asthma may be due to abnormal cross-linking between adjacent mucin oligomers (**Fig. 2**).[6]

The core mucin proteins are heavily decorated by sugar moieties forming a bottle-brush structure. Serine and threonine are prominent among these sugars. Studies of the core proteins in mucins have been hampered as antibodies to the core mucin proteins may bind poorly because of the carbohydrate coat.

Between the epithelium and the mucus layer is periciliary fluid, or airway surface fluid (ASF). While ASF was once thought to be a simple iso-osmolar, low density, Newtonian liquid, it is now known to contain a complex network of membrane-bound mucins attached to the epithelium microvilli and cilia, including MUC1 and MUC16.[7] The nature of the interaction between this ASF network and the overlying mucus layer is an area of active investigation. It is thought that the hydration of the airway surface liquid is largely regulated by ion channels in the epithelial surface including the CF transmembrane ion regulator channel, the calcium activated chloride channel, and the epithelial sodium channel.[8]

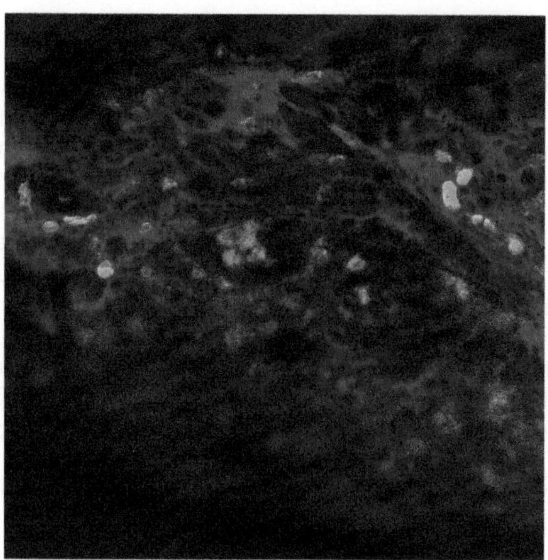

Fig. 2. Confocal micrograph of a plastic bronchitis cast showing dense mucin polymers in red but no copolymers of DNA and F-actin. DNA, pseudo-color green, is only stained within the nuclei of inflammatory cells.

Mucus clearance is determined, in part, by cilia or airflow acting on the mucus and by the interaction between the mucous layer and the epithelium below. These, in turn, are influenced by the biophysical and surface properties of the mucous layer.[9]

Rheology is the study of the deformation and flow of matter under an applied stress. It is used to characterize material behavior as liquid, solid, or gel-like. An ideal, or Newtonian, liquid responds to an applied stress by an induced deformation with energy loss. The amount of deformation relative to the energy loss determines the loss modulus (viscosity) of the substance. An ideal, or Hookian, solid responds to an applied stress by energy storage and release of this stored energy when the stress ceases. This storage modulus is called elasticity. The complex modulus, also known as mechanical impedance, is the vector sum of viscosity and elasticity and is sometimes referred to as the rigidity factor. A viscoelastic substance or gel, like mucus, responds to an applied stress by initially storing energy and, with continued stress, it will flow like a liquid. When the stress is removed, the stored energy is released. The elastic behavior of mucus is important for ciliary transport as it allows the kinetic energy of beating cilia to be used for mucus transport. In the absence of elasticity, this interaction would be inefficient. Conversely, a viscous component is needed to prevent the elastic mucus from snapping back between ciliary beats and it allows the mucus to flow after secretion from submucosal glands.[10]

For a gel, viscosity and elasticity are not static measures but vary with the energy or stress that is applied. Many gels have an increase in viscosity as the shear rate increases; this is called shear thickening. Some gels will have a decrease in viscosity with applied stress but will thicken when the stress is removed. This reversible shear thinning, or thixotropy, is characteristic of paints which can be spread with an applied stress (like brushing) and then rapidly thicken after the stress is removed, preventing the paint from running off. Some gels have a sudden and dramatic decrease in viscosity that is permanent and caused by irreversible breaking of polymeric bonds under stress. This is called apparent yield stress.[11] The sudden yielding of the polymeric structure may enhance bulk transport by cough.

Viscoelastic behavior that is favorable for ciliary clearance may not be ideal for cough clearance. Ciliary clearance is most effective when there is a fairly low viscosity and preserved elasticity while cough clearance tends to be better with higher viscosity secretion and is less affected by elasticity.[12] However, it is the surface properties of the phlegm that most strongly determine the cough clearability of secretions.[13]

The principal surface properties of mucus or phlegm are the interfacial or surface tension and wettability as measured by the contact angle of a droplet of the secretion. Wettability and interfacial tension can be used to calculate the work of adhesion, which is the attractive force of a liquid or gel to a surface like the airway epithelium. Cohesivity is the tendency for a gel to remain attracted to itself and form threads when slowly stretched. This thread forming ability is called spinnbarkeit or spinnability, and is measured using a device called a Filancemeter. Spinnability can be mathematically transformed into cohesivity, and the product of adhesivity and cohesivity is called tenacity. The tenacity of mucus appears to be the strongest determinant of its cough clearability in vitro.[14]

MUCIN SECRETION AND MUCUS CLEARANCE

Mucus secretion is often stimulated by infectious and inflammatory mediators as protective response. There are a variety of pathways involved in mucin secretion, including stimulation of chloride channels,[15] activation of the epithelial growth factor receptor,[16] cell stress, and environmental challenges such as exposure to hyperosmolarity.[17] Surface goblet cells are not directly innervated but they can rapidly degranulate and release mucin to environmental stress. Secretion from the serous cells and mucous cells in the submucosal gland is under receptor-mediated response and neurogenic control, and, therefore, can be modulated by agents like muscarinic antagonists.

Most of the factors that stimulate mucin secretion also stimulate ciliary beating; although faster ciliary beating does not necessarily lead to faster mucociliary transport.[18] Although the term mucus hypersecretion is frequently used for secretion retention in the airways, secretion retention can be due to impaired ciliary function or to mucus hypersecretion that overwhelms the ciliary clearance mechanism. Ciliary dysfunction can be congenital or acquired with acquired ciliary dysfunction often resulting from airway infection or inflammation. Persons with primary ciliary dyskinesia (PCD) who have congenital ciliary dysfunction usually have less lung disease than persons with CF,[19] suggesting that cough is an important clearance mechanism for patients with PCD and that defective mucociliary clearance is probably not the most important factor contributing to lung disease in CF.

The biophysical properties of mucus are modified by secretion hydration, the degree of polymerization of the mucous gel, and additional polymeric constituents such as DNA and F-actin copolymers associated with chronic inflammation and neutrophil necrosis. This secondary network is extremely tenacious and contributes to the poor cough clearability of CF sputum.[20]

Just as it is difficult to know if there is mucus hypersecretion based on secretion retention, it is also true that the volume of sputum expectorated is a poor indicator of the effectiveness of an intervention meant to improve mucus clearance. This is due to temporal changes in the rate of secretion clearance, variable dilution of expectorated sputum with saliva, reticence to expectorate, weakness contributing to a poor expiratory airflow and cough, and reduction in the volume of phlegm because of therapy leading to less sputum expectorated. With the possible exception of short-term acute interventions, expectorated sputum volume is a poor indicator of the degree of impairment or improvement. In addition, the color and texture of sputum do not indicate whether there is hypersecretion or infection.[21]

Cough clearance depends on the properties of the phlegm and the cough. An explosive cough with a large volume of air and rapid airflow is more likely to shear secretions and propel them in the airway. This is associated with effective vocal cord closure and preserved muscle strength. Both of these can be compromised in persons with neuromuscular weakness or patients who receive sedative or paralytic agents. Secretions that are viscous and exhibit apparent yield stress may be easier to propel by cough. It is also easier to cough while sitting or standing upright perhaps because this presents a greater profile of the secretion droplet to the cough airflow.[22]

Because phlegm adherence to the epithelial surface is one of the strongest determinants of cough impairment, there may be a role of mucolytics in unsticking secretions from the epithelium, thus breaking adhesive bonds. Abhesive (the opposite of adhesive) drugs that reduce secretion stickiness can be effective in promoting cough clearance and improving pulmonary function. There is evidence that surfactant phospholipids reduce the surface tension of airway mucus in the proximal airway and make the ciliary beating more effective at propelling mucus.[23] It has been demonstrated that there is surfactant dysfunction and an increase in sputum tenacity associated with diseases such as chronic obstructive pulmonary disease (COPD) and CF.[24]

UPPER AND LOWER AIRWAY MUCUS

Combined upper and lower airway diseases have been well described in persons with asthma, CF, and COPD, and the severity of upper airway disease is often related to the severity of lower airway disease.[25,26] Because of the common nature of infection and inflammation, it is likely that this response also includes an increased volume of secretions. There are few data evaluating the biophysical properties and transport properties of nasal secretions and lower respiratory secretions in the same subjects who have upper airway and lung disease. Therefore, it is not known if inflammation and infection in both locations is associated with similar changes in secretion biophysical and transport properties. It is also not clear if the lower airway disease or nasal airway disease precedes one another, of if these occur more or less simultaneously.

THERAPY FOR MUCUS CLEARANCE DISORDERS

Given the various ways that mucus can be cleared from the airway and the changes in airway secretions associated with inflammation and infection, different medications have been proposed for improving mucus clearance. Collectively, these are referred to as mucoactive medications.[27]

Mucolytics

By definition, mucolytics are drugs that decrease the viscoelasticity of secretions by severing polymers. Classic mucolytics, such as N-acetylcysteine, cleave disulfide bonds connecting mucin oligomers and, thus, reduce the viscoelasticity of disulfide-linked proteins such as mucin. The classic mucolytics do not have an effect on the secondary DNA–F-actin polymer network and, therefore, there are not useful for the treatment of diseases such as CF, chronic bronchitis, or bronchiectasis. Mucin secretion is defensive and mucin can neutralize some proinflammatory mediators (eg, cytokines and reactive oxygen species), and mucin may inhibit bacterial biofilm formation. Thus the severing of mucin bonds may be disadvantageous to the host.[28]

The peptide mucolytics are meant to hydrolyze the DNA polymer network, the F-actin polymer network, or both. The example in clinical use is dornase alfa, which hydrolyzes DNA polymers. Dornase is now routinely used for treating CF airway disease but it is ineffective for treating diseases where there is phlegm without a significant DNA component (eg, COPD and asthma).[29]

Drugs such as thymosin beta 4 can depolymerize the F-actin network and act as a peptide mucolytics. Thymosin beta 4 also appears to synergize with dornase in breaking down the secondary network.[30] These drugs are under development for diseases like bronchiectasis and CF:

1. Expectorants are drugs that are meant to improve cough clearability by improving the hydration and volume of secretions. The consumption of large volume of liquids is ineffective as an expectorant and most traditional expectorant medications are also ineffective.[31] Among the more interesting modern expectorants are the hyperosmolar medications such as 7% saline aerosol, used to treat CF,[32] and dry powder mannitol, which is in clinical testing for the therapy of bronchiectasis and CF.[33] These medications draw fluid into the airway, but they do not appear to add fluid to the mucous layer. Thus, their function may be to unstick the secretions from the airway surface. These medications induce coughing, which can contribute to their effectiveness, and they are potent mucin secretagogues. Increased mucus secretion may be beneficial in patients with CF.[34]
2. The mucokinetic agents are thought to improve ciliary beat frequency or power and include drugs like the beta agonist bronchodilators. These have a small effect on improving mucociliary clearance; however, their greatest benefit may be in improving expiratory airflow and, therefore, cough effectiveness in patients with narrowed airways.[31]
3. Mucospissic medications such as tetracycline can increase the viscosity of secretions—perhaps by increasing polymer crosslink density. Although not used clinically, theoretically these may improve clearance of secretions in patients with very thin mucus, such as those who have bronchorrhea. They may also be useful in decreasing droplet formation and reducing the risk of spreading airborne microorganisms with coughing.[35]
4. Abhesive drugs can decrease the tenacity of secretions, dramatically improving cough clearance. Examples, discussed earlier, are the aerosol surfactants.[24]
5. Mucoregulatory medications are meant to decrease chronic mucus hypersecretion associated with airway inflammation. Among the best studied of these are the macrolide antibiotics. These down-regulate the hyperinflammatory response through immunomodulation that is principally mediated through the extracellular-regulated kinase or extracellular-regulated kinase 1/2 pathway.[36] Anticholinergic medications can reduce submucosal gland secretions by blocking cholinergic signaling through muscarinic receptors. Although these agents can produce dry mouth, there is no evidence that they dehydrate mucus secretions.[37]

SUMMARY

A variety of mucoactive medications are used to treat chronic lung disease. When evaluating the role of the cough, it must be considered as an important protective mechanism. Therefore, it may be more important to improve the effectiveness of cough than to suppress or eliminate a chronic cough in patients with chronic lung disease.

REFERENCES

1. Voynow JA, Rubin BK. Mucus, mucins, and sputum. Chest 2009;135:505–12.
2. Thomas B, Rutman A, O'Callaghan C. Disrupted ciliated epithelium shows slower ciliary beat frequency and increased dyskinesia. Eur Respir J 2009;34:401–4.
3. Rubin BK. Mucus, phlegm, and sputum in cystic fibrosis. Respir Care 2009;54: 726–32.
4. Thornton DJ, Rousseau K, McGuckin MA. Structure and function of the polymeric mucins in airways mucus. Annu Rev Physiol 2008;70:459–86.
5. Sharma P, Dudus L, Nielsen PA, et al. MUC5B and MUC7 are differentially expressed in mucous and serous cells of submucosal glands in human bronchial airways. Am J Respir Cell Mol Biol 1998;19:30–7.
6. Sheehan JK, Richardson PS, Fung DC, et al. Analysis of respiratory mucus glycoproteins in asthma: a detailed study from a patient who died in status asthmaticus. Am J Respir Cell Mol Biol 1995;13:748–56.
7. Davies JR, Kirkham S, Svitacheva N, et al. MUC16 is produced in tracheal surface epithelium and submucosal glands and is present in secretions from normal human airway and cultured bronchial epithelial cells. Int J Biochem Cell Biol 2007;39:1943–54.
8. Matsui H, Randell SH, Peretti SW, et al. Coordinated clearance of periciliary liquid and mucus from airway surfaces. J Clin Invest 1998;102:1125–31.
9. Rubin BK, Fink JB, Henke MO. Mucus-controlling drug therapy. In: Doug Gardenhire, editor. Rau's respiratory care pharmacology. 7th edition. Philadelphia (PA): Elsevier Press; 2008. p. 162–90.
10. King M, Rubin BK. Mucus rheology, relationship with transport. In: Takishima T, editor. Airway secretion: physiological bases for the control of mucus hypersecretion. New York: Marcel Dekker, Inc; 1994. p. 283–314, chapter 7.
11. Basser PJ, McMahon TA, Griffith P. The mechanism of mucus clearance in cough. J Biomech Eng 1989;111:288–97.
12. Hassan AA, Evrensel CA, Krumpe PE. Clearance of viscoelastic mucus simulant with airflow in a rectangular channel, an experimental study. Technol Health Care 2006;14:1–11.
13. Albers GM, Tomkiewicz RP, May MK, et al. Ring distraction technique for measuring surface tension of sputum: relationship to sputum clearability. J Appl Phys 1996;81:2690–5.
14. Rubin BK. Surface properties of respiratory secretions: relationship to mucus transport. In: Baum G, editor. Cilia, mucus, and mucociliary interactions. New York: Marcel Dekker, Inc; 1998. p. 317–24, chapter 32.
15. Clunes MT, Boucher RC. Front-runners for pharmacotherapeutic correction of the airway ion transport defect in cystic fibrosis. Curr Opin Pharmacol 2008;8:292–9.
16. Burgel PR, Nadel JA. Roles of epidermal growth factor receptor activation in epithelial cell repair and mucin production in airway epithelium. Thorax 2004; 59:992–6.
17. Kishioka C, Okamoto K, Kim J-S, Rubin BK. Hyperosmolar solutions stimulate mucus secretion in the ferret trachea. Chest 2003;124:306–13.
18. Katz I, Zwas T, Baum GL, et al. Ciliary beat frequency and mucociliary clearance. What is the relationship? Chest 1987;92:491–3.
19. Bush A, Payne D, Pike S, et al. Mucus properties in children with primary ciliary dyskinesia: comparison with cystic fibrosis. Chest 2006;129:118–23.
20. Rubin BK. Mucus structure and properties in cystic fibrosis. Paediatr Respir Rev 2007;8:4–7.

21. Rubin BK. Designing clinical trials to evaluate mucus clearance therapy. Respir Care 2007;52:1348–61.
22. Ragavan AJ, Evrensel CA, Krumpe P. Interactions of airflow oscillation, tracheal inclination, and elasticity significantly improve mucus clearance during simulated cough. Chest, in press. PMID:19762551.
23. Allegra L, Bossi R, Braga P. Influence of surfactant on mucociliary transport. Eur J Respir Dis Suppl 1985;142:71–6.
24. Anzueto A, Jubran A, Ohar JA, et al. Effects of aerosolized surfactant in patients with stable chronic bronchitis. A prospective randomized controlled trial. JAMA 1997;278:1426–31.
25. Kim J-S, Rubin BK. Nasal and sinus involvement in chronic obstructive pulmonary disease. Curr Opin Pulm Med 2008;14:101–4.
26. Robertson JM, Friedman EM, Rubin BK. Nasal and sinus disease in cystic fibrosis. Paediatr Respir Rev 2008;9:213–9.
27. Rubin BK, Tomkiewicz RP, King M. Mucoactive agents: old and new. In: Wilmott Robert W, editor. The pediatric lung. Basel (Switzerland): Birkhäuser Publishing, Ltd; 1997. p. 155–79, chapter 7.
28. Henke MO, Renner A, Huber RM, et al. MUC5AC and MUC5B mucins are decreased in cystic fibrosis airway secretions. Am J Respir Cell Mol Biol 2004; 31:86–91.
29. Rubin BK. Who will benefit from DNase? Pediatr Pulmonol 1999;27:3–4.
30. Kater A, Henke MO, Rubin BK. The role of DNA and actin polymers on the polymer structure and rheology of cystic fibrosis sputum and depolymerization by gelsolin or thymosin beta 4. Ann N Y Acad Sci 2007;1112:140–53.
31. Rubin BK. Mucolytics, expectorants, and mucokinetic medications. Respir Care 2007;52:859–65.
32. Donaldson SH, Bennett WD, Zeman KL, et al. Mucus clearance and lung function in cystic fibrosis with hypertonic saline. N Engl J Med 2006;354:241–50.
33. Daviskas E, Anderson SD, Gomes K, et al. Inhaled mannitol for the treatment of mucociliary dysfunction in patients with bronchiectasis: effect on lung function, health status and sputum. Respirology 2005;10:46–56.
34. Henke MO, Gerrit J, Germann M, et al. MUC5AC and MUC5B mucins increase in cystic fibrosis airway secretions during a pulmonary exacerbation. Am J Respir Crit Care Med 2007;175:816–21.
35. Zayas G, Valle JC, Alonso M, et al. A new paradigm in respiratory hygiene: modulating respiratory secretions to contain cough bioaerosol without affecting mucus clearance. BMC Pulm Med 2007;13(7):11.
36. Shinkai M, López-Boado Y, Rubin BK. Clarithromycin has an immunomodulatory effect on ERK-mediated inflammation induced by P. aeruginosa flagellin. J Antimicrob Chemother 2007;59:1096–101.
37. Kishioka C, Okamoto K, Kim JS, et al. Regulation of secretion from mucous and serous cells in the excised ferret trachea. Respir Physiol 2001;126:163–71.

Cough and Swallowing Dysfunction

Milan R. Amin, MD[a,*], Peter C. Belafsky, MD, MPH, PhD[b]

KEYWORDS

- Cough • Cough reflex • Dysphagia
- Swallowing • Aerodigestive tract

The cough reflex is a highly developed and essential airway protective mechanism. The primary developmental obstacle for evolution from aquatic to earth subsistence was the ability to protect the lower airway from the incursion of liquid and food. Thus, in order of phylogenetic importance, the three functions of the larynx are airway protection, respiration, and phonation.[1] Reflexive glottic closure has evolved into one of the primary methods of airway protection. Stimulation of peripheral afferents innervated by the internal branch of the superior laryngeal nerve (SLN) triggers the laryngeal adductor response (LAR). The LAR is a rapid stimulation of the thyroarytenoid muscles in response to ipsilateral SLN stimulus.[2] Its purpose is to protect the airway from invading food and liquid from above. Bilateral stimulation of the SLN results in sphincteric closure of the glottis at three different levels: (1) aryepiglottic folds, (2) false vocal folds, and (3) true vocal folds.[3]

The LAR can be measured clinically with laryngopharyngeal sensory testing.[4] An air pulse stimulus can be administered to the laryngeal mucosa innervated by the SLN through a specialized endoscope and the magnitude of the stimulus necessary to elicit the LAR is measured. The importance of the LAR has been established. Individuals with dysphagia and an absent LAR aspirate thin liquid nearly 94% of the time in comparison to an aspiration rate of 17% for individuals with an intact LAR.[5] Once a food or liquid bolus has penetrated the laryngeal defenses, the cough reflex provides the final protective mechanism to expel the invading material.

Viewed from a mechanical perspective, coughing involves several important coordinated actions (**Fig. 1**). The initial phase typically involves inhalation. During this phase, the vocal folds are fully abducted, allowing for deep, rapid inflow of air.

[a] Department of Otolaryngology/Head and Neck Surgery, New York University School of Medicine, NYU Voice Center, 550 First Avenue, HCC, Suite 3C, New York, NY 10016, USA
[b] Department of Otolaryngology/Head and Neck Surgery, University of California, Davis, CA, USA
* Corresponding author.
E-mail address: milan.amin@nyumc.org (M.R. Amin).

Otolaryngol Clin N Am 43 (2010) 35–42
doi:10.1016/j.otc.2009.12.001

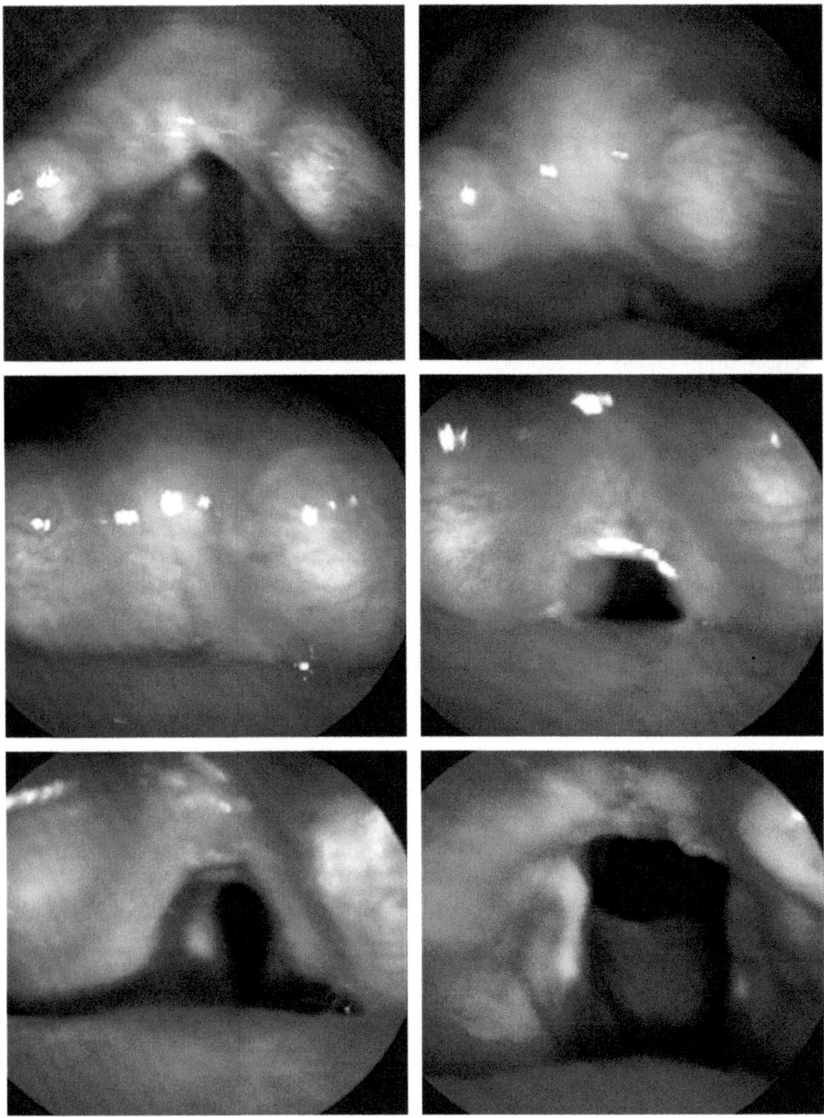

Fig. 1. Sequence of cough, demonstrating glottic closure followed by the explosive release of air.

The second phase consists of forceful exhalation against a closed glottis. Maximal adduction of the vocal folds and contraction of the aryepiglottic folds results in sphincteric closure of the glottis and supraglottis. During this phase, pressure is built up in the subglottis. This pressure results in narrowing of the upper trachea to up to one-sixth of its normal diameter, allowing for airflow rates nearing the speed of sound through this segment.[6] Structurally, the appearance of the larynx at this point is similar to that seen during the oropharyngeal phase of deglutition. However, the epiglottis is not retroverted, as the larynx remains in a low position. Additionally, the pressures generated at the glottic and subglottic levels are different during these two tasks. During swallowing, pressure generated at the glottic level from vocal cord closure is significantly higher than during cough. Conversely, subglottic pressure is much higher with a cough than with a swallow.[7] The third phase of the cough involves violent ejection of the air from the lungs after release of the laryngeal muscles. This release of air allows for the expulsion of secretions, mucus, or foreign material from the tracheobronchial tree. Passage of the air produces sound through the vibration of mucosa along the trachea, larynx, and vocal tract.

The cough reflex arc is initiated in sensory nerve endings and receptors located in the respiratory epithelium throughout the tracheobronchial tree. There are a few receptor types that are believed to trigger the cough reflex: mechanoreceptors, nociceptors, and so-called cough receptors. Mechanoreceptors respond to mechanical stimuli. This may be due to pressure on the mucosa (as may occur with aspirating a piece of food) or stretching of the mucosa (as may occur in the lungs with bronchospasm). Nociceptors respond to irritant or proinflammatory chemicals such as capsaicin, bradykinin, and citric acid that come in contact with the mucosa. In addition to these two receptor types, recent evidence has supported the presence of a separate primary receptor called the cough receptor, which responds to punctuate mechanical stimuli, low chloride solutions, and acids. This last receptor type is believed to exist largely in the larynx and trachea.[8–10]

Regardless of the trigger, the suprathreshold stimulation of the respiratory mucosa results in an afferent signal, which ultimately results in the cough sequence. The reflex arc involves afferent neurons traveling in the vagus nerve, which converge on the cough center, located in the medulla at the nucleus tractus solitarius. These neurons directly trigger efferent neurons, which bilaterally innervate the laryngeal adductor muscles (from the nucleus ambiguus via the vagus nerve), intercostal muscles, abdominal wall, diaphragm, and pelvic floor (in the cervical and thoracic spinal cord via phrenic and spinal motor nerves).

Here, there are overlaps with the swallowing sequence. The same afferent and efferent pathways used for coughing are used for a swallowing sequence. The different outcome (cough versus swallow) may be due to a difference in the initial trigger (food bolus in the oropharynx versus direct stimulation of the laryngeal mucosa) or different signaling based on the sensory receptors or afferent nerves. Additionally, though the neural anatomy is similar, there may be some important differences in the functional aspect of the signaling pathways. A recent article that examined the role of the internal branch of the superior laryngeal nerve found that blockade of this nerve alters laryngeal closure during swallowing, but does not affect voluntary closure during cough. Jafari and colleagues[11] concluded that this nerve might be involved in providing feedback to central neural pathways involved in laryngeal closure during the pharyngeal phase of swallowing.

Laryngeal closure is an important component of the cough reflex. Closure allows for buildup and release of subglottic pressure. The inability to close the glottis or supraglottis, as occurs with vocal fold paralysis, may result in a weak or ineffective cough, allowing secretions to accumulate in the trachea and lower airways, especially in otherwise weak or compromised patients. In addition, the presence of vocal fold paralysis in a patient has been found to increase the incidence of aspiration by 15% when compared with other patients referred for dysphagia evaluation.[12] This can be a critical issue, especially in patients with compromised pulmonary function.[13] Improving glottal closure, therefore, is an important consideration in preventing aspiration, restoring pulmonary function, and preventing deterioration.

Glottal insufficiency is typically addressed by vocal fold injection augmentation or laryngeal framework surgery. Both of these interventions aim to statically move the vocal fold toward the midline to allow for glottal closure. Whereas such procedures are commonly performed and successful outcomes have been reported,[14–17] there is, as yet, no large-scale, carefully performed study demonstrating benefit from glottal closure procedures alone for dysphagia resulting from unilateral vocal fold paralysis or paresis.

COUGH AND DYSPHAGIA

Cough is a brainstem-mediated, protective mechanism that functions, in part, to evict aspirated food and liquid from the lower respiratory tract. Oropharyngeal dysphagia with associated laryngeal penetration or aspiration should, therefore, be included in the differential diagnosis of persons with chronic cough. Symptoms and findings that suggest that the cough is associated with penetration or aspiration include increased cough with thin—as opposed to thick—liquids, a history of stroke or progressive neurologic disease, a history of oropharyngeal dysphagia, a history of head and neck cancer or head and neck surgery, the presence of a wet vocal quality, hoarseness, and coughing with meals as opposed to after meals. Postcibal cough is typically a sign of gastroesophageal or esophagopharyngeal reflux.[18] Some patients with a hypersensitive larynx also report coughing with meals and it is important to differentiate persons with a hypersensitive larynx from persons with oropharyngeal dysphagia who are at risk for aspiration. Alternative names for the hypersensitive larynx include vocal cord dysfunction and paradoxic vocal fold motion impairment. Patients with a hypersensitive larynx often report dyspnea or stridor with inspiration, excessive throat clearing, disproportionate throat mucus, neck tightness, intermittent dysphonia, and cough with spicy foods, vinegar, second hand tobacco, and perfumes. They are frequently diagnosed with asthma but fail treatment with inhaled corticosteroids and beta-agonists. The disorder is more prevalent in young overachieving female athletes. Cough attributable to vocal cord dysfunction is successfully treated with respiratory retraining. The goal of respiratory retraining is to create a rhythmic pattern by focusing on breathing with minimal expiratory force.[19] If the history suggests that cough may be due to laryngeal penetration or tracheal aspiration, a diagnostic workup is indicated.

FUNDAMENTALS OF SWALLOW ASSESSMENT

The oropharyngeal stage of swallowing may be evaluated by a clinical bedside assessment, endoscopy, or fluoroscopy. The bedside swallow evaluation involves administering a patient ice chips, water, or food and monitoring for cough, wet vocal quality, or voice change. Cervical auscultation and pulse oximetry may be added to increase diagnostic sensitivity. The predictive value of the bedside swallow evaluation is limited, however. Recent research has focused on improving the accuracy of bedside examinations. The assessment of voluntary cough strength (through measures of airflow dynamics) appears to demonstrate promise in improving sensitivity and specificity for the identification of aspirators.[20]

The gold standard swallowing assessment, however, has traditionally been the videofluoroscopic swallow evaluation (VSE) or modified barium swallow.[21] The VSE involves administering the patient barium sulfate under real-time fluoroscopic video recording. The rheology of the barium may be manipulated to test for aspiration with thin liquid or a variety of different viscosities. Aspiration with solid food can also be evaluated by adding barium to paste, puree, and solid food consistencies. The degree of laryngeal penetration and aspiration can be quantified with a validated penetration and aspiration scale (PAS).[22] Cough during the study is easily visualized and its association with aspiration is noted. An alternative to the VSE is the flexible endoscopic evaluation of swallowing or FEES. If the LAR is assessed with an air pulse stimulator during the FEES, the examination is referred to as a flexible endoscopic evaluation of swallowing with sensory testing or FEESST. A FEES and FEESST are performed in an unsedated patient sitting upright in an examination chair. A small caliber endoscope is passed through the nasal cavity and positioned in the pharynx above the tip of the epiglottis (**Fig. 2**). The entire examination is recorded for later slow-motion playback. The larynx is evaluated for lesions, masses, and edema. Pooling of saliva is a major risk factor for swallowing impairment, and aspiration and its presence in the pyriform sinuses is noted (**Fig. 3**). Vocal fold mobility is evaluated by having the patient perform the "eee-sniff maneuver." Having the patient say "eee" maximally adducts and sniffing maximally abducts the vocal folds. The presence of glottal insufficiency is a major risk factor for aspiration.[23] Nearly one quarter of patients with a paralyzed vocal fold will aspirate.[24] Laryngeal sensation is assessed with elicitation of the LAR with an air pulse stimulator or with the tip of the laryngoscope placed onto the aryepiglottic fold. An absent LAR is a significant risk factor for aspiration.[5]

Pharyngeal strength is assessed with the pharyngeal squeeze maneuver. The patient is instructed to say a forceful "eee." The examiner evaluates for movement of the lateral hypopharyngeal walls with the maneuver. An absent pharyngeal squeeze maneuver is also a predictor of aspiration.[25] The patient is then administered food and liquid of different consistencies impregnated with food coloring. The presence of penetration and aspiration during FEES can also be quantified with the PAS.[26] The ability of VSE and FEES to identify penetration and aspiration has been determined to be equal.[26,27] If a diagnostic study identifies an association between cough and

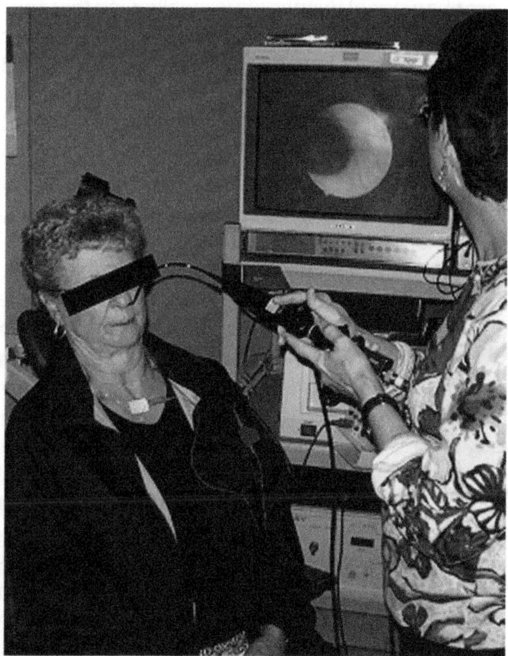

Fig. 2. Positioning during FEES.

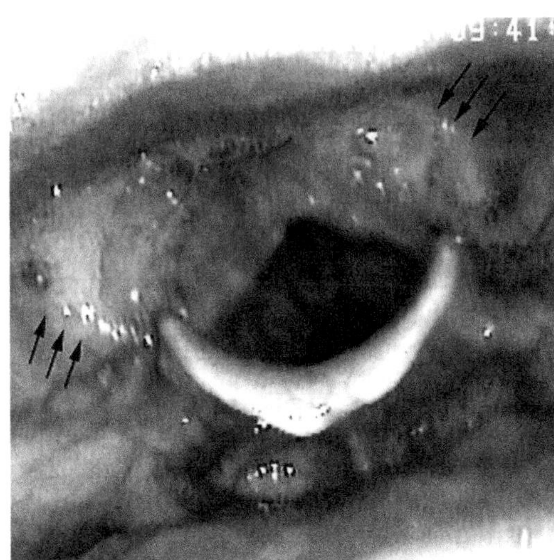

Fig. 3. Pooling of secretions in the pyriform sinuses (*black arrows*) during endoscopy and endoscopic evaluation of swallowing (FEES) is a significant risk factor for swallowing impairment, laryngeal penetration, and tracheal aspiration.

laryngeal penetration or tracheal aspiration, swallowing therapy is often successful at improving function, enhancing swallowing safety, and alleviating the cough.

FUNDAMENTALS OF SWALLOWING THERAPY

First-line therapy for oropharyngeal dysphagia is swallowing therapy. Depending on the individual needs and the cognitive ability of the patient, swallowing therapy typically focuses on the introduction of various swallowing maneuvers. Simply tucking the chin during deglutition shifts the epiglottis posteriorly, narrows the laryngeal vestibule, and improves airway protection.[28] A head turn to the side of a unilateral weakened pharynx or paralyzed vocal fold can encourage a food bolus to travel down the contralateral unaffected side and improve swallowing safety and reduce swallowing associated cough. The patient may be coached in a supraglottic swallowing maneuver. This maneuver is performed by having the patient take a breath and hold it while swallowing. A prophylactic cough is then performed to expel any contents that may have been aspirated during the swallow. An effortful swallow may increase lingual contraction force and assist with bolus transit through the hypopharynx. Motor exercises are often prescribed as an adjunct to swallowing maneuvers. These exercises can improve range of motion, laryngeal elevation, tongue base retraction, and upper esophageal sphincter opening.[29]

If swallowing therapy fails to limit the penetration and aspiration, the rheology of the food may be manipulated. If the patient is at risk for aspiration with thin liquids, simply adding a thickener can improve swallowing safety and alleviate cough during meals. If solids prove difficult, a soft mechanical or puree diet may be prescribed.

If conservative management is unsuccessful in mitigating the dysphagia and aspiration, surgery may be considered. Surgical procedures shown to improve swallowing function in certain individuals include esophageal dilation, cricopharyngeus myotomy, medialization laryngoplasty, laryngohyoid suspension, vocal fold closure, and total laryngectomy.[30–33] If the dysphagia is profound, nonoral enteral tube feeding may be recommended. Whereas this may not eliminate aspiration of secretions, it decreases the overall burden of aspirate, lessening the risk of developing pneumonia.

SUMMARY

This article reviewed the relationship between cough and swallowing. Given that cough is often an indication of microaspiration, patients presenting with cough should be screened for possible swallow impairment. If the initial screening reveals possible aspiration, a more comprehensive swallow assessment as outlined should be initiated.

Conversely, in patients with known swallow impairment, attention should be paid to their cough reflex. A weak cough can put individuals at increased risk of morbidity. Assessment and treatment of glottal closure problems may improve the cough and help to mitigate problems related to chronic aspiration.

REFERENCES

1. Sasaki CT. Laryngeal physiology for the surgeon. San Diego (CA): Plural Publishing Inc; 2007.
2. Ludlow CL, Van Pelt F, Koda J. Characteristics of late responses to superior laryngeal nerve stimulation in humans. Ann Otol Rhinol Laryngol 1992;101:127–34.
3. Sasaki CT, Hundal J, Ross DA. Laryngeal physiology. In: Fried MP, Ferlito A, editors. The larynx. 3rd edition. San Diego (CA): Plural Publishing Inc; 2007. p. 101–12.
4. Aviv JE, Martin JH, Kim T, et al. Laryngopharyngeal sensory discrimination testing and the laryngeal adductor reflex. Ann Otol Rhinol Laryngol 1999;108(8):725–30.
5. Aviv JE, Spitzer J, Cohen M, et al. Laryngeal adductor reflex and pharyngeal squeeze as predictors of laryngeal penetration and aspiration. Laryngoscope 2002;112(2):338–41.
6. Ross B, Gramiak R, Rahn H. Physical dynamics of the cough mechanism. J Appl Phys 1955;8(3):264–8.
7. Shaker R, Dua KS, Ren J, et al. Vocal cord closure pressure during volitional swallow and other voluntary tasks. Dysphagia 2002;17(1):13–8.
8. Canning BJ, Mazzone SB, Meeker SN, et al. Identification of the tracheal and laryngeal afferent neurones mediating cough in anaesthetised guinea-pigs. J Physiol 2004;557(Pt 2):543–58.
9. Wong CH, Matai R, Morice AH. Cough induced by low pH. Respir Med 1999;93: 58–61.
10. Fontana GA, Lavorini F, Pistolesi M. Water aerosols and cough. Pulm Pharmacol Ther 2002;15:205–11.
11. Jafari S, Prince RA, Kim DY, et al. Sensory regulation of swallowing and airway protection: a role for the internal superior laryngeal nerve in humans. J Physiol 2003;550(Pt 1):287–304.
12. Leder SB, Ross DA. Incidence of vocal fold immobility in patients with dysphagia. Dysphagia 2005;20(2):163–7.
13. Rubin BK. Physiology of airway mucus clearance. Respir Care 2002;47(7):761–8.
14. Pou AM, Carrau RL, Eibling DE, et al. Laryngeal framework surgery for the management of aspiration in high vagal lesions. Am J Otol 1998;19:1–7.
15. Laccourreye O, Paczona R, Ageel M, et al. Intracordal autologous fat injection for aspiration after recurrent laryngeal nerve paralysis. Eur Arch Otorhinolaryngol 1999;256:458–61.

16. Woodson G. Cricopharyngeal myotomy and arytenoid adduction in the management of combined laryngeal and pharyngeal paralysis. Otolaryngol Head Neck Surg 1997;116:339–43.
17. Abraham MT, Bains MS, Downey RJ, et al. Type I thyroplasty for acute unilateral vocal fold paralysis following intrathoracic surgery. Ann Otol Rhinol Laryngol 2002;111(8):667–71.
18. Belafsky PC, Rees CJ, Rodriguez K, et al. Esophagopharyngeal reflux. Otolaryngol Head Neck Surg 2008;138(1):57–61.
19. Murry T, Tabaee A, Aviv JE. Respiratory retraining of refractory cough and laryngopharyngeal reflux in patients with paradoxical vocal fold movement disorder. Laryngoscope 2004;114(8):1341–5.
20. Smith Hammond CA, Goldstein LB, Horner RD, et al. Predicting aspiration in patients with ischemic stroke. Chest 2009;135(3):769–77.
21. Bours GJ, Speyer R, Lemmens J, et al. Bedside screening tests vs. videofluoroscopy or fibreoptic endoscopic evaluation of swallowing to detect dysphagia in patients with neurological disorders: systematic review. J Adv Nurs 2009;65(3): 477–93.
22. Rosenbek JC, Robbins JA, Roecker EB, et al. A penetration-aspiration scale. Dysphagia 1996;11(2):93–8.
23. Fang TJ, Li HY, Tsai FC, et al. The role of glottal gap in predicting aspiration in patients with unilateral vocal paralysis. Clin Otolaryngol Allied Sci 2004;29(6): 709–12.
24. Bhattacharyya N, Kotz T, Shapiro J. Dysphagia and aspiration with unilateral vocal cord immobility: incidence, characterization, and response to surgical treatment. Ann Otol Rhinol Laryngol 2002;111(8):672–9.
25. Fuller SC, Leonard R, Aminpour S, et al. Validation of the pharyngeal squeeze maneuver. Otolaryngol Head Neck Surg 2009;140(3):391–4.
26. Colodny N. Interjudge and intrajudge reliabilities in fiberoptic endoscopic evaluation of swallowing (FEES) using the penetration-aspiration scale: a replication study. Dysphagia 2002;17(4):308–15.
27. Aviv JE. Prospective, randomized outcome study of endoscopy versus modified barium swallow in patients with dysphagia. Laryngoscope 2000;110(4):563–74.
28. Welch MV, Logemann JA, Rademaker AW, et al. Changes in pharyngeal dimensions effected by chin tuck. Arch Phys Med Rehabil 1993;74(2):178–81.
29. Mepani R, Antonik S, Massey B, et al. Augmentation of deglutitive thyrohyoid muscle shortening by the Shaker Exercise. Dysphagia 2009;24(1):26–31.
30. Wang AY, Kadkade R, Kahrilas PJ, et al. Effectiveness of esophageal dilation for symptomatic cricopharyngeal bar. Gastrointest Endosc 2005;61(1):148–52.
31. Kelly JH. Management of upper esophageal sphincter disorders: indications and complications of myotomy. Am J Med 2000;108(Suppl 4a):43S–6S.
32. Flint PW, Purcell LL, Cummings CW. Pathophysiology and indications for medialization thyroplasty in patients with dysphagia and aspiration. Otolaryngol Head Neck Surg 1997;116(3):349–54.
33. Kos MP, David EF, Aalders IJ, et al. Long-term results of laryngeal suspension and upper esophageal sphincter myotomy as treatment for life-threatening aspiration. Ann Otol Rhinol Laryngol 2008;117(8):574–80.

Vocal Cord Dysfunction, Paradoxic Vocal Fold Motion, or Laryngomalacia? Our Understanding Requires an Interdisciplinary Approach

Kent L. Christopher, MD[a,*],
Michael J. Morris, MD[b]

KEYWORDS

- Vocal cord dysfunction • Paradoxic vocal fold motion
- Paradoxic vocal cord motion • Laryngoscopy • Dyspnea
- Inspiratory stridor • Asthma • Laryngomalacia

A HISTORICAL PERSPECTIVE

Periodic occurrence of laryngeal obstruction (POLO) was first described in an 1842 medical textbook by Dunglison,[1] who noted a disorder of the laryngeal muscles in hysteric females that he termed, *hysteric croup*. In the textbook, *Principles and Practice of Medicine,* Austin Flint[2] described a similar syndrome in two male adults and termed the condition, *laryngismus stridulus*. MacKenzie, however, reported the first evidence of abnormal vocal fold motion visualized by laryngoscopy in 1869. He noted paradoxic closure of the vocal folds with inspiration in hysteric patients.[3] Sir William Osler,[4] in the 1902 edition of *The Principles and Practice of Medicine,* further expanded on this syndrome as he described "spasm of the muscles may occur with violent inspiratory efforts and great distress, and may even lead to cyanosis . . . Extraordinary cries may be produced, either inspiratory or expiratory." Little additional information was published until the 1970s when Patterson and colleagues described a 33-year-old woman with 15 hospital admissions for what they named, *Munchausen's stridor*.[5] Since then, more than 70 different terms have been coined over the past 30 years to describe abnormal movement of the true vocal folds.[6] Many of these terms have been used

The opinions or assertions contained herein are the private views of the authors and are not to be construed as reflecting the Department of the Army or the Department of Defense.

[a] Department of Medicine, University of Colorado Health Sciences Center, 9086 East Colorado Circle, Denver, CO 80231, USA
[b] Division of Pulmonary Disease/Critical Care, Department of Medicine, University of Colorado Health Sciences Center, Denver, CO, USA
* Corresponding author.
E-mail address: drkchristopher@comcast.net (K.L. Christopher).

Otolaryngol Clin N Am 43 (2010) 43–66
doi:10.1016/j.otc.2009.12.002

primarily to describe abnormal vocal fold movement in the absence of other medical diseases (**Table 1**).

There are several proposals to categorize VCD more fully and essentially classify all glottic movement disorders into one definition. Andrianopoulos and colleagues equated paradoxic vocal fold motion, paroxysmal VCD, episodic paroxysmal laryngospasm, and irritable larynx syndrome as the same entity.[7] A distinction was made between differing associated causes, such as gastroesophageal reflux disease, primary dystonias, psychogenic causes, and disorders of central nervous system affecting the vocal folds. The use of the term, *irritable larynx syndrome*, by Morrison and colleagues proposed a unifying hypothesis of VCD and laryngospasm in the presence of a sensory trigger. This definition, however, eliminates an identifiable psychiatric diagnosis as the cause.[8] Additionally, the hypothesis of solely an irritable or hyperresponsive state is contrary to recent data demonstrating reduced laryngeal irritability with sensory stimuli in the presence of laryngopharyngeal reflux.[9] It is apparent that neither of these classifications adequately describes the full-spectrum episodes of laryngeal dysfunction.

The two terms most frequently encountered in the literature and used extensively in clinical practice are *paradoxic vocal fold motion (PVFM)*[10] and *vocal cord dysfunction (VCD)*[11] (discussed later). PVFM is most likely to be selected by otolaryngologists and speech pathologists. In contrast, pulmonologists, allergists, psychiatrists, and psychologists are generally drawn to VCD. Do these terms represent exactly the same disorder with one common origin? Are different terms used simply because of different specialty educational paths? Alternatively, is the endoscope used to visualize a limited number of end-organ laryngeal responses without fully understanding a spectrum of causes that are literally hidden from sight? Addressing these and other important issues calls for an interdisciplinary team approach. Scientists prefer to answer the

Table 1
Historical terms for periodic occurrence of laryngeal obstruction

Term	Author	Year
Munchausen's stridor	Patterson R	1974
Pseudoasthma	Dailey RH	1976
Nonorganic upper airway obstruction	Cormier YF	1980
Functional upper airway obstruction	Appelblatt NH	1981
Factitious asthma	Downing ET	1982
Vocal cord dysfunction	Christopher KL	1983
Spasmodic croup	Collett PW	1983
Emotional laryngeal wheezing	Rodenstein DO	1983
Psychogenic upper airway obstruction	Barnes SD	1986
Episodic laryngeal dyskinesia	Ramirez JR	1986
Exercise-induced laryngospasm	Liistro G	1990
Functional laryngeal obstruction	Pitchenik AE	1991
Psychogenic stridor	Lund DS	1993
Functional laryngeal stridor	Smith ME	1993
Episodic paroxysmal laryngospasm	Gallivan GJ	1996
Irritable larynx syndrome	Morrison M	1999
Paradoxic vocal fold motion	Patel NJ	2004

Data from Morris MJ, Christopher KL. Diagnostic criteria for the classification of vocal cord dysfunction, submitted for publication.

questions by being "splitters" rather than "lumpers." It may be beneficial, however, to engage in a two-step process: first lumping, then splitting.

FOCUSING ON THE BIG PICTURE

A reasonable first step might be to lump VCD, PVFM, and other similarly presenting disorders into an umbrella classification based on the presence of POLO. Inclusion would be based on unifying chief complaints resulting from episodes of laryngeal obstruction, endoscopic findings, and general commonalities in the characteristics of the clinical presentation. Speculation regarding specific cause would likely bog down the process of classification at this level, and the authors recommend that the issue is best addressed at the second step, the splitting stage. That general grouping, as outlined, may improve understanding of what should be "in the box." As a wise colleague once stated, "...if you don't think about it, you can't diagnose it." Similarly, grouping should not be overly inclusive. Thinking too much "out of the box" and pulling in diseases and disorders that do not fit will keep involved clinicians in Babylon, perpetually mumbling about disjointed terms and concepts. As with the splitting second step, the umbrella level of the classification system should be dynamic—changing as the collaborative knowledge base expands.

To get the process off the ground, the authors propose that VCD, PVFM, and intermittent arytenoid region prolapse (IARP) have clinical similarities and can be justifiably lumped into an umbrella classification. The authors have selected the term, *IARP*, rather than laryngomalacia based on the observations of Bittleman.[12] The term, *laryngomalacia*, was avoided due to potential confusion with the neonate and infant population with presumed congenital abnormalities.

The authors conclude that VCD, PVFM, and IARP can be lumped into a classification of POLO manifested by chief complaints of noisy breathing and dyspnea. Secondary symptoms including, but not limited to, cough, chest tightness, throat tightness, and changes in voice may be present. Limitations of current diagnostic technology (eg, pulmonary function testing and diagnostic radiology) make endoscopic examination the gold standard[13] for documenting the presence and characteristics of the laryngeal obstruction. A fixed obstructive airway lesion should be excluded. One or more recurring precipitating factors are usually identifiable by history; interrelationships between multiple precipitating factors in a given patient can be perplexing. Patients are predominately, but not exclusively, female; adolescent and young adult age groups seem to be predisposed. Periodic symptoms have often occurred over many months to years, and complaints have been refractory to prior prescribed medical therapy (eg, asthma medications and hyposensitization). During a symptomatic period, a patient's noisy breathing is usually reported on physical examination as "stridor" or "wheeze" (which may not be accurate). Physical examination documentation is often sparse regarding how stridor or wheeze relates to the breathing cycle. Close attention by experienced ears frequently raises suspicion that the noisy breathing is generated at the level of the larynx. Patients may present across the spectrum from appearing to be in extremis during an episode; alternatively, they may have complaints out of proportion to objective findings. Because repetitive episodes are characteristically transient or self-limiting in nature, acute symptoms and physical examination findings should resolve when the POLO resolves. Endoscopy during an asymptomatic period usually assists by confirming the periodic nature of the laryngeal obstruction. Similarly, a more complete and comprehensive endoscopic examination can be performed when patients are asymptomatic, facilitating exclusion of some disorders that otherwise are in the differential diagnosis. Additionally, identification of more subtle endoscopic findings (eg, consistent with gastroesophageal reflux disease, laryngopharyngeal reflux, and rhinogenic disorders) can facilitate the transition to the second phase (the splitting phase) where specific causes and associated disorders can be pursued.

The features (discussed previously) are generally characteristic among the three entities in the umbrella classification. POLO can be at the level of the glottis, supraglottic area, or both. Glottic disorders in this proposed POLO classification are VCD and PVFM. IARP is presented as a supraglottic disorder.

WHAT DIAGNOSES ARE IN THE DIFFERENTIAL?

Any pulmonary disorder that presents with periodic noisy breathing, dyspnea, and secondary complaints, such as cough, could be considered in the differential diagnosis. Asthma has historically been at the top of the list. Chevalier Jackson's axiom is often quoted[14]: "not all that wheezes is asthma." Even after his death in 1958, the hunt for asthma masqueraders marches onward. Today, use of the statement that "all that wheezes is not POLO" is avoided; however, VCD, PVFM, and IARP should rank somewhere below asthma in the differential diagnosis for dyspnea and wheezing, particularly with regard to similarities to asthma in clinical presentation.

It is recognized by the pulmonary and allergy communities that too many patients are diagnosed with asthma without objective lung function testing by spirometry. Unfortunately, this can be a double-edged sword. Under specific circumstances, pulmonary diagnostic tools may confuse more than assist in excluding asthma; this can occur initially or when evaluating for coexistent disease after one of the POLO disorders is confirmed. These pitfalls are discussed later.

There are laryngotracheal mass lesions that may occasionally appear to be episodic at some point in their clinical course, but the obstruction does not resolve. As the progressive disease increases to critical airway occlusion, patients may experience cyclic increases in dyspnea and noisy breathing. For example, they may be in greater distress due to exertion, increased ventilatory requirements from any cause (eg, pneumonia), and airway inflammation. Cessation of exertion, reduction in ventilatory requirement, and treated airway infection or systemic disease flair (eg, relapsing polychondritis) may transiently improve symptoms. It is well recognized that airway-obstructing lesions may be benign by histology but malignant by course. An entity that requires special mention is idiopathic laryngotracheal stenosis,[15,16] particularly because of its predilection, as with POLO disorders, for young- to middle-aged women and similar presentation with exertional dyspnea and noisy breathing.

Important categories of laryngeal manifestations of diseases and disorders that should be considered in the differential diagnosis are illustrated in **Table 2**. The categories of neurogenic, vocal fold paresis and paralysis, and laryngospasm have different characteristics, presentations, and endoscopic findings from the POLO disorders. There are a variety of entities within each category. The conditions listed in **Table 2** are discussed in articles elsewhere in this issue.

HOW DO WE ADDRESS COUGH?

As discussed previously, cough is a complaint in the overall POLO population. Unfortunately, the literature has been inherently limited by a paucity of adequate studies. Lack of agreement on terms and concepts, absence of a structured scientific approach, and small sample sizes have made clinical investigation difficult. The authors' recent literature review (Morris MJ, MD and Christopher KL, MD, unpublished data, 2009), however, can offer insight regarding the overall prevalence of reported

Table 2
Laryngeal disorders not consistent with the periodic occurrence of glottic obstruction classification

Disorder	Examples of Conditions
Neurogenic	Brainstem compression Upper motor neuron injury Lower motor neuron injury Movement disorders Adductor laryngeal breathing dystonia
Vocal fold paralysis	Head and neck malignancy Chest surgery Idiopathic
Vocal fold paresis	Prolonged intubation
Laryngospasm	Intubation Airway manipulation Immunoglobulin E mediated Nocturnal aspiration

Data from Morris MJ, Christopher KL. Diagnostic criteria for the classification of vocal cord dysfunction, submitted for publication.

cough in the POLO population. Data are likely to be conservative as cough may have been present but not reported in the respective articles.

A total of 355 articles was reviewed (Morris MJ, MD and Christopher KL, MD, unpublished data, 2009); 67 articles were excluded that contained duplicate data or discussed laryngospasm, vocal cord paresis or paralysis, primary neurologic syndromes, or other glottic disorders that were not consistent with POLO. The final series of articles (n = 288) concerning POLO included 159 case reports, 37 retrospective studies, 21 prospective studies, 74 review articles, and 18 letters to the editor or editorials. In the few reports and collectively small numbers of patients with IARP, symptoms other than dyspnea and noisy breathing were not common; cough was rarely described. The review found symptoms (Morris MJ, MD and Christopher KL, MD, unpublished data, 2009) were reported in 1020 patients with VCD (64% of total); symptoms were chronic in 860 patients (85%) and acute in 151 patients (15%). Dyspnea was the predominant symptom in 73% of patients followed by wheeze (36%) and stridor (28%), with collective noisy breathing at 64%. Less common symptoms included cough (25%), chest tightness (25%), throat tightness (22%), and changes in voice (12%).

More than 3 years ago, Brugman[6] reviewed the symptoms of patients identified as having VCD from the published literature and noted a higher prevalence of symptoms. Dyspnea (95%), wheeze (51%), stridor (51%), and cough (42%) were the predominant findings.[6] In summary, with shortfalls of literature review in mind, in 85% of patients with VCD, symptoms were chronic, and cough was reported in 25%. In an earlier review of what could have been a slightly different population, cough was present in 42%. It would be reasonable to conclude that the conservative prevalence of cough is in the range of 25% to 42%. Further light may be shed on cough as the three POLO entities are split in terms of how they differ from each other.

DIFFERENCES AMONG PERIODIC OCCURRENCE OF LARYNGEAL OBSTRUCTION DISORDERS

POLO disorders can be placed into the three separate categories (**Table 3**). Furthermore, each of the three categories (psychogenic, exertional, and irritant) is composed

Table 3
Categories of periodic occurrence of glottic obstruction

Category	Conditions
Irritant	Intrinsic Gastroesophageal reflux disease Rhinogenic (sinusitis, rhinitis/postnasal drip) Extrinsic Chemical irritants Olfactory/visual stimuli
Exertional	At maximal exercise Athletic competition Exercise in general
Psychological	Other components (anxiety disorder, stress, depression) Somatoform disorder Conversion disorder Psychiatric illness History of sexual abuse Mass psychogenic illness

Data from Morris MJ, Christopher KL. Diagnostic criteria for the classification of vocal cord dysfunction, submitted for publication.

of several entities. The irritant category is subdivided into extrinsic and intrinsic conditions.

Because most agree that endoscopy is the diagnostic study of choice (Morris MJ, MD and Christopher KL, MD, unpublished data, 2009) for identifying POLO, how do descriptions differ between VCV, PVFM, and IARP? That information may assist in sorting out the three categories and their subcomponents in the future.

ENDOSCOPIC EVALUATION

Although characteristic endoscopic findings are discussed, it is difficult to determine relative frequency, as the literature review (Morris MJ, MD and Christopher KL, MD, unpublished data, 2009) demonstrates that endoscopy was not performed in 38% of patients. Inspiratory adduction was reported in 32% of those articles that described endoscopic findings. Descriptions were usually just the acknowledgment of "paradoxical vocal fold movement" or "vocal cord dysfunction" or referred to acronyms. Respiratory phase of the obstruction was frequently undefined (inspiratory, expiratory, or both). If inspiratory obstruction was noted (eg, PVFM), there was usually no statement as to whether or not expiratory findings were entirely normal.

The presence of inspiratory adduction is key to the diagnoses of PVFM and VCD. Additionally, concomitant expiratory obstruction can be seen in VCD. Inspiratory supraglottic obstruction is the major finding in IARP. For the purpose of this article, an overall concept of characteristic findings is constructed, drawing attention to key references when possible, and putting laryngoscopic findings in perspective based on the authors' experiences.

For the long term, development of an interdisciplinary POLO endoscopic classification system integrating various clinical experiences (otolaryngology, pulmonary, allergy, and speech pathology) would be a worthwhile pursuit. Defined protocols and uniform descriptors and integration of additional endoscopic testing (eg, stroboscopy and exercise laryngoscopy) may facilitate the process of targeting POLO categories, conditions (see **Table 3**), and exclusions in the differential diagnosis (see **Table 2**).

Primary care clinicians must become better educated regarding the importance of flexible laryngoscopic examination in patients with suspected laryngeal disease. They need to be aware that, as with any procedure, trained professionals should perform flexible laryngoscopy. Additionally, flexible laryngoscopy is well tolerated with minimal risk when performed properly.

As discussed previously, the endoscopic examination of POLO subjects is frequently normal when patients are symptom-free. Patient maneuvers (eg, sniff and established phonatory tasks) performed during routine examination may confirm normal abductor and adductor function and voice, thus facilitating exclusion of some disorders listed in **Table 2**. A forced expiratory vital capacity maneuver followed by a forced inspiratory vital capacity maneuver simulates generation of a flow-volume loop (FVL) and may be helpful. Pulmonary function and provocation testing are discussed later.

Ancillary endoscopic findings suggestive of a condition in the irritant category (see **Table 3**) are discussed in articles elsewhere in this issue. There still is much to learn about the origins in many conditions within each of the three POLO categories. A patient may present with conditions in more than one category. Co-existent but unrelated disorders must be objectively differentiated, and additional information in the presence of nonspecific endoscopic findings must be sought. The psychological category is the great imitator of conditions in the other two categories and is discussed.

What degree of obstruction is required with PVFM, VCD, or IARP? The critical obstruction (percent obstruction) required to produce symptoms in fixed obstructive lesions in a variety of "tubes" (eg, trachea and carotid artery) is easier to predict. Variable airway obstructions are more difficult to assess and depend on their timing relative to the breathing cycle. Inspiratory and expiratory glottic or supraglottic dynamic obstruction affects work of breathing and respiratory physiology in different ways.

PARADOXIC VOCAL FOLD MOTION

In PVFM, the true vocal folds do not abduct in a normal fashion during inspiration. The true vocal folds paradoxically and symmetrically adduct toward the midline during inspiration,[3,10] producing glottic obstruction. In those individuals with an isolated inspiratory abnormality, the endoscopic characterization is appropriate. PVFM, however, does not adequately describe glottic obstruction that also occurs on exhalation, as the true vocal folds normally adduct to some degree during quiet breathing. Abnormal expiratory adduction is not truly paradoxic because movement is not in the opposite direction of normal.

The PVFM on inspiration first described in hysteric patients in 1869 by MacKenzie[3] was a major finding. Furthermore, Osler[4] added clinical insight by documenting that noisy breathing ("extraordinary cries") and dyspnea ("great distress") could be on inspiration and expiration. The term PVFM does not encompass POLO disorders that also occur on exhalation. Taken at face value, PVFM is a straightforward and literal endoscopic descriptor; however, its use usually implies additional meaning to an examiner. A significant problem arises when endoscopic diagnoses, such as PVFM and VCD, are bantered about in a cavalier fashion.

VOCAL CORD DYSFUNCTION

The comments made regarding the term PVFM should be underscored and amplified when discussing VCD. Similarly, taken at face value, VCD is the most endoscopically nondescript term in the POLO classification. When looking at the original description of VCD, however, it is defined in the context of a disorder presenting as asthma[11] and defines more than one specific endoscopic abnormality. One author of this article (KLC) was the team leader and pulmonologist for the interdisciplinary team in that publication[11]; the team included an otolaryngologist, speech pathologist, pulmonary physiologist, and psychiatrist.

Clinical presentation and other diagnostic testing are discussed later. Endoscopic findings[11] are shown in **Fig. 1**. All subjects had normal laryngeal function and anatomy when laryngoscopy was performed during an asymptomatic period (see **Fig. 1**A). During a typical episode (see **Fig. 1**B) of complaints of dyspnea and noisy breathing, each had almost complete adduction of the true vocal folds; the glottis narrowed to a small posterior diamond-shaped chink.[11] The false vocal folds bunched together, obscuring visualization of the laryngeal ventricles. The arytenoids tended to be maintained at a lateral position with failure to adduct. These abnormalities were seen on inspiration (see **Fig. 1**B) and expiration (see **Fig. 1**C.) The moderate expiratory obstruction (see **Fig. 1**C) is contrasted to more severe expiratory obstruction (see **Fig. 1**D).

Fig. 2A shows a side-by-side view of the inspiratory glottic aperture under asymptomatic conditions (see **Fig. 1**A) and during symptoms (see **Fig. 1**B). Similarly, **Fig. 2**B illustrates a composite view from left to right comparing the inspiratory glottic aperture during symptoms (see **Fig. 1**B), a pronounced expiratory reduction in glottic area (see **Fig. 1**D), and a more moderate reduction in expiratory glottic aperture (see **Fig. 1**C).

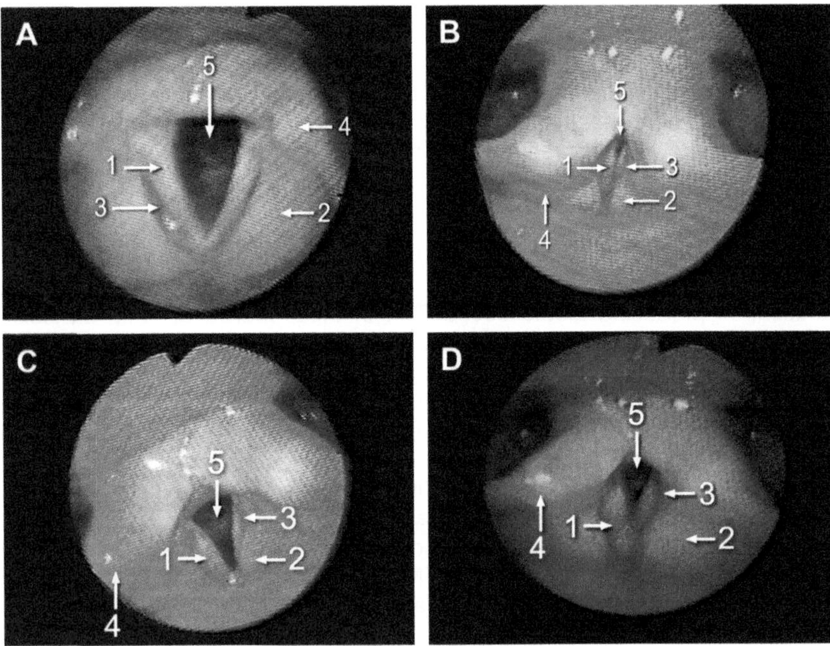

Fig. 1. Representative photographs obtained during laryngoscopy. (*A*) The findings in a patient during inspiration in a symptom-free period. (*B*) Inspiratory findings during an episode of noisy breathing and dyspnea. (*From* Christopher KL. Understanding vocal cord dysfunction: a step in the right direction with a long road ahead [editorial]. Chest 2006;129:842–3; with permission.) (*C*) Expiratory findings with moderate obstruction during an episode of noisy breathing and dyspnea. (*D*) Expiratory changes with more severe obstruction. 1, True vocal fold; 2, false vocal fold; 3, laryngeal ventricle; 4, arytenoid; 5, glottis.

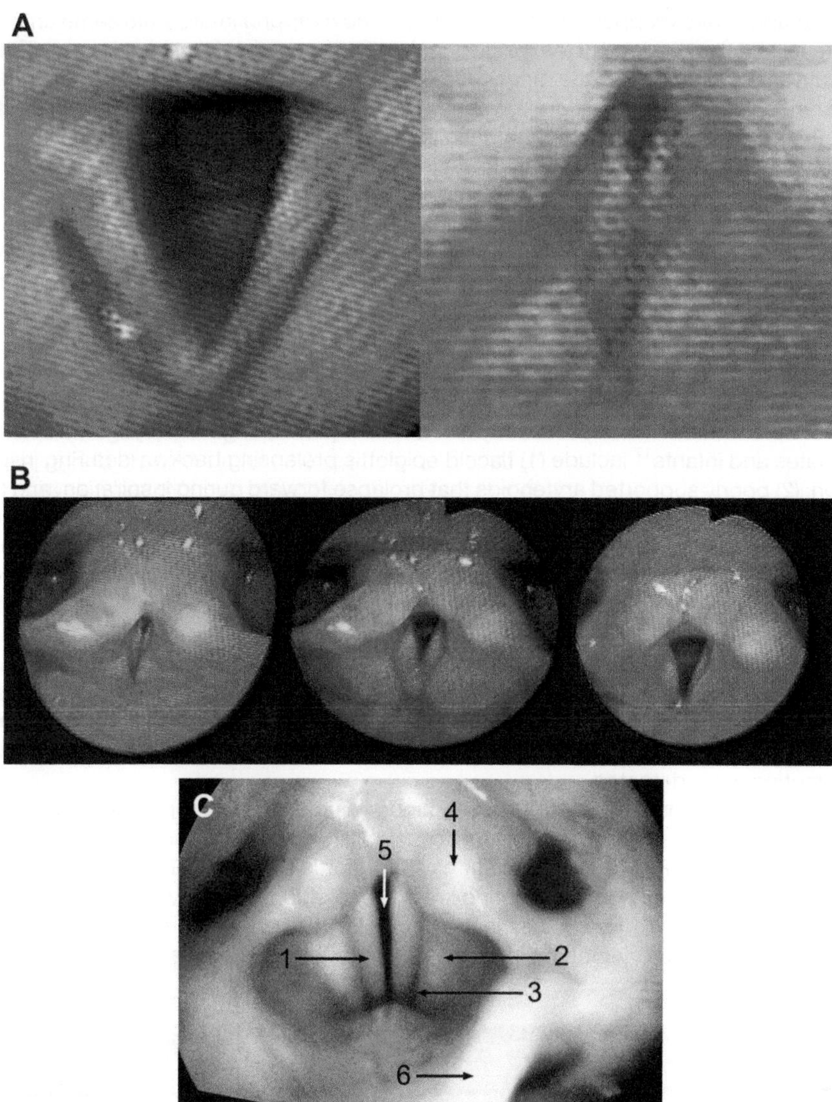

Fig. 2. (*A*) A side-by-side view of the inspiratory glottic aperture under asymptomatic conditions (see **Fig. 1**A) and during symptoms (see **Fig. 1**B). Similarly, (*B*) illustrates a composite view from left to right comparing the inspiratory glottic aperture during symptoms (see **Fig. 1**B), a pronounced expiratory reduction in glottic area (see **Fig. 1**D), and a more moderate reduction in expiratory glottic aperture (see **Fig. 1**C). Photographs were cropped similarly and then sized to approximately the same anteroposterior length at the level of the glottic opening. The approximate comparison gives readers a relative understanding of the magnitude of inspiratory and expiratory obstruction. Laryngeal function was different when patients were asked to reproduce their noisy breathing while they were asymptomatic (*C*). 1, True vocal fold; 2, false vocal fold; 3, laryngeal ventricle; 4, arytenoid; 5, glottis; and 6, epiglottis. (*From* Christopher KL, Wood RP, Eckert C, et al. Vocal cord dysfunction presenting as asthma. N Engl J Med 1983;308:1566–70.)

Photographs were cropped similarly and then sized to approximately the same anteroposterior length at the level of the glottic opening. The approximate comparison provides a relative understanding of the magnitude of inspiratory and expiratory obstruction.

Laryngeal function was different when patients were asked to reproduce their noisy breathing while they were asymptomatic (see **Fig. 2**C). Function was identical to that observed when normal and asthmatic subjects performed the same task of generating noisy breathing. The true vocal folds adducted but were bowed together, and the posterior diamond-shaped chink and bulging of the false vocal folds (described previously) were not observed. During this time, the arytenoids were fully adducted. This inspiratory adduction of the true vocal folds meets a criterion for PVCM, but was entirely volitional.

INTERMITTENT ARYTENOID REGION PROLAPSE

Clinical presentation is discussed later. Endoscopic findings in laryngomalacia in neonates and infants[17] include (1) flaccid epiglottis prolapsing backward during inspiration, (2) poorly supported arytenoids that prolapse forward during inspiration, and (3) short aryepiglottic folds.

Collective observations are different in adolescents and young adults and are most commonly seen during strenuous exercise.[18] Findings 1 and 3 are generally not present. The following are examples of observations in laryngomalacia that may be better defined as IARP.

Endoscopic examination with exercise in this POLO disorder was first described in 1994 by Bittleman and colleagues[12] and findings are shown in **Fig. 3**. Pre-exercise flexible laryngoscopy was unremarkable (see **Fig. 3**A). After peak exercise, "abnormal motion of the arytenoid region" was noted (see **Fig. 3**B). No abnormalities of true vocal fold motion were detected.

Bent and colleagues[19] evaluated continuous flexible laryngoscopy during maximal bicycle ergometry in normal subjects to establish normal function as a basis for comparison to IARP. There was dilation of the glottis during inspiration and expiration.[19] The vocal folds adducted during "restful expiration" but moved to a fixed position during "heavy exertion." The inspiratory glottic size appeared to remain "slightly larger" than "expiratory glottic size even during maximal exercise." The vocal folds

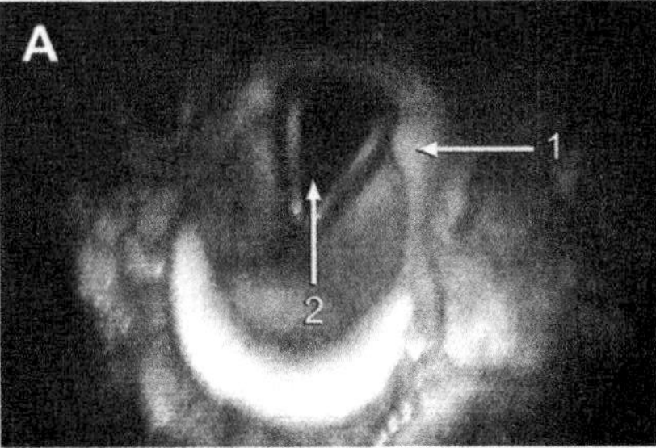

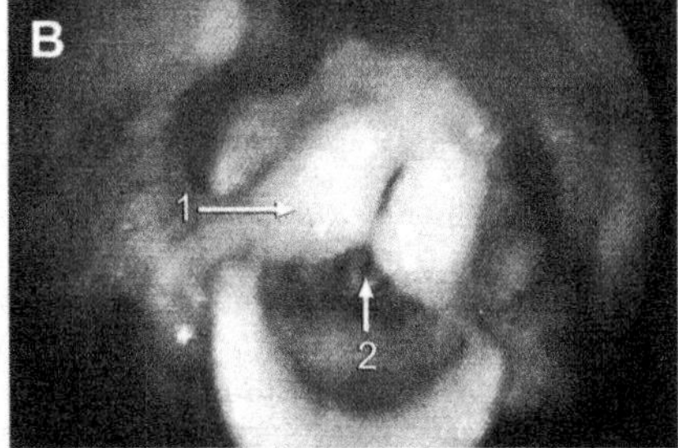

Fig. 3. Flexible laryngoscopy was obtained when a 16-year-old female basketball player became dyspenic with stridor during a maximal exercise bicycle study. Pre-exercise laryngoscopic examination was unremarkable (*A*). Immediately after maximal exertion (*B*), abnormal movement of the arytenoid region caused obstruction of the airway during inspiration. 1, Arytenoid region; 2, glottic opening. (*From* Bittleman DB, Smith RJ, Weiler JM. Abnormal movement of the arytenoid region during exercise presenting as exercise-induced asthma in an adolescent athlete. Chest 1994;106:615–6; with permission.)

were observed to elongate during inspiration at maximal exercise, changing the entire glottis to a diamond shape and further increasing endolaryngeal area.[19]

Smith and coworkers[18] described the endoscopic findings before and during continuous laryngoscopy with maximal bicycle exercise in an adolescent with "laryngomalacia" (IARP). During peak exercise, abnormal motion of the arytenoid region occurred with prolapse over the glottis. Anterior and medial movement of the arytenoid region, including aryepiglottic folds, partially obstructed the glottic opening; these findings were concurrent with the onset of dyspnea. The simultaneous production of stridor was thought to have resulted from the observation of vibration of the corniculate cartilages.[18] Smith and coworkers[18] demonstrated graphically that medial and anterior motion was not symmetric. Pinho and colleagues[20] made a similar observation. Endoscopy showed intermittently symmetric arytenoid motion alternating with asymmetric motion with both causing prolapse over the glottic opening. Pinho and colleagues presented an image[20] in which the left arytenoid region has moved across the midline and is positioned anterior to the right.

Heimdal and colleagues reported results of four patients with IARP obtained during continuous laryngoscopic endoscopy during a maximum exercise test.[21] Only at peak exercise levels did four subjects demonstrate "inspiratory synchronous medial motion of the dorsal part of the aryepiglottic folds." In addition, inspiratory adduction of the true vocal folds was present. Heinle and coworkers[22] also used continuous laryngoscopy during exercise. Six patients had laryngomalacia as a single observation and six subjects demonstrated laryngomalacia and PVFM. A word of caution is appropriate. Bjornsdottir and colleagues[23] noted supraglottic obstruction can obscure vision of the true vocal folds. Consequently, full assessment at the glottic level may be difficult.

THE THREE CATEGORIES OF PERIODIC OCCURRENCE OF LARYNGEAL OBSTRUCTION

The three categories for POLO (as defined in **Table 3**) are irritant (intrinsic and extrinsic), exertional, and psychological. Specific underlying conditions in the irritant category are presented in articles elsewhere in this issue. The presence of cough in those disorders also is discussed. Although unconfirmed, the authors suspect that cough is more common in the irritant category than the other two. Other articles in this issue discuss presentation, diagnosis, and management. Speech therapy may be a treatment option in several conditions in the categories; speech therapy is presented in another article. VCD or PVFM is used at the articles authors' discretion.

For the purpose of this article, the authors use VCD rather than PVFM for consistency and simplicity, knowing well that in some instances PVFM may also be appropriate.

Exertional

Exercise in fit individuals, roles of maximal exertion, and athletic competition

The term, *laryngomalacia*, implies a cause that has not been confirmed, especially in adolescents and young adults.[18] Consequently, the authors prefer the descriptive term, *IARP*, for this supraglottic POLO disorder. The entity was first described,[24] however, as "laryngomalacia" in 1900. In neonates and infants, it has been considered a transient, benign cause of inspiratory stridor[25] that usually resolves by the age of 2 years.[27] It has often been described as a congenital disorder but could represent a certain phase of normal development of the larynx.[17]

There is another distinct disorder[12,18,19,21–23] in adolescents and young adults that usually occurs in fit athletic women. These individuals present with shortness of breath, noisy breathing, and supraglottic obstruction during strenuous exercise. Based on studies cited previously, dyspnea and supraglottic obstruction are linked in time to onset of the obstruction. Stridor may result, at least in part, from corniculate vibration.[18] Obstruction is thought to be due to hyperpnia and tachypnea characteristic of exercise with accompanying substantial negative inspiratory pressure drawing the tissues together.[18] A Venturi effect from the Bernoulli principle has also been postulated.[18] Previously defined laryngoscopic findings and symptoms often disappear shortly after exercise ceases or level of exertion decreases.[26] Anxiety and panic also have been associated as well; hyperventilation may play a role.[20,27]

Exercise was first recognized as a cause of VCD in 1984 in a 32-year-old female runner with wheezing during exercise treated for 10 years as exercise-induced asthma. Methacholine challenge testing (MCT) was negative and postexercise FVLs showed characteristic flattening of the inspiratory limb.[28] Several more case reports over the next decade described a similar clinical presentation.[29–34] In 1996, McFadden reported a series of seven elite athletes with a "choking" sensation during exercise, normal baseline PFT, and negative bronchoprovocation testing. The diagnosis of VCD was made on the basis of laryngoscopy or the characteristic flattening of the postexercise FV.[35] A similar study, published the same year by Landwehr and colleagues, diagnosed seven adolescent athletes with VCD on the basis of postexercise inspiratory FVL flattening.[36] These first case series demonstrated an important characteristic of exercise-induced VCD in that many patients are highly competitive or elite athletes. Stress of competition and parental pressure to excel may have been issues. Rundell and Spiering evaluated 370 athletes for evidence of VCD by the presence of inspiratory stridor and found a prevalence of 5% in this population. Laryngoscopy was not done in this patient cohort so supraglottic collapse or other disorders may have been present in an unknown percentage of these patients.[37] Sullivan and coworkers[38] reported the successful treatment of 20 highly competitive female adolescent athletes with exercise-induced VCD by a program that included counseling and speech therapy. The other group in which exercise-induced VCD is common is active duty military personnel who are required to exercise regularly. A study of active duty military patients with exertional dyspnea found 12% of the patients had VCD precipitated by exercise.[39] Similarly, two other Army tertiary care facilities reported that 52% of their 176 VCD patients had exercise-induced symptoms.[40] The use of exercise tidal FVL in conjunction with cardiopulmonary exercise testing in 26 patients found inspiratory flow limitation in 74% of these patients.[41] In the general population, Diamond and coworkers[42] reported 11% of patients in a suburban pulmonary practice had VCD precipitated by exercise, and a recent case series of 49 patients found that 59% of patients were diagnosed with exercise-induced VCD.[42,43]

The primary differential diagnosis for exercise-induced VCD is exercise-induced bronchospasm (EIB). Morris and colleagues' military study and Rundell and Spiering's elite athlete study reported EIB as the primary cause of symptoms (35% and 53%, respectively).[37–39] Two recent studies (one included self-reported poorly controlled symptoms without laryngoscopy post exercise) specifically evaluated previously diagnosed EIB patients and found an 11% to 26% incidence of VCD.[44,45] The cause of VCD during exercise remains unexplained and unstudied. To date, there have been no prospective investigations to determine the mechanism of exercise-induced VCD. Few studies specifically associate VCD with EIB and in most cases, exercise testing or bronchoprovocation testing for asthma is negative.

A reduction of the expiratory glottic aperture in some forms of intrathoracic airway disease (eg, chronic obstructive pulmonary disease and asthma) has been reported. It is thought to serve much like the expiratory retard effect of pursed lips breathing in reduction of the work of breathing by maintaining a level of hyperinflation that mechanically keeps the airways dilated.[46,47] This compensatory reduction in glottic aperture, however, has not been reported to cause paradoxic inspiratory closure of the vocal folds or upper airway obstruction. Isolated expiratory obstruction as a cause of POLO with noisy breathing and dyspnea has been reported in two case studies,[48,49] but prospective studies have not been done.

Exercise in general

VCD is seen across the spectrum of intensity of exertion. Episodes precipitated by exercise can be seen in 18% of patients.[13] VCD frequently presents as noisy breathing and dyspnea that can occur at any level of exertion and is often confused with EIB characteristic of asthma.

Cough

According to previously described data, cough is encountered in approximately 25% to 42% of glottic POLO disorders. Assessment of the percent frequency of the exertion category relative to purely psychological or irritant categories is totally speculative due to inadequate data. The authors' clinical experience suggests that cough is present in this category but probably not as commonly as in irritant or psychological categories.

Psychological

The initial case reports of POLO emphasized the dominant underlying psychological disorders in these patients. The initial terminology—*hysteric croup, Munchausen's stridor*, and *emotional laryngeal wheezing*—suggested psychological disorders as the cause.[1,5,48]

In the 1983 original description coining the term VCD,[11] a psychiatrist team member interviewed and performed a battery of tests, including the Minnesota Multiphasic Personality Inventory, and established a psychological diagnosis for each of the patients. In four of five patients, psychiatric diagnoses were made before the presence of VCD was determined. Each patient had difficulty expressing anger, sadness, and fear and had various degrees of secondary gain from respiratory illness. A variety of psychiatric disorders were identified. The underlying diagnosis, however, was conversion disorder, a category under somatoform disorder. According to *Diagnostic and Statistical Manual of Mental Disorders, 4th Edition* diagnostic standards,[50] conversion disorder involves unexplained symptoms or deficits affecting voluntary motor (eg, vocal fold) or sensory function that suggest a neurologic or general medical condition (eg, asthma). Psychological factors are judged to be associated with the symptoms or deficits. As indicated in **Fig. 2**C, patients were not able to consciously reproduce VCD findings seen during a spontaneous episode, suggesting origin on a subconscious level; this is consistent with a conversion disorder in which patients are unaware of their psychological problem. Intentional laryngeal obstruction is consistent with a factitious disorder, however, and fits the PVFM description but not original VCD descriptors. Based on the model of somatoform disorder health care cost studies, Makita and Parker[51] demonstrated high outpatient health care use in establishing the diagnosis and management of VCD in military personnel and their dependents.

In a recent prospective study evaluating psychological disorders in 45 VCD patients, investigators described a classic conversion profile on Minnesota Multiphasic Personality Inventory-2 testing in 40% of patients and 30% with elevated scores suggesting conversion, but 25% of patients were without psychopathology.[52] Lacy and McManie[53] performed a review of 48 VCD cases from the literature from 1965 to 1994. They described 45 cases in which a psychiatric disorder was reported. The majority (52%) of patients were diagnosed with a conversion disorder, 13% had a major depression, 10% had a factitious disorder or Munchausen's stridor, 4% had a obsessive-compulsive disorder, and the remaining 4% had a adjustment disorder. Underlying all these diagnoses was the presence of significant emotional stress.[53]

The Lacy and McManis review commented that the increased female-to-male ratio, history of multiple hospitalizations, and numerous psychological symptoms in conversion disorder correlate with the findings in VCD.[53] Emotional stress is frequently mentioned as a common precipitant of psychogenic VCD and may play an important role in exercise-induced symptoms. Several studies highlight the importance of emotional stressors as a primary trigger in psychogenic VCD. Gavin and colleagues[54] conducted a case-control study of pediatric VCD and asthma patients and found that VCD patients tended to have significantly higher levels of anxiety and more anxiety-related diagnoses. Other stressors, such as competitive sports, are noted more frequently as triggers in exercise VCD.[35,55] It has also been reported that stressful situations, such as a combat environment, may trigger VCD.[56]

Depression has been a common underlying associated psychiatric diagnosis in many VCD patients and major depression may be a component of a conversion disorder.[57–60] Major depression or dysthymia was present in 13% of VCD patients in the review by Lacy and McManis.[53] Other large studies evaluating psychiatric disorders reported similar findings, with 33% to 40% of VCD patients having major depression.[54,61] In addition to psychological counseling, the use of antidepressants may be indicated to control VCD symptoms. Freedman conducted a retrospective chart review of 47 cases of VCD and described 14 patients with a reported history of sexual abuse and five patients with suspected childhood sexual abuse.[62] Two other case reports reported a history of sexual abuse in association with other psychiatric disorders, such as depression.[57] Newman and colleagues' and Husein and colleagues' studies reported a history of abuse in 38% of their patient cohorts.[52,63]

One of the striking features from Newman and colleagues' series is the association of VCD with underlying psychiatric disorders.[63] Nine patients had prior psychiatric hospitalizations and 73% had a psychiatric diagnosis.[63] A comparison of 12 adolescent VCD patients with asthma controls found eight patients had significant psychiatric diagnoses, including major depression, separation anxiety, overanxious disorder, and dysthymia disorder.[54]

As one of the author's Kent L. Christopher, MD, recalls (unpublished data, 1983), patient histories in the original description of VCD.[11] There were unlikely precipitators (eg, various metered-dose inhaled bronchodilators and subcutaneous epinephrine) and triggers, however, that were not confirmed to cause symptoms by challenges (eg, yellow dye food challenge). Selner and colleagues[64] and Tomares and coworkers[65] reinforced the importance of objective provocation testing of presumed exposures that are suspected of causation. **Box 1** lists findings that suggest the presence or possibility of a psychological POLO disorder.

VOCAL CORD DYSFUNCTION AND MASS PSYCHOGENIC ILLNESS

Fourteen adolescent high school girls who developed an audible inspiratory noise and dyspnea were evaluated by an interdisciplinary team and the health department.[66] Environmental studies did not demonstrate an environmental noxious chemical or biologic agent. Initially, stridor intensity increased when subjects were in the presence of other affected friends. Stridor was documented on flexible laryngoscopy to be due to

Box 1
Factors suggesting an underlying psychological disorder

- Findings resolve when patient distracted
- Findings resolve when patient phonates
- Episode relieved by placebo administration
- Symptoms and findings induced or relieved by suggestion
- Episode resolves with helium, even after gas withdrawn
- Episode reproduced by placebo challenge
- Absence of response when blinded to exposure to presumed agent
- Findings resolve with hypnosedative administration
- Episodes absent during monitored sleep
- History of sexual abuse
- Respiratory complaints out of proportion to objective findings
- History of psychiatric illness

the findings of VCD with posterior chink and IARP. The presence of findings in individual patients was not presented (ie, one abnormality or both).

COUGH

As discussed previously, cough is encountered in approximately 25% to 42% of POLO disorders in the glottic category. Assessment of the percent frequency of the psychological category relative to purely exertional or irritant categories is speculative due to inadequate data. As discussed in an article elsewhere in this issue, somatization disorder, or perhaps undifferentiated somatoform disorder, is a potential cause of chronic cough but only by exclusion. Because psychological VCD can present as a conversion disorder (in the somatoform category), it is not a stretch to consider that psychological cough may also be present. This concept is consistent with the authors' clinical experience.

HYPOTHESES FOR ORIGIN OF SOME LARYNGEAL DISORDERS

Some disorders of the upper airway may be primarily characterized by laryngeal hyperresponsiveness.[67] Bucca and colleagues[68] evaluated 441 patients with cough, wheeze, or dyspnea without documented asthma or bronchial obstruction. Extrathoracic airway hyperresponsiveness was determined by a 25% fall in maximal mid-inspiratory flow and was found in 67% of patients. Disease associations included postnasal drip and pharyngitis in 55%, laryngitis in 40%, and sinusitis in 30% of patients.[68] The presence of laryngeal hyperresponsiveness may be explained by these inflammatory conditions but is not the sole reason for paroxysmal vocal cord adduction. Ayres and Gabbott suggested that an altered autonomic balance maintained by activity of more central brain regions (medulla, midbrain, and area 25 of the prefrontal cortex) may play a role in abnormal glottic movement.[67] A combination of laryngeal hyperresponsiveness from an initial inflammatory component and alerted autonomic balance may lead to an exaggeration and perseveration of the laryngeal response in lung protection. Thus, an inflammatory condition or central input from emotional stresses may lead to symptomatic episodes. The hypothesis in irritant-associated VCD is that direct stimulation of sensory nerve endings in the upper or lower respiratory tract may initiate local reflexes that lead to paradoxic laryngeal closure.[69] Morrison used the term, *neural plasticity*, in describing the pathogenesis of "irritable larynx syndrome." It is suggested that repeated noxious stimulation leads to permanent alteration of the cell genome, thus brainstem laryngeal controlling neuronal networks are held in a perpetual hyperexcitable state.[8] An alternative hypothesis could be proposed that there is a learned Pavlovian-like conditioned response to repeated perceived environmental dangers. Despite the many hypotheses on laryngeal pathophysiology, there is minimal prospective evidence defining the specific role of laryngeal hyperresponsiveness or alteration in autonomic balance leading to VCD. Psychological disorders do not fit into the hypotheses.

PULMONARY DIAGNOSTICS

Flow-volume Relationship

The most common causes of a blunted or truncated inspiratory flow-volume curve are (1) inadequate instruction, (2) suboptimal effort, and (3) inability to perform proper technique.

A reported characteristic finding in VCD, however, is inspiratory FVL truncation consistent with a variable extrathoracic obstruction, as described by Miller and Hyatt.[70] In symptomatic patients, this common pulmonary function test can be helpful in suggesting the diagnosis of VCD but does not rule out the diagnosis in asymptomatic individuals, as results may be normal.[11] **Fig. 4**A (right) illustrates the FVL in an asymptomatic patient. The expiratory relationship of flow to volume is normal and the expiratory/inspiratory ratio (E/I) is normal. The illustration on the left was obtained when the same patient was symptomatic. The expiratory flow to volume relationship is normal. The inspiratory flow is limited (blunted or truncated) and the E/I is elevated, however, suggesting the presence of a variable extrathoracic obstruction.

The review by Morris[13] of the 1500 cases in the published literature revealed 28% of reported VCD patients had FVL truncation on spirometry. More importantly, the predictive value of FVL in diagnosing VCD has not been evaluated in a prospective manner. In a recent retrospective review of abnormal inspiratory FVL, 36% of patients

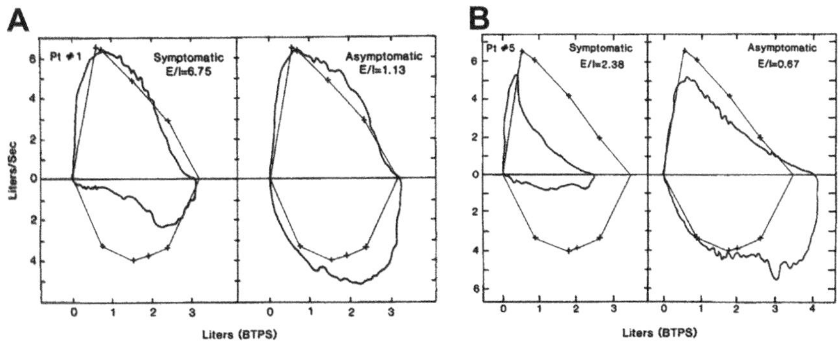

Fig. 4. The maximum inspiratory and expiratory flow-volume relationship was measured in two patients uring asymptomatic and symptomatic periods. Thin lines connecting crosses show predicted values; bold lines indicate actual measurements (*A, B*). (*From* Christopher KL, Wood RP, Eckert C, et al. Vocal cord dysfunction presenting as asthma. N Engl J Med 1983;308:1566–70. Copyright © 1983, Massachusetts Medical Society. All rights reserved.)

had VCD.[71] The usual prevalence in VCD patients in larger studies is 20% to 25%. In a prospective study of VCD in exertional dyspnea, Morris showed 20% of patients had an abnormal FVL at rest. Newman and colleagues reported a 23% incidence of abnormal FVL in asymptomatic patients with documented VCD whereas Perkner and coworkers reported 25% of patients with irritant-associated VCD had inspiratory FVL truncation at baseline.[63,69] Higher numbers were reported in several abstracts of 56% in community-based setting to 79% in a military setting.[40,42]

Expiratory flow restriction is not specific for obstruction localized to the lower tracheobronchial tree (ie, asthma). One pitfall of spirometry and the FVL is that the expiratory component of VCD with vocal fold adduction without bronchoconstriction may mimic asthma and lead to misdiagnosis of combined disease. VCD, often on a psychological basis, has expiratory obstruction and inspiratory obstruction (see **Fig. 1**C, D). An asymptomatic patient (see **Fig. 4**B, right) has a normal FVL except for mild expiratory flow limitation. In contrast, **Fig. 4**B (left) was obtained when the same patient was symptomatic. There is marked inspiratory flow limitation. The expiratory flow is substantially reduced with a concave appearance. These expiratory findings (and reduced forced expiratory volume in the first second of expiration [FEV_1]) are typical of asthma. On the basis of this test, it could be concluded that the patient has VCD and asthma. This patient was in the original VCD series where negative inhalation challenge and exercise testing ruled out the presence of asthma.[11] A misdiagnosis of asthma can creep back as "confirmed" coexistent asthma if a clinician is not aware of the pitfalls of spirometry and the FVL. The method of confirmation is not clear in many of those articles in the literature that describe asthma as coexistent with VCD.

Methacholine Inhalation Challenge

A totally negative bronchprovocation test (eg, standardized MCT) can be useful in excluding the diagnosis of asthma. The use of bronchoprovocation testing to differentiate VCD from asthma has been questioned based on several studies demonstrating MCT as unreliable in VCD patients.[72,73]

Fig. 5A shows results of a MCT result obtained before referral. The decrease in FEV_1 of 40% relative to baseline at a moderate dose suggests the presence of bronchial hyperreactivity, but full spirometry and FVL results were not available. **Fig. 5**B shows baseline FVL with normal saline inhalation. A placebo inhalation challenge with five successive doses of normal saline was performed because of the suspicion of VCD mimicking asthma. She consented when told she might receive a placebo or methacholine. At the fourth placebo dose, she complained of dyspnea and developed inspiratory and expiratory noisy breathing. **Fig. 5**C shows limited inspiratory and expiratory flow. Finally, **Fig. 5**D illustrates markedly reduced inspiratory and expiratory flow during the fifth placebo dose. Flexible laryngoscopy showed marked inspiratory and expiratory obstruction similar to **Fig. 1**B and D. The significance of these findings are twofold:

1. VCD can mimic asthma on a bronchial hyperreactivity test that is often considered a gold standard.
2. In the presence of inspiratory and expiratory VCD, the FVL can mimic a fixed airway obstruction. Advanced preparation for physical examination and endoscopy during challenge testing may be helpful. The medical literature currently lacks any prospective study that adequately defines the relationship between VCD and asthma or uses multiple (or specific) measures to define the presence of airway hyperreactivity.

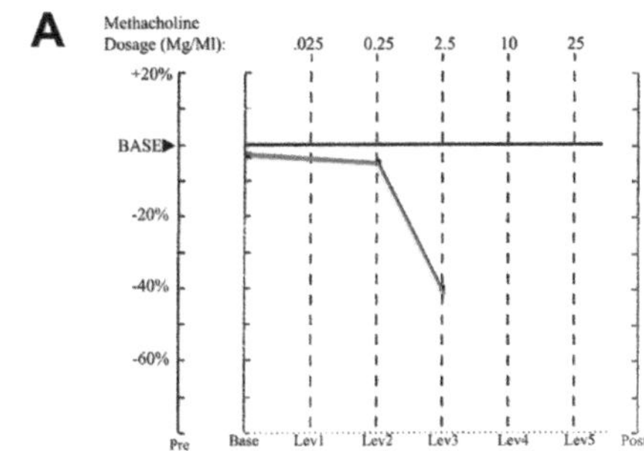

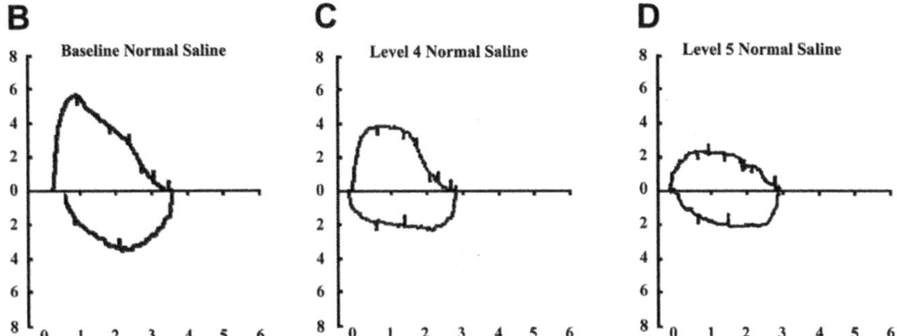

Fig. 5. Patient response to methacholine and placebo challenges. (*A*) Demonstration of MCT results before referral. Methacholine dose (mg/mL) is indicated on the horizontal axis and percent change in FEV_1 on the vertical axis. (*B–D*) Demonstration of flow-volume relationships obtained on a subsequent day while the patient became symptomatic during inhalation challenge with the fourth and fifth inhalations of normal saline placebo.

VOCAL CORD DYSFUNCTION MANAGEMENT

Treatment options for the acute and chronic presentations of VCD are not prospectively well validated and rely primarily on anecdotal reports and collective experience regarding most effective methods. In the authors' review (Morris MJ, MD and Christopher KL, MD, unpublished data, 2009), 665 patients (42% of overall) had various treatment options mentioned; few of these reports or studies prospectively evaluated VCD patients.

Acute Episodes

The acute management of VCD first requires establishing the correct diagnosis in patients during acute symptoms. In the absence of imminent respiratory failure, laryngoscopy is a rapid and safe procedure in most patients. Once recognized and correctly diagnosed, treatment should then be directed at acutely relieving airway obstruction. There may be minimal response with the use of inhaled bronchodilators, corticosteroids, and other asthma medications. These medications should be used initially, however, if underlying airway hyperreactivity is suspected or the diagnosis is unclear. Based on symptoms and definitive laryngoscopic evidence of VCD, the first management step is to reassure the patient that the condition is benign and self-limited; this approach has been reported in 33 patients (Morris MJ, MD and Christopher KL, MD, unpublished data, 2009). The authors' experience, however, backs this approach, as explaining VCD symptoms to many patients alleviates their concerns of "respiratory failure." Another reported measure that has been used effectively is sedation with benzodiazepines; in the authors' review (Morris MJ, MD and Christopher KL, MD, unpublished data, 2009), this method was used in 44 patients. Andrianopoulos and colleagues[7] reported the successful use of sedatives in five of the 27 VCD patients in their retrospective series. Heliox was originally reported by Christopher and colleagues[11] and has subsequently been recommended (reported in 19 patients) as an adjunct in the acute treatment and diagnosis of VCD.[74,75] A helium/oxygen mixture (eg, 80%/20% or 70%/30%) in acute VCD episodes had an immediate favorable response and often a sustained response after discontinuation.[11] Similar to other fixed upper airway disorders, reduction of air density decreases turbulent flow and reduces the work of breathing associated with upper airway obstruction; this may result in decreased anxiety and abort worsening VCD.

Despite the typically benign and self-limited episodes, the severity of the symptoms and impression of impending respiratory failure seen in some acute VCD episodes has led to emergent intubation or tracheostomy. A total of 68 patients (Morris MJ, MD and Christopher KL, MD, unpublished data, 2009) was reported to be emergently intubated and another 32 patients underwent tracheostomy (emergently and post intubation). Many case reports comment, after intubation, that stridor abates and the patients are "easy to ventilate"; patients are commonly extubated within 24 hours. Resolution of wheezing or stridor post intubation with normal airway pressures should prompt laryngoscopic evaluation for the presence of VCD. As with concerns about the presence of acute respiratory failure in any disease entity, arterial blood gases may be helpful in assessing compromise but may not be normal.

Maintenance Treatment

Speech therapy (reported in 17%) and psychotherapy (reported in 18%) have been the primary modalities used for chronic treatment to prevent recurrent symptoms (Morris MJ, MD and Christopher KL, MD, unpublished data, 2009). Speech therapy is extensively discussed in articles elsewhere in this issue.

Psychotherapy, Biofeedback, and Hypnotherapy

Psychotherapy or psychological counseling has been used extensively in the treatment of VCD and remains a primary treatment modality along with speech therapy. The cumulative VCD literature describes 43% of treated patients who underwent various forms of psychiatric therapy (Morris MJ and Christopher KL, unpublished data, 2009), but the effectiveness of psychotherapy in decreasing VCD episodes has not been studied. Studies include referral rates ranging from 30% to 90% for formal psychotherapy.[7,76] In patients who fit the diagnosis of psychogenic VCD, psychiatric evaluation in addition to speech therapy should be highly recommended.

Several specific methods as part of the overall psychotherapy plan have been advocated. The use of biofeedback was mentioned as a treatment option in 37 patients. There is only one prospective study investigating the utility of biofeedback training as a treatment for VCD. Nahmias evaluated[77] female patients diagnosed with "laryngeal dyskinesia" and provided electroencephalographic neurofeedback in five patients. The investigators were able to demonstrate a reduction in midmaximal flow ratio in two patients and normalization in the remaining three patients.[77] McFadden and Zawadski[35] found that four of the nine patients with exercise-induced VCD had rapid resolution of symptoms after basic biofeedback training. Ferris also used biofeedback in their series of nine patients in combination with counseling and antidepressants with good success.[76]

Hypnotherapy has been occasionally used as an adjunct to psychotherapy in the treatment of VCD.[78–80] A more general use of hypnosis in a pediatric pulmonary center for various disorders described improvement in 80% of patients. Use of hypnosis in 29 VCD patients who were taught self-hypnosis by their pediatric pulmonologists demonstrated symptom improvement in 31% of patients and VCD resolution in another 38 percent.[78] The investigators also describe its specific use in diagnosing VCD by using hypnotherapy to elicit symptoms and document the presence of inspiratory vocal cord adduction.

Other Treatment Options

Specific treatment for endogenous and exogenous irritant disorders is discussed in respective articles elsewhere in this issue. There is recent evidence in a 2006 series by Doshi and Weinberger[43] that anticholinergic inhalers were beneficial in controlling symptoms of exercise-induced VCD, but no additional studies have confirmed this finding.

Continuous positive airway pressure has been rarely used to treat patients with expiratory and inspiratory VCD, but experience is limited.[81,82] The use of botulinum toxin in VCD has appeal for temporizing or short-term control. The experience with it is also limited and reported in approximately 24 patients.[31,81,83,84]

SUMMARY

This article presents disorders of POLO resulting in noisy breathing and dyspnea and a variety of secondary symptoms, such as cough. The POLO supraglottic disorder, termed IARP, has historically been called laryngomalacia. PVFM and VCD are POLO glottic disorders. The three categories of POLO of glottic origin are defined as irritant (with intrinsic and extrinsic components), exertional, and psychological. Each of the three glottic disorder categories is composed of several conditions, also discussed. Clinical presentation of POLO disorders are examined.

Flexible laryngoscopy is identified as the diagnostic gold standard. Classic POLO endoscopic findings are presented:

(1). In IARP, there is bilateral, and usually symmetric, movement of the arytenoid area medially and anteriorly; prolapse on the glottic aperture associated with strong inspiratory efforts produces laryngeal obstruction;
(2). In PVCM, the true vocal folds adduct during inspiration, thus compromising the glottic aperture; obstruction must be limited to inspiration to meet the condition of paradoxic motion; and
(3). VCD can be limited to inspiration or present as inspiratory and expiratory obstruction.

Similar to PVFM, the true vocal folds adduct toward the midline. Additional findings can be seen, however; the anterior portion of the true vocal folds demonstrates complete or near complete adduction, but the posterior portion has incomplete adduction, leaving a small, posterior, diamond-shaped chink. Other characteristic features are bunching of the false vocal folds and the tendency for the arytenoids to remain out laterally to a variable degree with failure to fully adduct. The same findings are often seen on exhalation. Prior observation suggests that subjects with VCD are not able to consciously reproduce the findings seen during an episode.

Cough in POLO disorders is addressed. The relative value and pitfalls of provocation testing and spirometry with FVLs are identified. The differential diagnosis for POLO disorders is discussed, particularly with respect to asthma and laryngeal disorders.

Hypotheses for causes are presented and the importance of an interdisciplinary approach and prospective scientific studies stressed.

REFERENCES

1. Dunglison RD. The practice of medicine. Philadelphia: Lea and Blanchard; 1842. 257–258.
2. Flint A. Principles and practice of medicine. Philadelphia: Lea and Blanchard; 1842. 267–268.
3. MacKenzie M. Use of laryngoscopy in diseases of the throat. Philadelphia: Lindsey and Blackeston; 1869. p. 246–250.
4. Osler W. Hysteria. In: Osler W, editor. The principles and practice of medicine. 4th edition. New York: Appleton; 1902. p. 1111–22.
5. Patterson R, Schatz M, Horton M. Munchausen's stridor: non-organic laryngeal obstruction. Clin Allergy 1974;4:307–10.
6. Brugman SM. What's this thing called vocal cord dysfunction? Chest online. Available at: www.chestnet.org/education/online/pccu/vol20/lessons25_27/print26.php. Accessed June, 2009.
7. Andrianopoulos MV, Gallivan GJ, Gallivan KH. PVCM, PVCD, EPL and irritable larynx syndrome: what are we talking about and how do we treat it? J Voice 2000;14:607–18.
8. Morrison M, Rammage L, Emami AJ. The irritable larynx syndrome. J Voice 1999; 13:447–55.
9. Cukier-Blaj S, Bewley A, Aviv JE, et al. Paradoxical vocal fold motion: a sensory-motor laryngeal disorder. Laryngoscope 2008;118:367–70.
10. Kellman RM, Leopold DA. Paradoxical vocal cord motion: an important cause of stridor. Laryngoscope 1982;92:58–60.
11. Christopher KL, Wood RP, Eckert C, et al. Vocal cord dysfunction presenting as asthma. N Engl J Med 1983;308:1566–70.
12. Bittleman DB, Smith RJ, Weiler JM. Abnormal movement of the aryteniod region during exercise presenting as exercise-induced asthma in an adolescent athlete. Chest 1994;106:615–6.
13. Morris MJ, Perkins PJ, Allan PF. Vocal cord dysfunction: etiologies and treatment. Clin Pulm Med 2006;13:73–86.
14. Murrary DM, Lawlwe PG. All that wheezes is not asthma: paradoxical vocal cord movement presenting as severe acute asthma requiring ventilatory support. Anaesthesia 1998;53:1006–11.
15. Grillo HC. Management of idiopathic tracheal stenosis. Chest Surg Clin N Am 1996;6(4):811–8.
16. Ashiku SK, Mathisen DJ. Idiopathic laryngotracheal stenosis. Chest Surg Clin N Am 2003;13(2):257–69.
17. Nussbaum E, Maggi JC. Laryngomalacia in children. Chest 1990;98:242–4.
18. Smith RJ, Bauman NM, Bent JP, et al. Exercise-induced laryngomalacia, Pediatric exercise-induced laryngomalacia. Ann Otol Rhinol Laryngol 1995;104(7):537–41.
19. Bent JP, Miller DA, Kim JW, et al. Pediatric exercise-induced laryngomalacia. Ann Otol Rhinol Laryngol 1995;104(7):537–41.
20. Pinho SM, Tsuji DH, Sennes L, et al. Paradoxical vocal fold movement: a case report. J Voice 1997;11:368–72.
21. Heimdal JH, Roksund OD, Halvorsen T, et al. Continuous laryngoscopy exercise test: a method for visualizing laryngeal dysfunction during exercise. Laryngoscope 2006;116:52–7.

22. Heinle R, Linton A, Chidekel AS. Exercise-induced vocal cord dysfunction presenting as asthma in pediatric patients; toxicity of inappropriate inhaled corticosteroids and the role of exercise laryngoscopy. Pediatric Asthma Allergy Immunol 2003;16:215–24.
23. Bjornsdottir US, Gudmundsson K, Hjartarson H, et al. Exercise induced laryngochalasia: an imitator of exercise-induced bronchospasm. Ann Allergy Asthma Immunol 2000;83:387–91.
24. Thomson J, Turner AL. On the causation of stridor in infants. Br Med J 1900;2: 1561–3.
25. Ferguson CF. In: Pediatric laryngology, vol. 2. Philidelphia: WB Saunders; 1972. p. 1168.
26. Richter GT, Rutter MJ, deAlarcon A, et al. Late-onset laryngomalacia. Arch Otolaryngol Head Neck Surg 2008;134(1):75–80.
27. Nagai A, Kanemura T, Konno K. Abnorman movement of the arytenoid region as a cause of upper airway obstruction. Thorax 1992;47:840–1.
28. Lakin RC, Metzger WJ, Haughey BH. Upper airway obstruction presenting as exercise-induced asthma. Chest 1984;86:499–501.
29. Balasubramaniam SK, O'Connell EJ, Sachs MI, et al. Recurrent exercise-induced stridor in an adolescent. Ann Allergy 1986;57(243):287–8.
30. Fallon KE. Upper airway obstruction masquerading as exercise-induced bronchospasm in an elite road cyclist. Br J Sports Med 2004;38:9–11.
31. Garibaldi E, LeBlance G, Hibbett A, et al. Exercise-induced paradoxical vocal cord dysfunction: diagnosis with videostroboscopic endoscopy and treatment with Clostridium toxin. J Allergy Clin Immunol 1993;91(A236):200.
32. Kivity S, Bibi H, Schwarz Y, et al. Variable vocal cord dysfunction presenting as wheezing and exercise-induced asthma. J Asthma 1986;23:241–4.
33. Schmidt M, Brugger E, Richter W. Stress-inducible functional laryngospasm: differential diagnostic considerations for bronchial asthma. Laryngol Rhinol Otol 1985;64:461–5.
34. Wood RP II, Jafek BW, Cherniack RM. Laryngeal dysfunction and pulmonary disorder. Otolaryngol Head Neck Surg 1986;94:374–8.
35. McFadden ER, Zawadski DK. Vocal cord dysfunction masquerading as exercise-induced asthma a physiologic cause for "choking" during athletic activities. Am J Respir Crit Care Med 1996;153:942–7.
36. Landwehr LP, Wood RP II, Blager FB, et al. Vocal cord dysfunction mimicking exercise-induced bronchospasm in adolescents. Pediatrics 1996;98:971–4.
37. Rundell KW, Spiering BA. Inspiratory stridor in elite athletes. Chest 2003;123: 468–74.
38. Sullivan MD, Heywood BM, Beukelman DR. A treatment for vocal cord dysfunction in female athletes: an outcome study. Laryngoscope 2001;111: 1751–5.
39. Morris MJ, Deal LE, Bean DR, et al. Vocal cord dysfunction in patients with exertional dyspnea. Chest 1999;116:1676–82.
40. Perello MM, Gurevich J, Fitzpatrick T, et al. Clinical characteristics of vocal cord dysfunction in two military tertiary care facilities. Am J Respir Crit Care Med 2003; 167:A788.
41. Parker JM, Mooney LD, Berg BW. Exercise tidal loops in patients with vocal cord dysfunction. Chest 1999;118:256S.
42. Diamond E, Kane C, Dugan G. Presentation and evaluation of vocal cord dysfunction. Chest 2000;118(Suppl):199S.

43. Doshi DR, Weinberger MM. Long-term outcome of vocal cord dysfunction. Ann Allergy Asthma Immunol 2006;96:794–9.
44. Abu-Hasan M, Tannous B, Weinberger M. Exercise-induced dyspnea in children and adolescents: if not asthma then what? Ann Allergy Asthma Immunol 2005;94: 366–71.
45. Seear M, Wensley D, West N. How accurate is the diagnosis of exercise induced asthma among Vancouver school children? Arch Dis Child 2005;90: 898–902.
46. Higenbottam T. Narrowing of the glottis opening in humans associated with experimentally induced bronchoconstriction. J Appl Phys 1980;49:403–7.
47. Collett PW, Brancatisano AP, Engel LA. Changes in the glottic aperture during bronchial asthma. Am Rev Respir Dis 1983;128:719–23.
48. Rodenstein DO, Francis C, Stanescu DC. Emotional laryngeal wheezing: a new syndrome. Am Rev Respir Dis 1983;127:354–6.
49. Echternach M, Delb W, Verse T, et al. Does isolated expiratory vocal cord dysfunction exist? Otolaryngol Head Neck Surg 2008;138:805–6.
50. American Psychiatric Association. Diagnostic and statistical manual of mental disorders. 4th edition. Washington, DC: American Psychiatric Association; 1994.
51. Mikita J, Parker J. High levels of medical utilization by ambulatory patients with vocal cord dysfunction as compared to age- and gender-matched asthmatics. Chest 2006;129:905–8.
52. Husein OF, Husein TN, Gardner R, et al. Formal psychological testing in patients with paradoxical vocal fold dysfunction. Laryngoscope 2008;118:740–7.
53. Lacy TJ, McManis SE. Psychogenic stridor. Gen Hosp Psychiatry 1994;16: 213–23.
54. Gavin LA, Wamboldt M, Brugman S, et al. Psychological and family characteristics of adolescents with vocal cord dysfunction. J Asthma 1998;35:409–17.
55. Powell DM, Karanfilov BI, Beechler KB, et al. Paradoxical vocal cord dysfunction in juveniles. Arch Otolaryngol Head Neck Surg 2000;126:29–34.
56. Craig T, Sitz K, Squire E. Vocal cord dysfunction during wartime. Mil Med 1992; 157:614–6.
57. Brown TM, Merritt WD, Evans DL. Psychogenic vocal cord dysfunction masquerading as asthma. J Nerv Ment Dis 1988;176:308–10.
58. Geist R, Tallett SE. Diagnosis and management of psychogenic stridor caused by a conversion disorder. Pediatrics 1990;86:315–7.
59. Kattan M, Ben-Zvi Z. Stridor caused by vocal cord malfunction associated with emotional factors. Clin Pediatr 1985;24:158–60.
60. Skinner DW, Bradley PJ. Psychogenic stridor. J Laryngol Otol 1989;103:383–5.
61. Ramirez JR, Leon I, Rivera LM. Episodic laryngeal dyskinesia. Clinical and psychiatric characterization. Chest 1986;90:716–21.
62. Freedman MR, Rosenberg SJ, Schmaling KB. Childhood sexual abuse in patients with paradoxical vocal cord dysfunction. J Nerv Ment Dis 1991;179:295–8.
63. Newman KB, Mason UG, Schmaling KB. Clinical features of vocal cord dysfunction. Am J Respir Crit Care Med 1995;152:1382–6.
64. Selner JC, Staudenmayer H, Koepke JW, et al. Vocal cord dysfunction: the importance of psychologic factors and provocation challenge testing. J Allergy Clin Immunol 1987;79:726–33.
65. Tomares SM, Flotte TR, Tunkel DE, et al. Real time laryngoscopy with olfactory challenge for diagnosis of psychogenic stridor. Pediatr Pulmonol 1993;16: 259–62.

66. Powell SA, Chau TN, Gaziano MA, et al. Mass psychogenic illness presenting as acute stridor in an adolescent female cohort. Ann Otol Rhinol Laryngol 2007; 116(7):525–31.
67. Ayres JG, Gabbott PL. Vocal cord dysfunction and laryngeal hyperresponsiveness: a function of altered autonomic balance? Thorax 2002;57:284–5.
68. Bucca C, Rolla G, Brussino L, et al. Are asthma-like symptoms due to bronchial or extrathoracic airway dysfunction? Lancet 1995;346:791–5.
69. Perkner JJ, Fennelly KP, Balkissoon R, et al. Irritant-associated vocal cord dysfunction. J Occup Environ Med 1998;40:136–43.
70. Miller RD, Hyatt RE. Evaluation of obstructing lesions of the trachea and larynx by flow-volume loops. Am Rev Respir Dis 1973;108:475–81.
71. Sterner JB, Morris MJ, Sill JM, et al. Inspiratory flow volume curve evaluation for detecting upper airway disease. Respir Care 2009;54:461–6.
72. Perkins PJ, Morris MJ. Vocal cord dysfunction induced by methacholine challenge testing. Chest 2002;122:1988–93.
73. Guss J, Mirza N. Methacholine challenge testing in the diagnosis of paradoxical vocal fold motion. Laryngoscope 2006;116:1558–61.
74. Reisner C, Borish L. Heliox therapy for acute vocal cord dysfunction. Chest 1995; 108:1477.
75. Gose JE. Acute workup of vocal cord dysfunction. Ann Allergy Asthma Immunol 2003;91:318.
76. Ferris RL, Eisele DW, Tunkel DE. Functional laryngeal dyskinesia in children and adults. Laryngoscope 1998;108:1520–3.
77. Nahmias J, Tansey M, Karetzky MS. Asthmatic extrathoracic upper airway obstruction: laryngeal dyskinesia. Niger J Med 1994;91:616–20.
78. Anbar RD. Hypnosis in pediatrics: applications at a pediatric pulmonary center. BMC Pediatr 2002;2:11.
79. Smith MS. Acute psychogenic stridor in an adolescent athlete treated with hypnosis. Pediatrics 1983;72:247–8.
80. Caraon P, O'Toole C. Vocal cord dysfunction presenting as asthma. Ir Med J 1991;84:98–9.
81. Lloyd RV, Jones NS. Paradoxical vocal fold movement: a case report. J Laryngol Otol 1995;109:1105–6.
82. Goldman J, Muers M. Vocal cord dysfunction and wheezing. Thorax 1991;46: 401–4.
83. Maillard I, Schweizer V, Broccard A, et al. Use of botulinum toxin type A to avoid tracheal intubation or tracheostomy in severe paradoxical vocal cord movement. Chest 2000;118:874–6.
84. Altman KW, Mirza N, Ruiz C, et al. Paradoxical vocal fold motion: presentation and treatment options. J Voice 2000;14:99–103.

Evidence for Sensory Neuropathy and Pharmacologic Management

Scott M. Greene, C. Blake Simpson, MD*

KEYWORDS

- Postviral vagal neuropathy • Chronic cough • Irritable larynx
- Laryngeal sensory neuropathy

Postnasal drip, cough-variant asthma, and gastroesophageal reflux disease are the cause of chronic cough in 86% of adult patients. This percentage increases to over 99% when evaluating immunocompetent nonsmokers with normal chest radiograph findings and no history of angiotensin-converting enzyme-inhibitor use.[1] Despite this, a significant number of patients continue to have unexplained cough after an exhaustive workup and failed empiric treatments. Recently, a body of literature has emerged supporting a sensory or motor neuropathy responsible for many of the previously refractory cases of chronic cough. First introduced by Morrison and colleagues[2] in 1999, the idea of the irritable larynx has been redefined throughout the years, holding various titles for the same suspected cause: postviral vagal neuropathy (PVVN), sensory neuropathic cough and laryngeal sensory neuropathy (LSN). Many recent studies not only identify the at-risk population, but the common presenting symptoms, potential pathophysiology behind vagal neuropathy, and several promising medical interventions. The purpose of this article is to emphasize that postviral vagal neuropathy may be a distinct and treatable cause of chronic idiopathic cough while reviewing common clinical presentations and potential treatments. See the article by Irwin elsewhere in this issue for another perspective of the role of sensory neuropathy in the unexplained chronic cough.

The idea of postviral neuropathies has been well studied in various other disease processes, such as Bell palsy, Guillain-Barré syndrome, and postherpetic neuralgias. Of interest to otolaryngologists is the small, but significant, subset of patients with treatment-resistant chronic cough that have been identified with clinical or objective evidence suggesting an underlying vagal neuropathy. PVVN is a condition of vagal nerve injury or dysfunction following an antecedent viral illness. Vagal neuropathy

The Department of Otolaryngology—Head and Neck Surgery, The University of Texas Health Science Center at San Antonio, 7703 Floyd Curl Drive, San Antonio, TX 78229, USA
* Corresponding author.
E-mail address: simpsonc@uthscsa.edu (C.B. Simpson).

Otolaryngol Clin N Am 43 (2010) 67–72
doi:10.1016/j.otc.2009.11.003
oto.theclinics.com

may affect the motor branches of the vagus nerve, resulting in vocal fold paralysis or paresis, or it may affect the sensory branches, inducing a throat tickle, globus sensation, excessive throat mucous, odynophonia, chronic cough, or laryngospasm. These symptoms may be aggravated by sensory stimuli such as laughing, prolonged phonation, and noxious stimuli, and has been described being elicited clinically by palpation at the cricoid level.[1,3,4]

In 2001, Amin and Koufman[5] first described the association of neuropathic cough and previous upper respiratory tract infection. They described a case report of five patients presenting over 5 years with similar symptoms consisting of chronic cough, globus, dysphagia, vocal fatigue, and effortful phonation, persisting long after resolution of their acute viral illness. Subsequent investigation through videostroboscopy and laryngeal electromyography (LEMG) revealed varied presentations: (1) vocal fold paresis, (2) neuropathy-induced laryngopharyngeal reflux disease, (3) dysphagia, and (4) neuropathic pain.

Two potential mechanisms by which viral infection may cause nerve injury have been described: (1) direct infection and inflammation of the nerve or (2) induction of a nonspecific inflammatory response that secondarily involves a nerve.[5] In either situation, viral involvement lowers the threshold of both the efferent and afferent arms, sensitizing the nerves to previously ignored stimuli. In 2009, Rees and colleagues[2] made clinical distinction between the motor and sensory components of vagal neuropathy. In a prospective cross-sectional series of 44 patients presenting with persistent cough, throat clearing, dysphonia, and vocal fatigue following a previous upper respiratory infection, 45% with motor and sensory neuronal involvement, 41% with isolated sensory nerve involvement, and 14% with isolated motor nerve involvement. Rees and colleagues[3] concluded "cough, throat clearing, and globus are considered primarily sensory symptoms while loss of voice and vocal fatigue are considered primarily motor symptoms," which all may be attributed to vagal nerve dysfunction. Unfortunately, it may never be possible to definitely establish this causal relationship, as vagal nerve biopsy remains the only means of definitive diagnosis. As more case studies and prospective analysis emerge, greater support appears for a clinical diagnosis of PVVN.

CLINICAL EVALUATION

In diagnosing PVVN, the clinician must maintain a high level of suspicion. As with all clinical diagnoses, a thorough history is essential in providing clues to this potential cause. Many algorithms, such as the anatomic diagnostic protocol, are available to help guide the clinician in assessing the patient.[2] Once the most common causes of chronic cough have been ruled out, further inquiry into potential viral illness surrounding the initial presentation of symptoms should be investigated. PVVN is usually associated with an acute onset of cough that persists long after the resolution of the concomitant viral symptoms. The majority of patients presenting with PVVN have previously been misdiagnosed. An average of 83 weeks from onset to diagnosis has been sited; therefore, patients may show significant frustration in the persistence of their symptoms.[3] Many of these patients have been treated with multiple rounds of antibiotics, proton pump inhibitors, and antihistamines well before presenting to the otolaryngologist. Although not all the literature agrees, the majority of recent studies suggest PVVN is more common in women, occurring most often in the fifth and sixth decade of life.[2] The vagus, supplying both the superior laryngeal nerve (SLN) and recurrent laryngeal nerve (RLN), allows for a multitude of presentations, many of which can be classified according the their primary symptoms: motor, sensory, or mixed motor-sensory dysfunction.

Motor Symptoms

Acute onset of "breathy dysphonia, vocal fatigue, effortful phonation, odynophagia, cough, globus, or dysphagia lasting long after the resolution of the acute viral illness" may represent the initial presentation of PVVN involving the efferent branches.[3] Whereas routine nasolaryngoscopy can appear both anatomically and functionally normal, videostroboscopy and LEMG may provide the only objective evidence of RLN or SLN dysfunction.[4] With primary motor branch involvement, stroboscopy may reveal reduced diadochokinesis of the vocal folds or axis deviation of the glottis. LEMG may also reveal the presence of polyphasic units, rapid-firing units, and reduced recruitment in the cricothyroid and thyroarytenoid muscles, providing further objective evidence for RLN or SLN paresis.[4]

Sensory Symptoms

When the sensory branches are mainly affected, the patient may not necessarily present with sharp pain or the classic burning ache associated with many of the other neuropathies, but may instead describe a tickle, dry patch, or globus most commonly found at the level of the cricoid. This sensation often precipitates a 20- to 30-second coughing spell.[3] Bastian and colleagues[5] describe this phenomenon as a "bogus tickle that leads to uncontrollable coughing." Excessive throat clearing is another well-recognized symptom within the literature. Tussive-like spells and laryngospasm have been reported, usually following exposure to specific aromatics such as perfume or household cleaning agents.

Viral-induced Laryngopharyngeal Reflux

Several studies have recognized symptoms consistent with laryngopharyngeal reflux (LPR) beginning with the onset of a previous viral illness.[6,7,8] Rees and colleagues[7] propose postviral LPR may be secondary to altered esophageal peristalsis and esophageal clearing or alternately an increase in symptoms through altered sensation in the throat due in part to preexisting reflux.

TREATMENT OPTIONS

Whereas several studies have provided objective evidence of vocal fold paresis following a previous viral illness, the majority of cases have been diagnosed through symptomatic presentation and taking a thorough history. At present, there is no standard of care for patients with suspected PVVN, but it has been recently suggested that treatment for PVVN be patient-specific and, therefore, tailored to individual presenting symptoms.[7] The patient's specific triggers that induce cough should be identified and patients should be educated on avoidance of suspected triggers. Vocal fold paralysis or paresis may be referred to a speech pathologist for vocal therapy and these patients should be counseled concerning their various surgical options, including medialization laryngoplasty and injection augmentation of the vocal folds.

PHARMACEUTICALS FOR TREATMENT OF PVVN

Pregabalin

Method of action

Pregabalin is a γ-aminobutyric acid (GABA) analog that strongly binds to the alpha(2)-delta site in the central nervous system tissues. Binding to the alpha(2)-delta subunit may be involved in pregabalin's effects on neuropathic pain. Pregabalin reduces the calcium-dependent release of several neurotransmitters, including glutamate, noradrenaline, and substance P, possibly by modulation of calcium channel function;

however, the exact mechanism of action is unknown. Currently, pregabalin has Food and Drug Administration (FDA) approval in the treatment of neuropathic pain, including postherpetic neuralgia, diabetic peripheral neuropathy, and fibromyalgia. Pregabalin is renally excreted unchanged in the urine, with a half-life of 6.3 hours.[9]

Advantages

Pregabalin shares many of the favorable qualities of gabapentin, including its rapid titration, rapid onset of activity, and minimal drug interactions. Advantages over gabapentin are greater absorption, increased bioavailability, and less dosing frequency.[10] Studies have shown equivalent efficacy to gabapentin at much lower doses of pregabalin in the treatment of neuropathic pain, therefore many believe pregabalin is likely to be associated with fewer dose-related adverse events.[11,12]

Disadvantages

Pregabalin is a pregnancy class C drug. Somnolence is the most common side effect demonstrated in studies, often potentiating the side effects of other sedating drugs. Other common side effects are dry mouth, peripheral edema, weight gain, and blurred vision and dizziness.

Dosing schedule

Patients were started at 75 mg twice a day and were then raised over 4 weeks to 150 mg twice a day if needed for symptomatic relief. In one patient, 150 mg three times a day was needed.

Evidence

Charts were reviewed for 12 consecutive patients prescribed pregabalin for symptoms of LSN. Outcomes were analyzed by reviewing pre- and posttreatment questionnaires.[10]

Gabapentin

Method of action

Gabapentin does not interact with GABA receptors, is not metabolized to a GABA agonist or to GABA, and does not inhibit GABA uptake or degradation. The mechanism of action is unknown. Gabapentin does, however, prevent pain-related behavior in response to a normally innocuous stimulus and exaggerated response to painful stimuli in animal models. Gabapentin is FDA approved in the treatment of seizure and postherpetic neuralgia, but has secured a long list of off-label uses within the clinical setting. Gabapentin is not metabolized and is entirely excreted renally unchanged with a half-life of 5 to 7 hours.[13]

Advantages

Gabapentin is normally well tolerated and has relatively few drug interactions. It does not change levels of other seizure medications. It is cleared by the kidney, so it does not interact at the level of the liver.

Disadvantages

Gabapentin is slowly absorbed (peak: 3 to 4 hours postdose) and, more importantly, plasma concentrations have been found to have a nonlinear relationship to increasing doses. Other disadvantages of gabapentin include a short half-life that requires a three times daily regimen.

Dosing schedule

Patients were instructed to begin dosing at 100 mg/d and to increase dosage up to 900 mg/d in divided doses over a 4-week period.

Evidence

Initially cited in a case report of five patients with suspected PVVN, the empiric use of gabapentin for intractable chronic cough has been accepted as a reasonable first-line treatment in many United States clinics.[4]

Amitriptyline

Method of action

Amitriptyline hydrochloride is a tricyclic antidepressant that also exhibits a sedative property. It promotes neuronal activity by blocking the membrane pump mechanism, which is responsible for the absorption of serotonin and norepinephrine in serotonergic and adrenergic neurons. Amitriptyline is FDA approved for the treatment of depression, but has been used off-label for many years for the treatment of headache, irritable bowel syndrome, pain syndromes, and postherpetic neuralgia. Amitriptyline is hepatically metabolized via P450 CYP2D6 and is renally excreted almost entirely in metabolite form. Amitriptyline has a half-life of 10 to 26 hours.[14]

Advantages

Amitriptyline is usually well tolerated and is considered to have a less adverse effect profile compared to many of the other tricyclic antidepressants. Amitriptyline is also dosed once daily.

Disadvantages

Heavy hepatic metabolism with the major metabolite, nortriptyline, excreted through the urine and feces.

Dosing schedule

Patients were treated with 10 mg everyday.

Evidence

A prospective randomized controlled study comparing the effectiveness of amitriptyline versus codeine-guaifenesin for select cases of suspected PVVN found that the majority of patients in the amitriptyline arm achieved complete response as defined by the investigators.[3] See the article by Irwin elsewhere in this issue that provides a perspective on the potential limitations of this study.

In a cohort of 12 consecutive patients with suspected PVVN, all patients had at least 40% reduction of self-reported symptoms, with most describing between 75% to 100% short-term relief.[6]

SUMMARY

PVNN, while a relatively new clinical diagnosis, has been observed and well described within the literature in recent years. As additional studies are reported, a growing body of anecdotal and empirical evidence suggests PVVN may be a distinct and treatable cause of idiopathic chronic cough. PVVN varies in presentation, but is most commonly seen in adult women with symptoms persisting long after resolution of an acute viral illness. Symptoms are classified according to the vagal branch most affected, either motor, sensory, or both. LPR has also been reported in association with suspected onset of viral neuropathy. At present, there is no standard of care for treating PVVN. This article highlights the efficacy, side effect profiles, and supporting evidence of the currently recommended pharmacological interventions. Future studies are needed to provide greater objective evidence as well as the potential pathophysiologic mechanism behind this elusive disease process.

REFERENCES

1. Irwin RS, Curley FJ, French CL. Chronic cough: the spectrum and frequency of causes, key components of the diagnostic evaluation, and outcome of specific therapy. Am Rev Respir Dis 1990;141:640–7.
2. Morrison M, Rammage L, Emami AJ. The irritable larynx syndrome. J Voice 1999; 13:447–55.
3. Jeyakumar A. Effectiveness of amatriptyline versus cough suppressants in the treatement of chronic cough resulting from postviral vagal neuropathy. Laryngoscope 2006;116:2108–12.
4. Lee B, Woo P. Chronic cough as a sign of laryngeal sensory neuropathy: diagnosis and treatment. Ann Otol Rhinol Laryngol 2005;114:253–7.
5. Bastian RW, Vaidya AM, Delsupehe KG. Sensory neuropathic cough: a common and treatable cause of cough. Otolaryngol Head Neck Surg 2006;135:17–21.
6. Amin MR, Koufman JA. Vagal neuropathy after upper respiratory infections: a viral etiology? Am J Otolaryngol 2001;22:251–6.
7. Rees CJ, Henderson AH, Belafsky PC. Postviral vagal neuropathy. Ann Otol Rhinol Laryngol 2009;118(4):247–52.
8. Irwin R, Boulet L, Cloutier M, et al. Managing cough as a defense mechanism and as a symptom: a consensus report of the American College of Chest Physicians. Chest 1998;144(2 Suppl Managing):133S–81S.
9. Pregabalin: In: DRUGDEX System [Internet database]. Greenwood Village, Colo: Thomson Reuters (Healthcare) Inc. Updated periodically.
10. Halum SL, Sycamore DL, McRae BR. A new treatment option for laryngeal sensory neuropathy. Laryngoscope 2009.
11. Freynhagen R, Strojek K, Griesing T, et al. Efficacy of pregabalin in neuropathic pain evaluated in a 12-week, randomised, double-blind, multicentre, placebo-controlled trial of fble- and fixed-dose regimens. Pain 2005;115(3):254–63.
12. Wesche D, Bockbrader H. A pharmacokinetic comparison of pregabalin and gabapentin. The Journal of Pain 2005;6(3)(Suppl 1):S29.
13. Gabapentin. In: DRUGDEX System [Internet database]. Greenwood Village, Colo: Thomson Reuters (Healthcare) Inc. Updated periodically.
14. Amitryptline. In: DRUGDEX System [Internet database]. Greenwood Village, Colo: Thomson Reuters (Healthcare) Inc. Updated periodically.

The Role of Voice Therapy in the Management of Paradoxical Vocal Fold Motion, Chronic Cough, and Laryngospasm

Thomas Murry, PhD[a,*], Christine Sapienza, PhD[b]

KEYWORDS

- Paradoxical vocal fold motion
- Gastroesophageal reflux disease
- Chronic cough • Laryngospasm

Gastroesophageal reflux disease (GERD), paradoxical vocal fold motion (PVFM), chronic cough (CC), and laryngospasm are significant medical problems that share many common signs and symptoms. However, they are treated differently by numerous disciplines, resulting in a plethora of outcomes, including acceptable responses, failed treatments, and partial responses. The varied characteristics associated with this triad of conditions are often severe, and usually clinicians focus on the most severe occurrences when patients are seen initially. Complaints of episodic choking, shortness of breath, and cough command attention from pulmonologists, allergists, and gastroenterologists. However, a growing body of evidence suggests that otolaryngologists and speech–language pathologists should provide the definitive and long-term management of patients who have these disorders.[1–4]

Regarding PVFM, the overwhelming impression derived from the literature from the past 25 years is that the various disease titles and descriptions confound the understanding of its pathophysiology and neuropathology. Is PVFM the same as CC that is refractory to standard medications? Is PVFM a result of a laryngospasm? Is laryngospasm prompted by severe episodes of upper respiratory irritation and CC? These

[a] Department of Otorhinolaryngology, Weill Cornell Medical College, 1305 York Avenue, 5th Floor, New York, NY 10021, USA
[b] Department of Speech and Hearing Science, University of Florida, Gainesville, FL 32601, USA
* Corresponding author.
E-mail address: thm7001@med.cornell.edu (T. Murry).

Otolaryngol Clin N Am 43 (2010) 73–83
doi:10.1016/j.otc.2009.11.004
oto.theclinics.com
0030-6665/10/$ – see front matter

circumferential questions show that no clear understanding exists of the symptoms associated with each of these conditions or their underlying mechanisms. **Table 1** presents further evidence that the definitions of these conditions somewhat overlap, creating difficulty in accurately defining them. A review of several journals produced the list of terms that contain descriptions that resemble each other and implicate CC, laryngospasm, or PVFM.

Although evidence may suggest that these three conditions have similar underlying mechanisms, they are often treated according to a standard set used by the specialist who initially sees the patient. This variation in treatment standards may result in misdiagnosis or failed or partial treatments. In the most unfortunate cases, it may result in the patient taking needless medications.

The occurrence of PVFM, CC, or laryngospasm clearly centers on symptoms that involve some degree of vocal fold adduction, either for an instant or up to several seconds. Highly variable conditions trigger this behavior, not only among patients but often within the same patient. This article briefly reviews the three conditions as they relate to a multidisciplinary team, including otolaryngologists and speech–language pathologists.

LARYNGOSPASM

Laryngospasm is a serious condition defined as a sudden-onset, rapid, and forceful contraction of the laryngeal sphincter, resulting in airway obstruction or complete glottic closure and apnea for up to 20 seconds.[5] Occurring in response to noxious stimuli, laryngospasm[5–8] may represent an abnormal excitation or loss of inhibition of the laryngeal closure reflex.[9] Known concomitant conditions that can lead to a laryngospasm include PVFM, vocal fold paralysis,[4] irritable larynx syndrome,[1] GERD,[6] and trigeminal neuralgia.[4]

Table 1
Terminology collected from recent literature describing symptoms associated with paradoxical vocal fold motion , chronic cough, or laryngospasm

	Paradoxical Vocal Fold Motion	Chronic Cough	Laryngospasm
Vocal cord dysfunction	X		X
Munchausen's stridor	X		
Functional airway obstruction	X	X	X
Paradoxical vocal cord dysfunction	X	X	X
Episodic paroxysmal laryngospasm	X		X
Adult onset asthma	X	X	X
Factitious asthma	X		
Paradoxical vocal fold movement	X	X	X
Breathing abnormalities	X	X	X
Psychogenic stridor	X	X	X
Irritable larynx syndrome	X	X	X
Laryngeal dyskinesia	X		X
Trigeminal neuralgia	X	X	X

The most commonly described signs and symptoms associated with laryngospasm in children and adults include (not necessarily in this order of frequency) choking, breathing disruptions, dysphagia, aspiration, dyspnea, episodes of complete airway obstruction, stridor (a continuous sound during inspiration), voice disorders (aphonia and dysphonia), cough, throat clearing, globus, and pain in the jaw area (presumed to represent a traumatic glossopharyngeal neuralgia). Many of these same signs are associated with PVFM and CC.

In a group of 10 individuals who had laryngospasm, Gallivan and colleagues[10] found evidence of various symptoms, including stridor, choking, allergies to foods, and cough. The vocal fold movement in these individuals was described as inspiratory adduction of the anterior vocal fold and a diamond-shaped posterior glottic gap.

PARADOXICAL VOCAL FOLD MOTION

PVFM is a laryngeal disorder that affects respiratory function through obstructing the airway in the closing or partial closing of the vocal folds during inspiration.[2,11] Furthermore, because of the closing motion of the vocal folds, PVFM can also impact voice production.[12,13] The paradoxical motion has been shown to occur primarily during inhalation but may also occur during both inhalation and exhalation.[14–18] The multiplicity of patients' complaints often leads to incorrect diagnoses and more importantly a series of failed treatments.

PVFM, sometimes referred to as *vocal cord dysfunction* [VCD], has been associated with CC and laryngospasm. Vertigan and colleagues[19] outlined the recent history of the relationship between CC and PVFM. Studies by several other investigators[4,11,20–22] indicate that a large number of individuals who had abnormal vocal fold motion complained of cough that continued for long periods. In a study using flexible endoscopy and stroboscopy, Treole and colleagues[22] described the paradoxical motion in patients complaining of cough, choking and shortness of breath while they were sitting comfortably and not talking or exercising.

CHRONIC COUGH

CC has been defined as cough that persists for longer than 8 weeks despite medical management. Although many individuals who require treatment for a cough respond to medical management, a percentage of individuals continue to cough despite medical intervention. Unlike cough that occurs with a flu or upper respiratory infection, CC is a dry-sounding cough occurring randomly throughout the day.[23,24] It may be triggered by various events, such as exposure to cold air, smoke, perfume, or soap powder, or activity such as walking, talking, or laughing. In one study, Vertigan and colleagues[3] observed that approximately 50% of individuals who had CC were habitual mouth breathers, suggesting a drying effect on the laryngeal tissues and creating an irritating trigger.

GERD and laryngopharyngeal disease (LPR) are believed to be the causative factors in more than one half of adults who have CC. However, cough and GERD/LPR are common conditions that affect adults and children, and they may have a high rate of coexistence, if only by chance.[23] GERD/LPR may be controlled with diet management, proton pump inhibitors, prokinetic agents, and antianxiety medications. However, pharmacologic agents alone do not stem the CC even when the GERD/LPR conditions are improved.[4,11] Moreover, CC is often accompanied by other conditions, such as hoarseness[25] and PVFM.[26] Thus, a need exists for a complete evaluation of the onset factors, especially when common treatment methods do not reduce the CC.

Patients who have CC are usually seen by a pulmonologist; however, when no pulmonary component is found, patients often must seek help from other specialists and try other medical management without success. Murry and colleagues[11] reported on 5 patients who had a history of CC and were ultimately diagnosed with PVFM who had an average duration of symptoms before diagnosis of 66 months (5.5 years) with a range of 5 to 158 months (>13 years).

These findings suggest that CC, PVFM, and laryngospasm may be overlapping conditions, which leads to the following questions: Is PVFM a response to cough? Is the laryngospasm a severe episode of PVFM? Is cough a response to the adductory vocal fold motion seen in PVFM? These questions suggest a focused laryngeal component to CC, laryngospasm, and PVFM, once pulmonary issues are ruled out. The terminology in **Table 1** may reflect the overlapping relationship among CC, PVFM, and laryngospasm. Clearly, as Andrianopoulos and colleagues[1] pointed out in the review of these conditions, a thorough diagnosis is critical to successful medical and behavioral management of these conditions.

Evaluation by the Speech–Language Pathologist

In the past, CC, PVFM, and laryngospasm were considered separate entities. More recently, however, the conditions have been shown to have many similarities and thus may be considered overlapping or associated. Because of close association among CC, PVFM, and laryngospasm, the overall management typically involves several specialists because the patient's complaints encompass breathing difficulties, swallowing abnormalities, dysphonia, and an overall degradation in quality of life. The evaluation of PVFM, CC, and laryngospasm consists of medical examinations and behavioral assessments. Other articles in this issue outline the medical evaluations and tests, including flexible endoscopy and a thorough head and neck examination by an otolaryngologist, pulmonary workup, and chest radiograph by a pulmonologist, and evaluation by a gastroenterologist, which may include esophagoscopy.

Equally important in the management of patients who have symptoms of PVFM, CC, and laryngospasm is the role of the speech–language pathologist. Christopher and colleagues[27] were among the first groups to identify the importance of the speech–language pathologist in the care of patients who have PVFM. Andrianopoulos and colleagues[1] studied a group of 27 patients and identified 51.8% who had episodic acute aphonia, 18.5% hoarseness, and 44.4 % dysphagia. However, these percentages vary widely depending on the presence of other conditions or diseases. For example, Cukier-Blaj and Murry[28] reported on 70 patients who had laryngospasm and laryngopharyngeal reflux and found the related signs and symptoms to include several patients who had both dysphonia and dysphagia. Their results are summarized in **Table 2**.

The speech–language pathologist provides critical assessment of the conditions surrounding these signs and symptoms and performs tests to determine the exact nature of the complaint. The components of the evaluation include patient self-assessment, perceptual assessment of the voice, instrumental assessment of voice and swallowing (if symptoms warrant), and trial therapy. The speech–language pathologist should have access to the laryngoscopic examination and pulmonary data. The flexible endoscopic examination should be noted for evidence of paradoxical motion during quiet breathing.[22] The spirometry tests should be noted for the flattened inspiratory curve often seen in patients who have PVFM.[11]

Several tools may be used to obtain the patient's perception of the problem. The Voice Handicap Index[29,30] or Voice Handicap Index-10 (VHI-10) provides valid and reliable assessments of patients' perception of voice severity. The Dyspnea Index[31]

Table 2
Common symptoms in a cohort of 70 consecutive patients who had laryngeal findings of PVFM

Symptoms	%
Throat clearing	80.0
Throat mucus	74.3
Hoarseness	68.6
Annoying cough	62.9
Something sticking in the throat	54.3
Breathing difficulties	48.6
Coughing after lying down	42.9
Heartburn/chest pain	42.9
Difficulty swallowing	28.6

offers additional information regarding patients' self-assessment of breathing difficulty.

At the initial evaluation, the SLP should focus on issues relating to the onset of the primary problem (eg, cough, shortness of breath, swallowing difficulty). Specifically, when and how did the primary problem begin? Often patients may not recall and they must be prompted regarding events, such as sickness, travel, new medications, and lifestyle changes. The speech–language pathologist should probe each issue to determine how the event may be related to the primary problem. Focusing on the primary problem is important because most patients have had the problem for a long time and tend to mention issues that may not be part of the primary problem. Once the primary problem onset has been established, the evaluation proceeds.

Identifying the triggers that cause the primary symptom (cough or shortness of breath) is important. Having a few different soap powders or perfumes in the office may be helpful. Other triggers that may be more subtle include speaking, swallowing rapidly, walking, running, or simply going from indoors to outdoors or vice versa.

Laryngeal palpation of the suprahyoid and infrahyoid muscle groups may help to identify excessive neck tension. Careful palpation during inhalation and exhalation may identify intrinsic or extrinsic laryngeal muscle tightness. Palpation during the initiation of phonation may identify an elevated laryngeal position. Observation of the shoulders and chest during quiet breathing and during speech may also reveal abnormal breathing patterns. Inspiration accompanied with shoulder lifting and chest tightening often brings on cough or shortness of breath associated with speaking.

Trial therapy should always be a part of the initial evaluation by the speech–language pathologist. Rhythmic breathing exercises as outlined later may produce a more relaxed breathing posture and cue the patient to understanding the nature of the problem. Alternatively, if the voice is dysphonic, voice exercises to modify voice production are appropriate during the trial therapy period. Previous studies have shown that approximately 35% of patients who have CC, PVFM, or laryngospasm complain of dysphonia, even if it is not the primary complaint.[3,12]

Instrumental assessment depends on the symptoms. If the patient's voice is dysphonic, acoustic analysis of the voice is helpful to establish baseline information of voice quality. Other instrumental assessments may include flexible endoscopy (if not already performed by the otolaryngologist), aerodynamic assessment during speech, and voice and spirometry, including careful study of the inspiratory phase of the flow volume loop.

Spirometry provides significant objective evidence of normal pulmonary function. Measures of forced vital capacity and other expiratory measures provide an indication of the health or disease of the lungs. Patients who are coughing, feel short of breath, or have chest tightness are seen routinely by a pulmonologist, and spirometric measures are usually obtained. A methacholine challenge test is also performed to help assess for the possibility of cough-variant asthma that usually presents with normal baseline spirometry. However, in many cases, spirometry only includes the expiratory measures, such as forced expiratory volume in one second or maximum voluntary ventilation and the maximum expiratory flow–volume loop. In particular, the flow–volume relationships diagnose the presence and can assess the effect of large (central) airway obstructions.

Several investigators have shown that patients who have PVFM have abnormal inspiratory loops in their spirometry. Several investigators, such as Altman,[4] Murry and colleagues,[11] and Hartnick,[31] have shown a flattened inspiratory loop in patients who have PVFM compared with a U-shaped inspiratory flow loop seen in normal subjects.

Exercise

Occasionally, it may be helpful to have the patient undergo a short period of exercise to determine if breathing patterns change or speech and voice become degraded after increased activity.[32] Rapid walking, step climbing, and pedaling a stationary bike may elicit the primary or secondary symptom.[33]

Once the evaluation by the speech–language pathologist is complete, the data should be reviewed with the otolaryngologist and others participating in the patient's care. A coordinated approach to treatment may include pharmacotherapy, inhalation therapy, or further referral based on the findings.

Speech–language pathologist treatment

Table 3 lists the possible treatments for CC, laryngospasm, and PVFM. This article focuses on behavioral treatments usually provided by a speech–language pathologist. Other articles in this issue address medical treatments.

Table 3
Origins of laryngospasm reported to be primarily related to either inflammatory or neuropathic conditions.

Condition	Origins
Inflammatory[a]	Cough
	Erosive esophagitis
	Gastroesophageal reflux disease
	Laryngeal pharyngeal reflux
	Sinus syndrome
	Sudden infant death syndrome
Neuropathic	Aberrant reinnervation
	Kennedy disease
	Laryngeal dystonia
	Laryngeal paralysis
	Paradoxical vocal fold motion
	Upper respiratory infection

[a] In some inflammatory conditions, neuropathy also cannot be ruled out, such as in sudden infant death syndrome and cough.

For any behavioral treatment option, the speech–language pathologist must list the goals of voice therapy and discuss the benefits and expectations with patients. They must always emphasize the role of patient compliance in determining the success or failure of therapy. Following these simple strategies will enhance therapy regardless of the technique.

Behavioral treatment

Clinicians have used various behavioral approaches in the treatment of laryngospasm. An assortment of respiratory-based treatments have been proposed. Christopher and colleagues[27] described the use of relaxation breathing techniques in patients who exhibited PVFM and asthma symptoms. Gay and colleagues,[33] Vertigan and colleagues,[3] and Murry and colleagues[11] modified the original protocol outlined by Blager and colleagues[34] in 1988. The treatment comprises a program of respiratory retraining and a series of graduated resistance breathing exercises used to control symptoms in patients diagnosed with PVFM who complained of choking, coughing, and shortness of breath.

In 1991, Pitchenik[32] first described the panting maneuver as another respiratory-based behavioral treatment. Improvement of symptoms and the measures of pulmonary function testing were reported with this maneuver. According to the investigator, when panting at functional residual capacity, significantly greater electromyographic activity in the posterior cricoarytenoid muscle and a sustained increase in the width of the glottis occurs compared with peak values of these measurements made during tidal breathing. Other treatments emphasizing the respiratory mechanism have been proposed, including the suggestion by Sperfeld and colleagues[35] for patients to rapidly change to an upright position and slow breathing to shorten the duration of laryngospasm.

The sequence of exercises used in the respiratory retraining program, listed in **Box 1**, is based on the early work of Christopher and colleagues.[27] Patients advance from low breathing effort to breathing against increased resistance.

Box 1
Sequence of exercises used in the respiratory retraining program

Quiet rhythmic breathing

Exhaling with shoulders relaxed and abdominal movement in and out consistent with continuous exhalation and inhalation.

Breathing with vocal resistance

Exhaling while sustaining one of several sounds (SH, F, or Z). Patients are asked to sustain the sound for increasing time lengths.

Pulsed exhalation

Patients are asked to produce a pulse of air using "Ha" or "Sha" followed by sniffing in through the nose with the mouth closed.

Abdominal focus at rest

Patients are asked to lie flat and put a small book on their stomach. They then focus on elevating the book on inhalation and lowering the book on exhalation. Once successful, they are given a straw to breathe through. As they squeeze the straw with their breaths, they increase the resistance while focusing on the abdominal movement. They can do the exercise while sitting and standing and lying down.

Inspiratory Muscle Strength Training for Paradoxical Vocal Fold Motion and Airway Limitation

One behavioral treatment option for PVFM with relatively short treatment duration (<6 weeks) is to use a respiratory muscle strength trainer. Respiratory muscle strength trainers are devices used to strengthen inspiratory or expiratory muscles, and their application to conditions affecting the voice were elucidated recently, particularly with regard to abductor vocal fold paralysis and PVFM and a behavioral strategy for enhancing the performance voice.

Several respiratory muscle strength training devices are on the market that can be used to strengthen the respiratory muscles, but they have distinct differences that should be realized. Resistive trainers have small orifices to breathe through that become progressively smaller as the treatment progresses. However, they are impacted by the breathing pattern, which means that patients can simply slow down their breathing to combat the increased resistance that has been imposed on them. Therefore, they will lessen the expected training outcome. In other words, clinicians have less control over the expected training effect.

On the other hand, pressure threshold load respiratory muscle trainers are not susceptible to variations in a patient's airflow rate, making them unique from the other devices. For example, when training with an inspiratory pressure threshold device, patients must overcome the threshold load by generating an inspiratory pressure sufficient to open the inspiratory spring-loaded valve within the device. The patient sustains the pressure level throughout the inspiration or expiration. If the patient does not generate the threshold pressure, the valve remains closed. Presently, the pressure threshold load respiratory muscle trainers are the recommended style of trainer for threshold loading as it provides near flow-independent resistance to inspiration or expiration. Several devices are on the market, including the Respironics Threshold IMT (Philips Healthcare, Andover, Massachusetts), the PowerBreathe (HaB International Ltd, Warwickshire, United Kingdom), the PowerLung (PowerLung, Inc, Houston, Texas), and Aspire Products EMST150 (Aspire Products, Gainesville, Florida). Product references are listed in the Appendix.

Patients who have upper airway resistance stemming from dynamic conditions such as PVFM seem to be candidates for inspiratory muscle strength training. Mathers-Schmidt and colleagues[36] studied an 18-year-old female patient who had PVFM that was induced with physical activity, particularly during soccer games. Using an inspiratory muscle strength training program, they examined outcomes on the patient's exertional dyspnea and exercise effort. Using a common therapy regime of respiratory training for 5 days per week, the patient completed five sets of 12 breaths through the training device set to 75% of the patient's maximum inspiratory pressure per session. Results showed normal laryngeal function occurring just after 5 weeks of inspiratory muscle strength training with no symptoms of PVFM occurring when playing soccer.

Inspiratory muscle strength training was also incorporated in a rower who had exercise-induced PVFM.[37] The results of this case study showed substantial improvement in inspiratory muscle strength training and complete reduction in PVFM during exercise.[38] The elimination of the PVFM is believed to be related to the principle of neural adaptation and crossover effects that accompany physical training.[39] The study by Baker and colleagues[39] of a19-year-old women who had bilateral abductor paralysis further explains the mechanism behind the outcomes of inspiratory muscle strength training on glottal airway. A well-known phasic relationship exists between diaphragmatic activity and the inspiratory activity of the posterior cricoarytenoid muscle (PCA).

During the inspiratory phase of breathing, PCA activity occurs slightly before the activity of the diaphragm and continues its contraction to a maximum point of mid-inspiration. When diaphragm stimulation is increased, through phrenic nerve stimulation or voluntary control of breathing depth, PCA activity increases in a coordinated manner. The pressure threshold–training program targets the inspiratory muscles through inducing a greater load to the inspiratory phase of breathing, thus increasing the motor drive to the diaphragm. This loading takes advantage of the known phasic relationship between the diaphragm and the PCA, increasing the drive to the diaphragm while also enhancing the motor activity of the PCA. The increased PCA activity results in increasing glottal aperture size during inspiration. The increased glottal aperture subsequently decreases the laryngeal airway resistance, providing a sensation of decreased effort during the inspiratory phase of breathing and thereby reducing the symptoms of PVFM.

SUMMARY

PVFM, CC, and laryngospasm share multiple signs and symptoms. Of critical importance is the focal point, namely the larynx and vocal folds. The role of the speech–language pathologist is to assess the behavioral manifestations associated with patient complaints, evaluate the medical data as they relate to the behavioral signs, and then treat patients with behavioral techniques of breath control based on findings that have been shown to ameliorate the symptoms. Working in conjunction with the medical members of the team, the speech–language pathologist is responsible for the behavioral management to reduce or eliminate the triggers for the condition.

APPENDIX 1. PRODUCT REFERENCES FOR RESISTANCE BREATHING DEVICES

1. Respironics Threshold IMT
   http://thresholdimt.respironics.com/
   Philips Healthcare
   3000 Minuteman Road
   Andover, MA 01810-1099
   Phone: 800-229-6417
   Online store: https://my.respironics.com/my/pub/my/login.action
2. PowerBreathe
   http://www.powerbreathe.com/
   HaB International Ltd. Northfield Road
   Southam, Warwickshire CV47 0RD, UK
   Phone: +44 (0) 1926 816100
   Fax: ++44(0) 1926 816101
   E-mail: enquiries@powerbreathe.com
3. PowerLung
   http://www.powerlung.com/region/us/
   PowerLung, Inc.
   10690 Shadow Wood Dr Ste 101
   Houston, Texas 77043
   Phone: 800-903-3087
   Fax: 713-465-5742
4. Aspire Products EMST150
   http://www.aspireproducts.org/about.html
   Aspire Products

P.O. Box 240
5745 SW 75th Street
Gainesville, FL 32608
Fax: 352-335-9080
E-mail: aspireproducts2@yahoo.com

REFERENCES

1. Andrianopoulos MV, Gallivan GJ, Gallivan KH. PVCM, PVCD, EPL, and irritable larynx syndrome: what are we talking about and how do we treat it? J Voice 2000;14(4):607–18.
2. Hicks M, Brugman SM, Katial R. Vocal cord dysfunction/paradoxical vocal fold motion. Prim Care 2008;35(1):81–103.
3. Vertigan AE, Theodoros DG, Gibson PG, et al. Voice and upper airway symptoms in people with chronic cough and paradoxical vocal fold movement. J Voice 2007;21(3):361–83.
4. Altman K, Simpson C, Amin M, et al. Cough and paradoxical vocal fold motion. Otolaryngol Head Neck Surg 2002;127:501–11.
5. Poelmans J, Tack J, Feenstra L. Paroxysmal laryngospasm: a typical but under-recognized supraesophageal manifestation of gastroesophageal reflux? Dig Dis Sci 2004;49:1868–74.
6. Maceri DR, Zim S. Laryngospasm: an atypical manifestation of severe gastro-esophageal reflux disease (GERD). Laryngoscope 2001;111:1976–9.
7. Sacre-Hazouri JA. When the cause of dyspnea is on larynx. Asthma of difficult control, resistant to treatment? Vocal cords dysfunction? Or both? Rev Alerg Mex 2006;53(4):150–61.
8. Wani MK, Woodson GE. Paroxysmal laryngospasm after laryngeal nerve injury. Laryngoscope 1999;109:694–7.
9. Sasaki CT, Suzuki M. Laryngeal spasm: a neurophysiologic redefinition. Ann Otol Rhinol Laryngol 1977;86:150–7.
10. Gallivan GJ, Hoffman L, Gallivan KH. Episodic paroxysmal laryngospasm: voice and pulmonary function assessment and management. J Voice 1996;10(1):93–105.
11. Murry T, Tabaee A, Aviv JE. Respiratory retraining of refractory cough and laryngopharyngeal reflux in patients with paradoxical vocal fold movement disorder. Laryngoscope 2004;114:1341–5.
12. Koufman JA. The otologic manifestations of gastroesophageal reflux disease (GERD): a clinical investigation of 225 patients using ambulatory 24 hour pH monitoring and an experimental investigation of the role of acid and pepsin in the development of laryngeal injury. Laryngoscope 1991;101:1–78.
13. Hoit JD, Lansing RW, Perona KE. Speaking-related dyspnea in healthy adults. J Speech Hear Res 2007;50:361–74.
14. Newman KB, Dubester SN. Vocal cord dysfunction: masquerade of asthma. Semin Respir Crit Care Med 1994;15(2):161–7.
15. Perkner JJ, Fennelly KP, Balkissoon R, et al. Irritant-associated vocal cord dysfunction. J Occup Environ Med 1998;40(2):136–43.
16. McFadden ER, Zawadski DK. Vocal cord dysfunction masquerading as exercise-induced asthma. a physiologic cause for "choking" during athletic activities. Am J Respir Crit Care Med 1996;153(3):942–97.
17. Reisner C, Nelson HS. Vocal cord dysfunction with nocturnal awakening. J Allergy Clin Immunol 1997;99:843–86.

18. Newman KB, Mason UG III, Schmaling KB. Clinical features of vocal cord dysfunction. Am J Respir Crit Care Med 1995;152(4):1382–6.
19. Vertigan AE, Theodoros DG, Winkworth AL, et al. Chronic cough: a tutorial for speech-language pathologists. J Med Speech-Lang Pathol 2007;15(3):189–206.
20. Vertigan AE, Theodoros DG, Gibson PG, et al. The relationship between chronic cough and paradoxical vocal fold movement: a review of the literature. J Voice 2006;20:466–80.
21. Milgrom H, Corsello P, Freedman M, et al. Differential diagnosis and management of chronic cough. Compr Ther 1990;16(10):46–53.
22. Treole K, Trudeau M, Forrest L. Endoscopic and stroboscopic description of adults with paradoxical vocal fold dysfunction. J Voice 1999;13:143–52.
23. Mello CJ, Irwin RS, Curley FJ. Predictive values of the character, timing, and complications of chronic cough in diagnosing its cause. Intern Med 1996;156(9):997–1003.
24. Chang AB, Lasserson TJ, Gaffney J, et al. Gastro-oesophageal reflux treatment for prolonged non-specific cough in children and adults. Cochrane Database Syst Rev 2006;(4):CD004823.
25. Patel NJ, Jorgensen C, Kuhn J, et al. Concurrent laryngeal abnormalities in patients with paradoxical vocal fold dysfunction. Otolaryngol-Head Neck Surg 2004;130:686–9.
26. Vertigan AE, Theodoros D, Winkworth A, et al. Perceptual voice characteristics in chronic cough and paradoxical vocal fold movement. Folia Phoniatr Logop 2007; 59:256–67.
27. Christopher KL, Wood RP II, Eckert RC, et al. Vocal-cord dysfunction presenting as asthma. N Engl J Med 1983;308(26):1566–70.
28. Cukier-Blaj S, Murry T. Laryngospasm. In: Jones H, Rosenbek J, editors. Encyclopedia of oropharyngeal dysphagia in rare conditions. San Diego (CA): Plural Publishing Inc; 2009. p. 281–93.
29. Jacobson BH, Johnson A, Grywalski C. The voice handicap index (VHI): development and validation. Am J Speech Lang Pathol 1994;6:66–70.
30. Rosen CA, Lee AS, Osborne J, et al. Development and validation of the Voice Handicap Index-10. Laryngoscope 2004;114(9):1549–56.
31. Hartnick C. Pediatric voice disorders. San Diego (CA): Plural Publishing Inc; 2008. p. 260–1.
32. Pitchenik AE. Functional laryngeal obstruction relieved by panting. Chest 1991; 100:1465–7.
33. Gay M, Blager F, Bartsch K, et al. Psychogenic habit cough: review and case reports. J Child Psychiatry 1987;48(12):483–6.
34. Blager FB, Gay ML, Wood RP. Voice therapy techniques adapted to treatment of habit cough: pilot study. J Commun Dis 1988;21:393–400.
35. Sperfeld AD, Hanemann CO, Ludolph AC, et al. Laryngospasm: an underdiagnosed symptom of X-linked spinobulbar muscular atrophy. Neurology 2005;64:753–4.
36. Mathers-Schmidt BA, Brilla LR. Inspiratory muscle training in exercise-induced paradoxical vocal fold motion. J Voice 2005;19(4):635–44.
37. Ruddy B, Sapienza CM, Davenport PD, et al. Inspiratory muscle strength training and behavioral therapy in a case of a rower with exercise induced paradoxical vocal fold dysfunction. Int J Pediatr Otorhinolaryngol 2004;68(10):1327–32.
38. Powers S, Howley E. Exercise physiology: theory and application to fitness and performance. Columbus (OH): McGraw-Hill; 2001.
39. Baker SE, Sapienza CM, Martin D, et al. Inspiratory pressure threshold training for upper airway limitation: a case of bilateral abductor vocal fold paralysis. J Voice 2003;17(3):384–94.

Occupational, Environmental, and Irritant-Induced Cough

Stuart M. Brooks, MD[a,b,*]

KEYWORDS

- Cough • Irritancy • World Trade Center
- Pungency • Evolution

The Occupational Safety and Health Administration defines an irritant as a chemical, which is not corrosive, but which causes a reversible inflammatory effect on living tissue by chemical action at the site of contact.[1] Important physical features of an irritant exposure are its intensity (massive versus low-moderate concentrations); differences in the chemical constituents (eg, halogenated versus nonhalogenated gas); vapor pressure in reference to the atmosphere (high, so higher levels in air); solubility in aqueous solution (determines upper versus lower airway involvement); molecular state (vapor, gas fume, dust); and degree of chemical reactivity (highly reactive chemicals tend to be more irritating).[2] **Table 1** provides common irritants in various occupations and environments.

RESPIRATORY TRACT EFFECTS OF IRRITANTS

The clinical and pathologic spectrum of chemically induced respiratory tract irritation ranges from neurogenically mediated alterations in regional blood flow, mucus secretion, and airway caliber to the initiation of cough.[3–6] There may just be the complaint of annoyance or the sensation of chest discomfort, burning, or pain. "Somesthesis," "chemesthesis," and "chemical nociception" are terms that describe the chemically induced sensations caused by an irritant.[7,8] The outcomes may depend on the location of the injury, especially following massive and high-level exposures. As such,

Some of the funding to support the subject of this report was received from the National Institute for Occupational Safety and Health.

[a] Department of Environmental & Occupational Health, College of Public Health, University of South Florida, 13201 Bruce B Downs Boulevard, Tampa, FL 33612, USA

[b] Divisions of Pulmonary, Sleep & Critical Care Medicine and Allergy & Immunology, College of Medicine, University of South Florida, Tampa, FL, USA

* Department of Environmental & Occupational Health, College of Public Health, University of South Florida, 13201 Bruce B Downs Boulevard, Tampa, FL 33612.

E-mail address: sbrooks@hsc.usf.edu

Otolaryngol Clin N Am 43 (2010) 85–96
doi:10.1016/j.otc.2009.11.013
0030-6665/10/$ – see front matter. Published by Elsevier Inc.
oto.theclinics.com

Table 1
Causes of irritation in various environments

Exposure	Agent or Process
Acids	Acetic, sulfuric, hydrochloric, hydrofluoric acid
Alkali	Bleach, calcium oxide, sodium hydroxide, World Trade Center dust
Gases	Chlorine, sulfur dioxide, ammonia, mustard, ozone, hydrogen sulfide, phosgene
Spraying	Spraying of paints and coatings
Explosion	Irritant gases, vapors and fume releases
Fire/pyrolysis	Combustion and pyrolysis products of fires, burning paint fumes, pyrolysis products of polyvinylchloride meat wrapping film
Confined spaces	Epichlorhydrin, acrolein, floor sealant, metal coating remover, biocides, fumigating aerosol, cleaning aerosol sprays, mixture of drain cleaning agents
Workplace	Glass bottle–making workers, popcorn-flavoring makers, second-hand tobacco smoke, chlorine gas puffs, pyrite dust explosion, locomotive and diesel exhaust, aerosols of metalworking fluids, aluminum smelter workers exposed to pot-room fumes, metal processing plant, pulp mill workers, shoe and leather workers exposed to the organic solvents, workers exposed to SO2 from apricot sulfurization, aldehydes including formaldehyde and glutaraldehyde, biologic dusts, tunnel construction workers, coke oven emissions, cleaning and disinfecting workers in the food industry, chili pepper pickers, cyanoacrylates

there may be corneal damage; swelling of the tongue; persistent rhinitis; closure of the glottis and larynx; sudden-onset asthma (reactive airways dysfunction syndrome); acute respiratory distress syndrome; or persistent bronchiolar obstruction (bronchiolitis obliterans).[3,9–17] **Box 1** summarizes outcomes from repeated lower levels of irritant exposures.[6,10,12,18–29]

ALLERGEN VERSUS IRRITANT

An allergen can cause an effect even in very low, nonirritating concentrations. In order for these effects to occur, there needs to be earlier repetitive exposures (usually for months or years) that bring about sensitization to the allergen. Allergy depends on this unique cellular sensitivity and involves immunologic mechanisms, unlike irritation. The irritant operates in a nonspecific manner to cause changes, whereas the allergen is distinctly different. The appreciation of irritation (ie, chemesthesis) affecting the eyes, nose, and throat is principally mediated by the trigeminal nerve (cranial nerve V). Pulmonary irritation is mainly under vagal (cranial nerve X) nerve control. Odor is detected by the olfactory nerve (cranial nerve I).[30,31]

ROLE OF ODOR

Some individuals report respiratory and other types of complaints, in some cases simulating asthma and often accompanied by coughing; the symptoms are professed to be caused by a low concentration of an irritant chemical recognized mainly by an odor.[32–38] "Pungency" refers to a sharp, bitter, or biting taste but can also be used to describe an irritating odor.[39–41] Unfortunately, the nose is not a sensitive discriminator for irritancy. Odor does not equate with toxicity. There may be magnitudes of

Box 1
Consequences of irritant exposures

Breathing pattern: apnea and slowed breathing rate

Upper airway: "pungency," rhinitis, or nasal obstruction; stinging or burning of eyes and mucous membranes; corneal damage; eye lacrimation; tongue or glottal swelling with obstruction; vocal cord dysfunction

Trachea and bronchi: Somesthesis, chemesthesis, and chemical nociception; cough or phlegm; bronchospasm; decrease in forced expiratory volume in 1 second; increased nonspecific airway hyperresponsiveness; irritant-induced asthma from repeated exposures; reactive airways dysfunction syndrome from high-level single exposure

Alveolar: Acute respiratory distress syndrome, chemical pneumonitis

Bronchiolitis obliterans

Adjuvant or enhancement: to an allergen

Chronic obstructive pulmonary disease: industrial bronchitis

Persistent cough

Noninvasive changes: Alteration in exhaled breath nitric oxide or changes in induced sputum parameters

differences between the detection concentration of an airborne odorant and the concentration causing pungency, irritation, or even significant toxicity.[7,31]

There seems to be so-called exceptionally chemically "sensitive" persons in the general population, however, and their prevalence may be greater than appreciated. As many as 15% to 30% of individuals who participate in focused surveys claim to be very sensitive to chemicals in their environment.[42–44] An administered telephone questionnaire to 4046 California subjects found that 15.9% reported being "allergic or unusually sensitive to everyday chemicals."[43] There was general homogeneity across race-ethnicity, geography, education, and marital status. Putting the study into perspective, a 15.9% prevalence of chemical sensitivity equates to approximately 4 million Californians. Meggs and colleagues[44] defined "chemical sensitivity" as becoming ill after smelling chemical odors, such as perfume, pesticides, fresh paint, and cigarette smoke; new carpets; or automobile exhaust. The study by Bell and colleagues[42] was even less precise. Their questionnaire queried about feeling ill from smelling multiple common environmental chemicals (eg, cacosmia). Kippen and colleagues[45] expanded the scope of defining the exposures but did not clearly define the response. In this latter study, patients attending an environmental and occupational health clinic were administered a questionnaire asking about 122 common environmental substances, such as aerosol, deodorant, cigarette smoke, diesel exhaust, fabric softener, marker pens, new carpeting, colognes or perfumes, and recent dry-cleaned clothes that caused symptoms. Symptoms were defined as awareness of discomfort or bothersome change; many of the complaints were a response to odors.[45] Although the clinical symptoms resemble asthma in some cases, all physiologic measurements including lung function testing, methacholine challenge, and skin prick tests were normal or negative. There is great controversy with those investigations using the very uncertain term chemical "sensitivity" to explain a "condition" based solely on self-reporting of symptoms and a perceived exposure recognized principally by an odor.

Several investigations report persons claiming increased sensitivity to odors and irritants and manifesting an enhanced cough reflex as defined by capsaicin challenge testing.[33,34,46,47] The interpretation of these studies is limited by the small subject population size, lack of customary standards for administration of cough challenges, and virtually no assessment of environmental or occupational exposures.[32,33,46] Overall, qualitative estimates of chemical sensitivity based solely on reports of illness caused by odors have little validity. This latter conclusion is likely one of the major reasons why there is such controversy over the diagnosis of multiple chemical sensitivity. The latter is a condition, perception, or circumstance where subjects complain of many symptoms following what seems to be an innocuous exposure; few if any show any objective laboratory findings.

OCCUPATIONAL, ENVIRONMENTAL, AND IRRITANT-INDUCED COUGH

Groneberg and associates[48] emphasized the role of occupational factors in the pathogenesis of chronic cough. Blanc and colleagues[49] reported that chili pepper workers continually exposed to capsaicin report chronic cough. Gordon and colleagues[50,51] investigated workers making glass bottles who were chronically exposed to a variety of irritants including hydrochloric acid aerosol. Symptomatic bottle workers reported a higher prevalence of nose and throat irritation complaints and cough. In a laboratory setting, greater cough sensitivity to citric acid and capsaicin aerosols was observed in symptomatic workers. The latent interval between starting work and first developing symptoms was typically 4 years. A persisting postinfectious cough occurs after viral and bacterial infections and is associated with disruption of epithelial integrity and widespread inflammation of the upper or lower airways.[52–54]

WORLD TRADE CENTER COUGH

A prototype for irritant-induced cough is epitomized by the events of September 11, 2001, when terrorist operatives of Al-Qaida's Osama Bin Laden commandeered four United States commercial airplanes and initiated an attack on the United States. Two of the planes were flown into the World Trade Center (WTC) towers causing their collapse. The destruction and collapse of the towers generated an intense, short-term exposure to inorganic dust, pyrolysis products, and other respirable materials. Nearly 3000 people died and an estimated 250,000 to 400,000 people in the vicinity of the WTC collapse were exposed to dust, debris, smoke, and chemicals.[55] Firefighters and other rescue workers were exposed to high levels of the dust and other particulate materials, especially during the first few days after the WTC collapse. The specific content of the dust was later measured by the United States Geological Survey, who collected dust samples from various WTC areas and from steel girder coatings of the WTC debris.[56] The leachate solutions of the dust showed alkaline pH values between 8.2 and 11.8, likely a result of the dissolution of concrete, glass fibers, gypsum, and other material in the dust. Following the WTC collapse, several respiratory illnesses were described among rescue workers, including what has been called "World Trade Center cough." There were other reports of conditions with persistent airway hyperreactivity, claimed reactive airways dysfunction syndrome, and acute eosinophilic pneumonia.[57–59] A high prevalence of rhinitis-sinusitis and gastroesophageal reflux disorder was also noted.

WTC cough presented as a persistent cough that developed after exposure to the WTC site and was accompanied by respiratory symptoms severe enough to require medical leave for at least 4 weeks.[59] WTC cough was more common in firefighters relegated to the highest exposure categories who reported to the WTC site on the morning of the collapse (<24 hours); a moderate level of exposure was selected for firefighters arriving within 2 days; and low exposure was designated for firefighters arriving between 3 and 7 days after the collapse. No exposure was appropriated for firefighters if they were not at the site during at least 2 weeks of the rescue operation. Within 24 hours after exposure, those firefighters with WTC cough reported having a productive cough with black-gray–colored sputum that was "infiltrated with pebbles or particles."[59] Nonspecific airway hyperreactivity was noted in about 25% of the tested firefighters with high levels of exposure, whether or not they had WTC cough.[58,60]

EVOLUTION OF IRRITANT-INDUCED COUGH

Over millions of years, primitive animals and then humans evolved adaptations that created a physiologic or biochemical advantage over disease or adaptations to protect against noxious environmental hazards. An evolutionary process resulted in the cough reflex, one of the most important human defensive adaptations; cough became a common symptom of various lung diseases.[61] Over millions of years, two types of human cough reflexes evolved to become adapted for different protective purposes. Presumably, both types use the same muscles and nerves to elicit a precisely timed, multifaceted, neuromuscular phenomenon distinguished by the concurrent and sequential coordination of muscular activity of the diaphragm; muscle groups of the chest wall, neck, and abdomen; and the laryngeal abductor and adductor muscles. **Fig. 1** summarizes information of two different types of cough reflexes.

Supposedly, one type of cough reflex evolved to prevent the harmful effects of the aspiration of gastric content into the lungs because the larynx moved in close proximity to the opening of the esophagus as human ancestors adapted phonation over olfaction beginning less than 10 million years ago.[62–64] This mechanosensory-type reflex, transduced mainly by laryngeal and tracheal Aδ fibers, generates immediate expiratory efforts, often referred to as the "expiration reflex."[63,65–67]

The second type of cough reflex is transmitted by unmyelinated sensory vagal C-fibers that occupy a dense neuronal plexus beneath the airway epithelium.[68,69] This type of cough was likely adapted by prehistoric humans who began living closely together in larger social groups, in poorly ventilated enclosures, and in close proximity to nonprimate animals. There was the possibility of contracting a contagious respiratory tract or parasitic infection or being exposed to gaseous-particulate irritant emanations that produced airway and distal lung inflammation or damage. This second type of cough reflex relied on primordial ionic channels, inherited from some ancient predecessor living hundreds of millions of years before, to create a chemosensory-type of cough reflex.[70,71] This cough response is analogous to the induced pain following tissue injury, and it is controlled by the identical transient receptor potential vanilloid cation channel (TRPV1).[65,72–74] The airways do not normally manifest nociceptive pain from a stimulus but the only consistent response that capsaicin and inflammation provoke in healthy human airways is cough.

The polymodal TRPV1 receptor acts both as a receptor in the traditional sense that it binds to high-affinity specific ligands and also is an ion channel.[75] TRPV1 is responsive to capsaicin ("capsaicin receptor") and inflammatory products (**Fig. 2**). TRPA1, referred to as the "irritant receptor," is an excitatory ion channel expressed by a subpopulation of unmyelinated afferent C fiber nociceptors that are possibly linked to TRPV1 and contribute to the transduction of the noxious stimuli.[76–78] TRPA1 has been found to be activated by a number of irritant chemicals including capsaicin; mustard oil (ie, isothiocyanate); acrolein; allicin; wasabi and horseradish; cinnamon oil; menthol; acrolein; formalin; diallyl disulfide; garlic (ie, 2-propenyl 2-propene

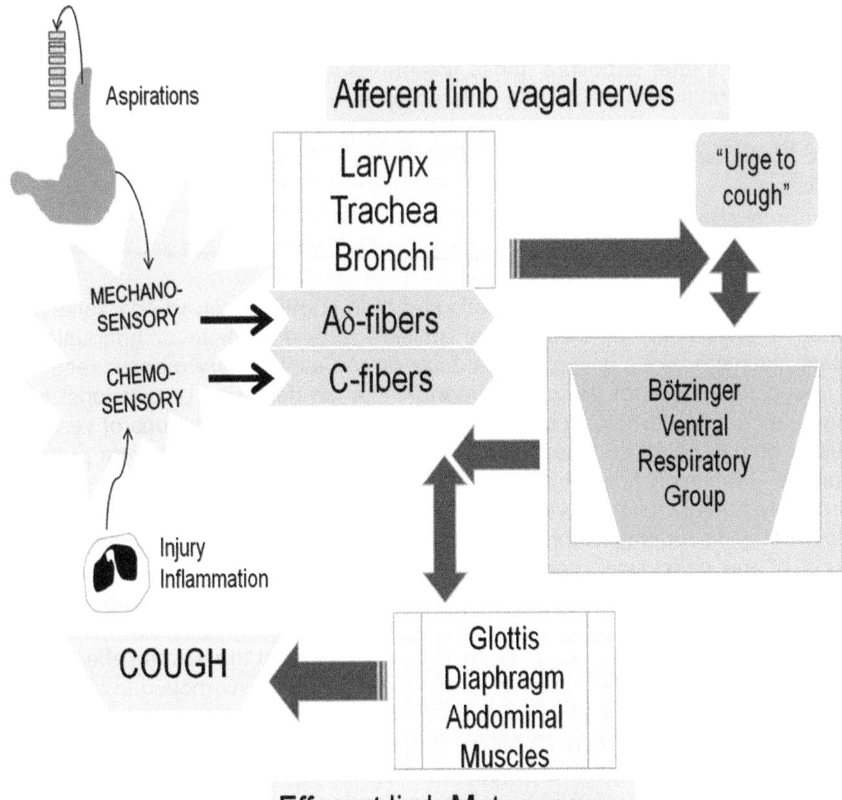

Fig. 1. Different types of cough reflex. The involuntary cough reflex provoked by mechanosensory-responsive Aδ fibers (guinea pig) was likely adapted by evolutionary ancestors of humans a few million to several hundred thousand years ago as the larynx moved in closer proximity to the esophageal opening. This type of cough reflex is relatively insensitive to chemical stimuli. The second type of involuntary cough reflex has a longer evolutionary history beginning with the "nociceptor" created 0.5 billion years ago. This type of cough travels through unmyelinated vagal sensory C-fibers that are normally quiescent but become activated or hyperactivated by tissue injury, inflammation, or by naturally occurring chemicals, such as capsaicin. The chemically sensitive cough reflex may have been a coevolutionary adaptation by animal and plant species tens of millions of years ago. Both types of cough reflex apply the same nerves and muscles as are used for breathing or perhaps a modification of functions originally created for other purposes.

thiosulfinate, allyl isothiocyanate, diallyl sulfides, ajoene, dithiines, and 4-hydroxy-2-nonea); and tetrahydrocannabinol.[78–81]

IRRITANT-INDUCED COUGH, A TRPPATHY

Groneberg and colleagues[82] determined the expression of TRPV-1 receptors in the airways of patients with chronic persistent cough of diverse causes and noted an enhanced capsaicin cough response. They obtained airway mucosal biopsies by flexible bronchoscopy in 29 patients with chronic cough and 16 healthy volunteers without a cough. When using an anti–TRPV-1 antibody, these investigators observed

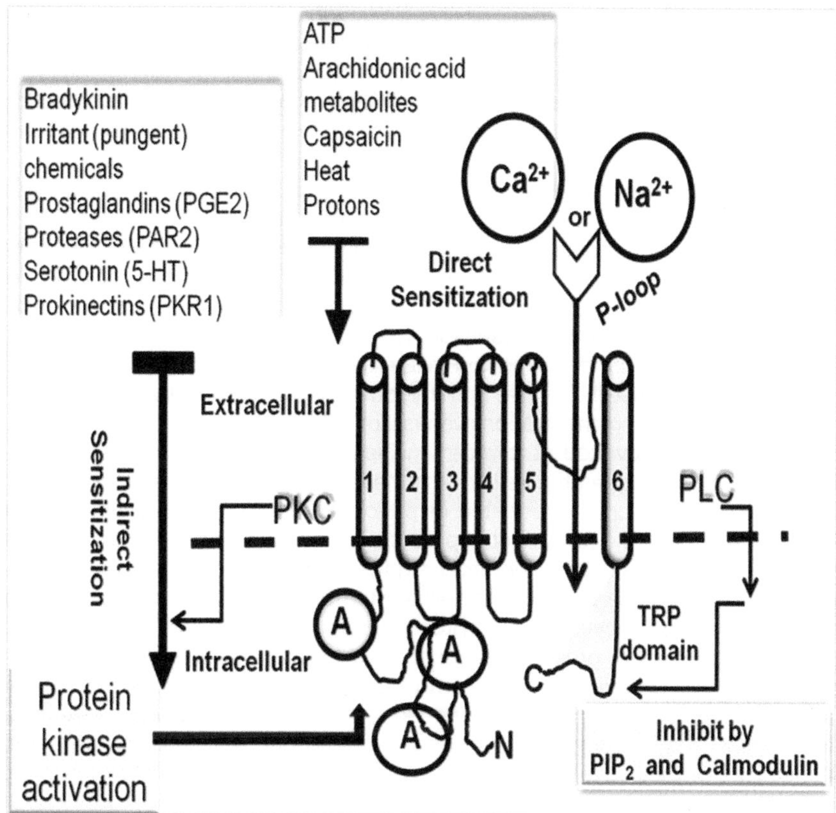

Fig. 2. Vanilloid subfamily of transient receptor potential (TRP). The TRPV1 channel is activated (directly or indirectly) by a variety of chemical and environmental signals.[85] The TRP structure includes a P loop that forms a central pore, a cytoplasmic N terminus, and a cytoplasmic C terminus. The N-terminal region of TRPV proteins usually contains three or more ankyrin motif repeats followed by a conserved transmembrane domain. There are amino acid residues in the transmembrane domain of the TRPV1 protein necessary and sufficient to confer vanilloid sensitivity.[80] Calcium entry through plasma membrane channels is recognized as a cellular signaling event to bring about a neuronal action potential propagation that leads to motor actions.

a phenotypic expression of airway nerves in patients with chronic cough that was changed; there was a fivefold greater expression of TRPV-1. TRPV-1 gene expression was found predominantly in nociceptive-like primary afferent neurons whose cell bodies resided in the dorsal root, trigeminal, and nodose ganglia. There was a significant correlation between capsaicin cough response and the number of TRPV-1–positive nerves within the airways of patients having persistent cough, suggesting that TRPV-1 receptors contributed to the enhanced cough reflex. Specific gene mutations that take place in TRP ion proteins to cause human-animal disorders and diseases have been referred to as “channelopathies” or “TRPpathies.”[80,83,84]

The precise role of the TRP receptors in the pathogenesis of the human pathologic cough has not been fully elucidated. A possible similar mechanism of cough that has been established in animals is suspected in humans but further investigations are necessary to better appreciate the role of TRPV1-TRPA1 in human disease.

A hypothesis to explain irritant-induced chronic cough in humans presumes that ionic channels are in some way altered (ie, TRPV1 or TRPA1) by repeated or prolonged exposures to various irritating gases, vapors, dusts, and fumes. The changes may be analogous to what has been claimed for TRPV1 channels and the dysfunctional sensation of pain that embraces neuropathic pain; hyperesthesia (enhanced sensitivity to touch or natural stimuli); hyperalgesia (abnormal sensitivity to pain); allodynia (exaggerated response to otherwise innocuous stimuli, either static or mechanical); and spontaneous burning pain.[80] Plausibly, the lungs manifest a TRPpathy in the form of a chronic cough and not as a syndrome of chronic pain. The persistent cough is construed to be the result of an upregulation of TRPV1 (and possibly of TRPA1) receptors caused by the repeated irritant exposure.[85] Animal investigations verify that the normally quiescent chemosensors are directly activated or even hyperactivated following lung injury or pulmonary inflammation.[62,64,74,86–88] The role of inflammation is central because it changes both the quantitative and qualitive features of the sensory nerves including the responsiveness of the nerve endings; the nerve (and TRPV1 receptor) is provoked at lower intensities of mechanical or chemical stimuli and there may be exaggerated reflex responses to innocuous stimuli.[5,89] Through an ionic channel mechanism, repeated or prolonged exposures to diverse irritating gases, vapors, dusts, and fumes could potentially lead to the development of persistent irritant-induced cough.[85] Laboratory studies confirm that airways inflammation incites the release of the products of cellular and tissue damage and inflammatory mediators including bradykinin, ATP, prostaglandin E_2, and nerve growth factor.[90] During such a complex process neuronal cells become sensitized and manifest greater electrical excitability. Nerve growth factor levels may increase and become a signaling mechanism in both an autocrine and paracrine manner.[91] Persistent oxidant stress may overwhelm pulmonary antioxidant defenses to perpetuate a biochemical- or molecular-induced persistent cough state.[92]

REFERENCES

1. US Department of Labor. The OSHA Hazard Communication Standard (HCS) Regulations (Standards–29 CFR). USA, Occupational Safety and Health Administration (OSHA). Appendix A to the Hazard Communication Standard, 1994.
2. Brooks SM, Truncale T, McCluskey J. Occupational and environmental asthma. In: Rom WN, Markowitz S, editors. Occupational and environmental medicine. 4th edition. Philadelphia (PA): Lippincott-Raven Publisher; 2006. p. 418–63.
3. Shusterman D. Review of the upper airway, including olfaction, as mediator of symptoms. Environ Health Perspect 2006;110(Suppl 4):649–53.
4. Gavett SH, Kollarik M, Undem BJ. Irritant agonists and air pollutants: neurologically medicated respiratory and cardiovascular responses. In: Foster WM, Costa DL, editors, Air pollutants and the respiratory tract, vol. 204. 2nd edition. Boca Raton (FL): Taylor and Francis Group; 2005. p. 195–232.
5. Groneberg DA, Quarcoo D, Frossard N, et al. Neurogenic mechanisms in bronchial inflammatory diseases. Allergy 2004;59(11):1139–52.
6. Morris JB, Symanowicz PT, Olsen JE, et al. Immediate sensory nerve-mediated respiratory responses to irritants in healthy and allergic airway-diseased mice. J Appl Phys 2003;94:1563–71.
7. Cometto-Muniz JE, Cain WS, Abraham MH, et al. Chemical boundaries for detection of eye irritation in humans from homologous vapors. Toxicol Sci 2006;9: 600–9.

8. Ferrer-Montiel A, Garcia-Martinez C, Morenilla-Palao C, et al. Molecular architecture of the vanilloid receptor: insights for drug design. Eur J Biochem 2004;271: 1820–6.
9. Schachter EN, Zuskin E, Saric M. Occupational airway diseases. Rev Environ Health 2001;16(2):87–95.
10. Brooks SM, Hammad Y, Richards I, et al. The spectrum of irritant-induced asthma: sudden and not-so-sudden onset and the role of allergy. Chest 1998; 113(1):42–9.
11. Brooks SM, Weiss MA, Bernstein IL. Reactive airways dysfunction syndrome (RADS): persistent asthma syndrome after high level irritant exposure. Chest 1985;88:376–84.
12. Brooks SM. Inhalation airway injury: a spectrum of changes. Clin Pulm Med 2007; 14:1–8.
13. Gautrin D, Bernstein IL, Brooks SM, et al. Reactive airways dysfunction syndrome, or irritant induced asthma. In: Bernstein IL, Chan Yeung M, Malo J-L, et al, editors. Asthma in the workplace. New York: Marcel Dekker; 2006. p. 581–630.
14. Olin AC, Granung G, Hagberg S, et al. Respiratory health among bleachery workers exposed to ozone and chlorine dioxide. Scandinavian journal of work. Environ Health 2002;28(2):117–23.
15. Kullman G, Boylstein R, Jones W, et al. Characterization of respiratory exposures at a microwave popcorn plant with cases of bronchiolitis obliterans. J Occup Environ Hyg 2005;2:169–78.
16. Akpinar-Elci M, Travis WD, Lynch DA, et al. Bronchiolitis obliterans syndrome in popcorn production plant workers. Eur Respir J 2004;24:298–302.
17. Boswell RT, McCunney RJ. Bronchiolitis obliterans from exposure to incinerator fly ash. J Occup Environ Med 1995;37:850–5.
18. Alarie Y. Sensory irritation by airborne chemicals. CRC Crit Rev Toxicol 1973;3: 299–363.
19. Vaughan R, Szewczyk JM, Lanos M, et al. Adenosine sensory transduction pathways contribute to activation of the sensory irritation response to inspired irritant vapors. Toxicol Sci 2006;93:411–21.
20. Tarlo SM. Workplace respiratory irritants and asthma. Occup Med 2000;15(2): 471–84.
21. Medina-Ramon M, Zock JP, Kogevinas M, et al. Asthma symptoms in women employed in domestic cleaning: a community based study. Thorax 2003;58(11): 950–4.
22. Gautrin D, Infante-Rivard C, Ghezzo H, et al. Longitudinal assessment of airway caliber and responsivenesss in workers exposed to chlorine. Am J Respir Crit Care Med 1999;160:1232–7.
23. Malo JL, Cartier A, Boulet LP, et al. Bronchial hyperresponsiveness can improve while spirometry plateaus two to three years after repeated exposure to chlorine causing respiratory symptoms. Am J Respir Crit Care Med 1994;150(4):1142–5.
24. Jorres R, Nowak D, Magnussen H, et al. The effect of ozone exposure on allergen responsiveness in subjects with asthma or rhinitis: short-term O3 increases bronchial allergen response with mild allergic asthma or rhinitis without asthma. Am J Respir Crit Care Med 1996;153:56–64.
25. Vagaggini B, Taccola M, Cianchetti S, et al. Ozone exposure increases eosinophilic airway response induced by previous allergen challenge. Am J Respir Crit Care Med 2002;166:1073–7.
26. Peden DB, Setzer RW Jr, Devlin RB. Ozone exposure has both a priming effect on allergen-induced responses and an intrinsic inflammatory action in the nasal

airways of perennially allergic asthmatics. Am J Respir Crit Care Med 1995; 151(5):1336–45.
27. Olin A, Ljungkvist G, Bake B, et al. Exhaled nitric oxide among pulpmill workers reporting gassing incidents involving ozone and chlorine dioxide. Eur Respir J 1999;14(4):828–31.
28. Ulvestad B, Lund MB, Bakke B, et al. Gas and dust exposure in underground construction is associated with signs of airway inflammation. Eur Respir J 2001;17(3):416–21.
29. Maniscalco M, Grieco L, Galdi A, et al. Increase in exhaled nitric oxide in shoe and leather workers at the end of the work-shift. Occup Med (Lond) 2004; 54(6):404–7.
30. Bandell M, Macpherson LJ, Patapoutian A. From chills to chilis: mechanisms for thermosensation and chemesthesis via thermoTRPs. Curr Opin Neurobiol 2007; 17:1–8.
31. Cometto-Muftiz JE, Cain WS. Relative sensitivity of the ocular trigeminal, nasal trigeminal and olfactory systems to airborne chemicals. Chem Senses 1995; 20(2):191–8.
32. Millqvist E, Lowhagen O. Placebo controlled challenges with perfume in patients with asthma-like symptoms. Allergy 1996;51:434–9.
33. Millqvist E, Bende M, Lowenhagen O. Sensory hyperreactivity: a possible mechanism underlying cough and asthma-like symptoms. Allergy 1998;53:1208–12.
34. Ternesten-Hasseus E, Farbrot A, Lowhagen O, et al. Sensitivity to methacholine and capsaicin in patients with unclear respiratory symptoms. Allergy 2002;57: 501–7.
35. Lee LY, Widdicombe JG. Modulation of airway sensitivity to inhaled irritants: role of inflammatory mediators. Environ Health Perspect 2001;109(Suppl 4):585–9.
36. Hausteiner C, Bornschein S, Hansen J, et al. Self-reported chemical sensitivity in Germany: a population-based survey. Int J Hyg Environ Health 2005;208:271–8.
37. Shusterman D. Odor-associated health complaints: competing explanatory models. Chem Senses 2001;26:339–43.
38. Schiffman SS. Livestock odors: implications for human health and well-being. J Anim Sci 1998;76:1343–55.
39. Prasad BCN, Kumar V, Gururaj HB, et al. Characterization of capsaicin synthase and identification of its gene (csy1) for pungency factor capsaicin in pepper (*Capsicum* sp). Proc Natl Acad Sci 2006;103:13315–20.
40. Blum E, Liu K, Mazourek M, et al. Molecular mapping of the C locus for presence of pungency in capsicum. Genome 2002;45:702–5.
41. Randle WM, Bussard ML. Streamlining onion pungency analyses. HortScience 1993;28:60.
42. Bell IR, Schwartz GE, Peterson JM, et al. Self-reported illness from chemical odors in young adults without clinical syndromes or occupational exposures. Arch Environ Health 1993;48:6–13.
43. Kreutzer R, Neutra RR, Lashuay N. Prevalence of people reporting sensitivities to chemicals in a population-based survey. Am J Epidemiol 1999;150:1–17.
44. Meggs WJ, Dunn KA, Bloch RM, et al. Prevalence and nature of allergy and chemical sensitivity in a general population. Arch Environ Health 1996;51:275–81.
45. Kippen HM, Hallman W, Kelly-McNeil K, et al. Measuring chemical sensitivity prevalence: a questionnaire for population studies. Am J Public Health 1998; 85:575–7.
46. Millqvist E, Lowhagen O, Bende M. Quality of life and capsaicin sensitivity in patients with sensory airway hyperreactivity. Allergy 2000;55:540–5.

47. Ternesten-Hasseus E, Bende M, Millqvist E. Increased capsaicin cough sensitivity in patients with multiple chemical sensitivity. J Occup & Environ Med 2002;44:1012–7.
48. Groneberg DA, Nowak D, Wussow A, et al. Chronic cough due to occupational factors. J Occup Med Toxicol 2006;1(3):1–10.
49. Blanc P, Liu D, Juarez C, et al. Cough in hot pepper workers. Chest 1991;99: 27–32.
50. Gordon SB, Curran AD, Turley A, et al. Glass bottle workers exposed to low-dose irritant fumes cough but do not wheeze. American Journal of Respiratory & Critical Care Medicine 1997;156(1):206–10.
51. Gordon SB, Curran A, Fishwick D, et al. Respiratory symptoms among glass bottle workers: cough and airways irritancy syndrome? Occup Med 1998;48(7): 455–9.
52. Braman SS. Postinfectious cough: ACCP evidence-based clinical practice guidelines. Chest 2006;129:138S–46S.
53. Ryan NM, Gibson PG. Extrathoracic airway hyperresponsiveness as a mechanism of post infectious cough: case report. Cough 2008;4:4–7.
54. Fujimura M, Myou S, Matsuda M, et al. Cough receptor sensitivity to capsaicin and tartaric acid in patients with mycoplasma pneumonia. Lung 1998;176(4):281–8.
55. Statement of Janet Heinrich Director, Health Care—Public Health Issues. Testimony before the subcommittee on national security, emerging threats, and international relations, representatives: health effects in the aftermath of the World Trade Center attack (9/8/04). Washington, DC: United States Government Accountability Office; 2004.
56. US Geological Survey. Open-file report 01-0429: World Trade Center USGS Bulk Chemistry Results. [Web page] 2001 Friday December 16, 2005. Available at: http://pubs.usgs.gov/of/2001/ofr-01-0429/chem1/index.htm. Accessed August 12, 2009.
57. Rom WN, Welden M, Garcia R, et al. Acute eosinophilic pneumonia in a New York City firefighter exposed to World Trade Center dust. Am J Respir Crit Care Med 2002;166:797–800.
58. Banauch GI, Alleyne D, Sanchez R, et al. Persistent hyperreactivity and reactive airway dysfunction in firefighters at the World Trade Center. American Journal of Respiratory & Critical Care Medicine 2003;168(1):54–62.
59. Prezant DJ, Weiden M, Banauch GI, et al. Cough and bronchial responsiveness in firefighters at the World Trade Center site. N Engl J Med 2002;347:806–15.
60. Banauch GI, Hall C, Weiden M, et al. Pulmonary function after exposure to the World Trade Center in the New York City fire department. Am J Respir Crit Care Med 2006;174:312–9.
61. Morice AH, Fontana GA, Sovijarvi ARA, et al. ERS Taskforce: the diagnosis and management of chronic cough. Eur Respir J 2004;24:481–92.
62. Poliacek I, Stransky A, Szerda-Przezestaszewska M, et al. Cough and laryngeal muscle discharges in brainstem lesioned anesthetized Cats. Physiol Res 2005; 54:645–54.
63. Widdicombe J, Fontana G. Cough: what's in a name? Eur Respir J 2006;28:10–5.
64. Mazzone SB. An overview of the sensory receptors regulating cough. Cough 2005;1(2):1–9.
65. Mazzone SB. Sensory regulation of the cough reflex. Pulm Pharmacol Ther 2004; 17:361–8.
66. Hadjikoutis S, Wiles CM, Eccles R. Cough in motor neuron disease: a review of mechanisms. QJM 1999;92(9):487–94.

67. Poliacek I, Rose MJ, Corrie LWC, et al. Short reflex expirations (expiration reflexes) induced by mechanical stimulation of the trachea in anesthetized cats. Cough 2008;4:1–9.
68. Undem BJ, Chuaychoo B, Lee M-G, et al. Subtypes of vagal afferent C-fibres in guinea-pig lungs. J Physiol 2004;556:905–17.
69. Undem BJ, Carr MJ. Pharmacology of airway afferent nerve activity. Respir Res 2001;2:234–44.
70. Woolf CJ, Ma Q. Nociceptors: noxious stimulus detectors. Neuron 2007;55:353–64.
71. Hucho T, Levine JD. Signaling pathways in sensitization: toward nociceptor cell biology. Neuron 2007;55:365–76.
72. Szallasi A. Vanilloid (capsaicin) receptors in health and disease. Am J Clin Pathol 2002;118:110–21.
73. Gatti R, Andre E, Amadesi S, et al. Protease-activated receptor-2 exaggerates TRPV1-mediated cough in guinea pigs. J Appl Phys 2006;101:506–11.
74. Adcock J. TRPV1 receptors in sensitization of cough and pain reflexes. Pulm Pharmacol Ther 2009;22:65–70.
75. Taylor-Clark T, Undem BJ. Transduction mechanisms in airway sensory nerves. J Appl Phys 2006;101:950–9.
76. Story GM, Gereau RW. Numbing the senses: role of TRPA1 in mechanical and cold sensation. Neuron 2006;50:177–9.
77. Bautista DM, Jordt S-E, Nikai T, et al. TRPA1 mediates the inflammatory actions of environmental irritants and proalgesic agents. Cell 2006;124:1269–82.
78. Bautista DM, Movahead P, Hinman A, et al. Pungent products from garlic activate the sensory ion channel TRPA1. PNAS 2005;102:12248–52.
79. Trevisani M, Siemens J, Matwrazzi S, et al. 4-Hydroxynonenal, an endogenous aldehyde, causes pain and neurogenic inflammation through activation of the irritant receptor TRPA1. PNAS 2007;104:13519–24.
80. Nilius B, Voets T, Peters I. TRP channels in disease. Sci STKE. 2005;295:1–9.
81. McNamara CR, Mandel-Brehm J, Bautista DM, et al. TRPA1 mediates formalin-induced pain. PNAS 2007;104:13525–30.
82. Groneberg DA, Niimi A, Dinh QT, et al. Increased expression of transient receptor potential vanilloid-1 in airway nerves of chronic cough. Am J Respir Crit Care Med 2004;170:1276–80.
83. Clapham DE. TRP channels as cellular sensors. Nature 2003;426:517–24.
84. Kiselyov K, Soyombo A, Muallem S. TRPpathies. J Physiol 2007;578(3):641–53.
85. Brooks SM. Irritant-induced chronic cough: a TRPpathy. Lung 2008;186:S88–93.
86. Canning BJ, Farmer DG, Mori N. Mechanistic studies of acid-evoked coughing in anesthetized guinea pigs. Am J Physiol Regul Integr Comp Physiol 2006;291: R454–63.
87. Canning BJ. Anatomy and neurophysiology of the cough reflex: ACCP evidence-based clinical practice guidelines. Chest 2006;129:33S–47S.
88. Bolser DC. Experimental models and mechanisms of enhanced coughing. Pulm Pharmacol Ther 2004;7:383–8.
89. Carr MJ, Undem BJ. Inflammation-induced plasticity of the afferent innervation of the airways. Environ Health Perspect 2001;109:567–71.
90. Nakatsuka T, Gu JG. P2X purinoceptors and sensory transmission. Pflufgers Arch-Eur J Physiol 2006;452:598–607.
91. Olgart C, Frossard N. Nerve growth factor and asthma. Pulm Pharmacol Ther 2002;15(1):51–60.
92. Kelly FJ. Oxidative stress: its role in air pollution and adverse health effects. Occup Environ Med 2003;60:612–6.

Reflux and Cough

Albert L. Merati, MD[a,b,c,*]

KEYWORDS

- Reflux • Cough • Otolaryngology
- Gastroesophageal reflux disease

Laryngopharyngeal reflux (LPR) and gastroesophageal reflux disease (GERD) continue to be important clinical entities in otolaryngology; reflux is one of the most common causes of cough[1] found in referral clinics. This content focuses on the relationship between reflux and cough and expands upon the discussions in other articles in this publication, such as "Cough: a Worldwide Problem" and "Unexplained Cough." It is also necessary to consider LPR and GERD when discussing other entities in this issue, because patients with troublesome cough may have reflux and rhinitis, for example, perhaps caused by underlying[2] autonomic dysfunction. Albeit somewhat artificial to completely separate them, the following sections will deal only with the entities of LPR and GERD and how cough may manifest as part of these disorders, how they can be identified, and how they may be treated.

Both LPR and GERD are quite common; it is estimated that 7% to 10% of Americans have reflux symptoms every day. Twenty percent suffer at least once a week, and up to 36% suffer once a month.[3,4] These include many familiar complaints such as heartburn, dysphagia, and dyspepsia, as well as nonspecific complaints commonly seen in otolaryngology practice, such as globus sensation, hoarseness, throat clearing, postnasal drip, and of course, cough, the topic of this article.

Within the otolaryngology community, the evidence[5] clearly reflects an increasing awareness in the diagnosis and treatment of reflux disorders. The direct cost of antireflux medical treatment (predominantly in the form of proton pump inhibitors, or PPIs) is staggering, estimated at over $14 billion annually. This cost estimate does not include the medical cost related to the clinic evaluation and diagnostic testing for this disorder, nor does it include any estimate of indirect costs related to loss of work productivity and effects on quality of life. There is also the possible cost of complications related to the use of PPIs such as osteoporosis and bacterial pneumonitis.[6–10]

[a] Department of Otolaryngology – HNS, University of Washington School of Medicine, St Louis, MO, USA
[b] Department of Speech and Hearing Sciences, College of Arts and Sciences, University of Washington, Seattle, WA, USA
[c] Box 356515, 1959 Northeast Pacific, Seattle, WA 98195, USA
* Department of Otolaryngology – HNS, University of Washington School of Medicine, St Louis, MO.
E-mail address: amerati@uw.edu

Otolaryngol Clin N Am 43 (2010) 97–110
doi:10.1016/j.otc.2009.12.003 **oto.theclinics.com**

In this article, the pathophysiology of reflux and, more specifically, reflux-associated cough, are discussed. Laryngeal inflammation and irritation, reflex cough, and concepts such as nonacidic reflux are discussed. Treatment options, including pharmacologic therapy and behavioral and speech–language interventions as well as surgery are presented.

PATHOPHYSIOLOGY OF REFLUX

At one point or another, most adults have had some complaint of heartburn; the pathophysiology of gastric contents flowing backward into the esophagus and even into the larynx and pharynx above is quite familiar in this sense. Ultimately, it is the failure of the lower esophageal sphincter (LES) to control this unwanted retrograde flow that is at the heart of gastroesophageal reflux. The digestive tract must maintain some capacity for retrograde flow, as it is depended upon for the urgent expulsion of gas or emesis when noxious elements are ingested or there is too much gas in the system. The LES cannot just be an unchangeable, static, one-way valve. Perhaps as a byproduct of this, pathologic reflux can and does occur. There are numerous potential mechanisms, however, by which reflux, GERD, and LPR may be related to cough, as listed in **Table 1**.

THE LES AND TRANSIENT LES RELAXATION

Fyke and colleagues[11] in 1956 often is credited with an early description and definition of the LES and its function. LES activity reflects a combination of dynamic and more static sphincteric characteristics. The latter include the fibers of the crural diaphragm that create the external sphincter. The more familiar dynamic component comes from the actual fibers of the muscular layer of the esophagus; together these two create the LES zone that is approximately 4 cm in length.[12,13]

Transient lower esophageal pressure relaxation (TLESR) is believed to be the key abnormality that leads to the pathologic reflux of gastric material (be it from the stomach or duodenum) into the esophagus. The LES is sensitive to intrathoracic and intra-abdominal pressure; as the crural fibers of the diaphragm contract on inspiration, the pressure in the external aspect of the sphincter rises. Cough itself, with its often violent changes in thoracic pressure, also can negatively impact the LES in this manner. In the normal state, the LES varies with inspiration, rising with diaphragmatic

Table 1
Relationships between GERD/LPR and cough

Action	Mechanism
Regurgitation of gastric contents to the laryngopharynx	Mechanical stimulation pH-sensitive stimulation Non-acidic reflux precipitating tissue change Enhanced cough sensitivity to other irritants
Gross and "micro" (or silent) aspiration	Aspiration pneumonia Chemical tracheitis and/or pneumonitis
Distal esophageal reflux	Vagal-mediated reflex
Esophago-bronchial reflex	Vagal-mediated Likely cough secondary to pulmonary exacerbation
Cough-induced reflux	Diaphragmatic/LES discoordination or relaxation

contraction due to the extrinsic force of the crural fibers.[14] As an example of the interrelatedness of the foregut and its derivatives, esophageal stimulation by distension will lead to a drop in LES pressure by the inhibition of the crural diaphragmatic fibers. It is possible that this reflex contributes to the pathophysiology of reflux by way of a positive feedback loop[15]; stimulation of the distal esophageal afferents in response to irritation or distension causes further decline in LES pressure and, perhaps, more reflux.

The dictum "no acid, no ulcer" that reflected the clinical mindset during the decades of surgical dominance of peptic disease probably is no longer accurate. With the advent of potent and effective medical therapy for acid suppression and advances in diagnostic technology, it now is believed that nonacidic reflux likely also plays a role in the pathogenesis of cough in some refractory patients. The presence of noxious nonacidic agents continues to be offered as an explanation of the PPI treatment failure in many cases. Indeed, there is growing evidence that the entity of nonacidic reflux is quite real and not uncommon; beyond that, its significance continues to be worked out.

The two principal nonacidic agents discussed here are bile and pepsin. Bile has been suspected as a source of laryngeal inflammation and irritation for decades. Some of the reluctance to accept bile as a notable contributor to reflux pathophysiology in the upper aerodigestive tract is because of some mixed messages from initial animal studies. In a superb study, Vaezi[16] demonstrated that bile indeed can injure the laryngeal epithelium but only in an acidic environment. In 2005, Sasaki was able to demonstrate histologic laryngeal injury in a rat model following bile exposure in a neutral environment.[17] Work in this area is ongoing.

The literature regarding pepsin, the principal proteolytic enzyme of the stomach, continues to grow. Although pepsin clearly is predominantly active in acidic pH and has been shown to cause laryngeal injury in this mileu,[16] pepsin retains its proteolytic activity up to a pH of 7, and can be reactivated.[18] Johnston found intraepithelial pepsin in the larynx of patients with the clinical diagnosis of LPR but not in controls (**Fig. 1**); in these same patients, pepsin was absent in their esophageal epithelium.[19] Furthermore, these patients had a depletion of intracellular carbonic anhydrase (type 3).

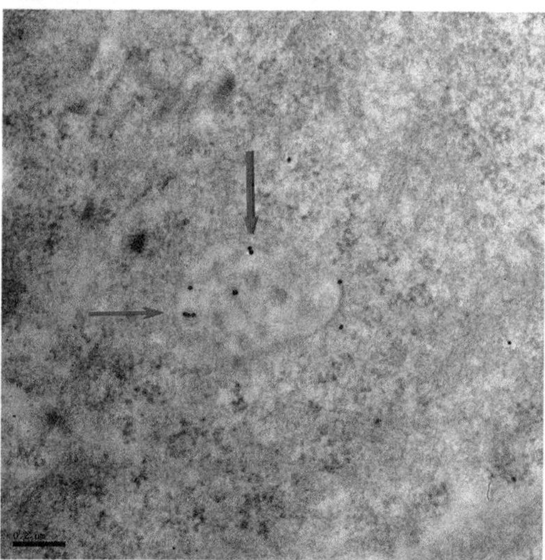

Fig. 1. Intravesicular pepsin within a laryngeal epithelial cell of a patient with LPR. *Arrows:* pepsin. *Bar* in bottom left corner: 0.2 microns. *Courtesy of* Nikki Johnston, Medical College of Wisconsin.

Pepsin is believed to be taken up into the laryngeal epithelium by an active, receptor-based mechanism.[20] Given that the focus of chemotherapy and even surgery for reflux disease over the past century has focused on the reduction of acid production and neutralization, the possibility that a nonacidic injurious agent may contribute to ongoing damage and symptomatology is a major paradigm shift. Individual variability in patients' ability to withstand or repair injury also may play a role in understanding LPR, GERD, and specific clinical situations related to these disorders, such as reflux-associated cough.

HOW DOES REFLUX AFFECT THE LARYNX AND UPPER AIRWAY?

The impact of reflux may occur by acute or chronic injury, and by noncontact effects (ie, reflex activation of laryngeal and lower airway responses leading to hoarseness or cough are two examples). Fundamentally, the basic event in reflux-associated cough is believed to be pathologic reflux rising up the esophagus, above the upper esophageal sphincter (UES), resulting in irritation of the larynx.[21] Nonacidic reflux also may act in this manner, as demonstrated by Patterson and colleagues[22] in a study of 37 cough patients, roughly half with asthma and half with cough without asthma. Each subject underwent esophageal impedance and pH probe testing off of acid-suppressive medication. The patients, in general, had some evidence of cough temporally related to reflux events (7 of 26 subjects). Although this fraction is relatively modest, this higher symptom-association group had a higher number and proportion of reflux episodes crossing the UES into the pharynx; there was no difference in the reflux event/symptom association group with regard to esophageal reflux events.

There is no doubt that reflux is a major contributing cause of other physical changes in the larynx, such as vocal fold nodules,[23] granulomata,[24] and pseudosulcus.[25,26] The more common, albeit less-specific findings of vocal fold edema and erythema are discussed in the section on clinical evaluation.

These physical changes in the larynx associated with reflux are mentioned here to demonstrate the macroscopic impact of pathologic reflux on the upper aerodigestive tract. In Koufman's[21] landmark 1991 Triological thesis, the disorder that had the highest association with reflux was airway stenosis; many of these patients have chronic cough as part of their clinical presentation. It is not known if the cough often associated with airway stenosis is related to the underlying reflux or by some impact on the lower airway, mucus retention, or generalized inflammation. There is also a strong association between idiopathic pulmonary fibrosis and reflux,[27] as another example of an upper airway disorder whose pathophysiology may result in end-organ changes. Beyond these gross physical changes at the larynx and upper airway, much of the derangement related to reflux and cough occurs at a more microscopic level.

COUGH: REFLUX OR REFLEX?

The mere presence of acid in the esophagus also may stimulate the glottis by way of the esophago-glottal reflex,[28] or perhaps the more central airways themselves.[29] Lang and the group at the Medical College of Wisconsin have reported that, based on their animal model, the main impact of acid reflux on the lower airway was to increase mucus secretion.[29] Furthermore, they postulated that the increase in mucus may act as a buffering agent against refluxed materials in the upper or lower airway.

Javorkova and colleagues[30] from Slovakia published a compelling study in 2008 that further elucidated the relationship between reflux and cough. Twenty-five patients with GERD were recruited and submitted to catheter infusions of acid or saline in a randomized, double-blind manner. Their cough response to inhaled capsaicin was measured in all test conditions. Interestingly, in the nine subjects who had pre-existing GERD with cough, sensitivity to experimental capsaicin exposure was heightened with esophageal acidification. The 15 GERD subjects without cough were not affected by esophageal acidification. Furthermore, this experiment also was run on 18 healthy volunteers; again, no increase in cough sensitivity to capsaicin occurred with esophageal acidification. This indicates that the presence of distal esophageal acidification can increase the reflux cough sensitivity to other, nonacidic and even exogenous agents. It is possible that this is a significant part of the pathophysiology of the irritable larynx syndrome[31] and certainly helps in understanding and managing cough patients.

Ferrari and colleagues[32] in Verona furthered the understanding of the mechanism of reflux-associated cough with a compelling experiment in asthmatic patients. In their work, 29 subjects with known asthma were challenged with methacholine and capsaicin before and after a short course of omeprazole (20 mg twice daily). Of the 29 patients, 17 had acidic reflux events in the distal esophagus; many but not all of the same were in the group of 17 who had proximal reflux events. Omeprazole treatment did not affect these subjects' reactivity to methacholine challenge, but the response to capsaicin was significantly diminished, but only in patients with pathologic reflux, predominantly in the proximal acid group. The authors concluded that, in asthmatics, omeprazole reduced cough sensitivity in those with proximal reflux without influencing bronchial responsiveness. Another example of the complex interrelation between cough and reflux is seen in a Polish study published in 2005.[33] Ziora and colleagues examined the citric acid cough threshold (CACT) in GERD patients before and after fundoplication. In the preoperative group, CACT was lower than seen in healthy volunteers, indicating that the reflux state increased the sensitivity to outside stimulants beyond whatever direct irritation is provided by the refluxate itself.

COUGH IN REFLUX: CLINICAL EVALUATION

As the understanding of reflux-associated disease of the upper aerodigestive tract evolved, the distinctions between patients with LPR and GERD became clearer. Perhaps the first and most critical point is that the absence of heartburn, the cardinal symptom of GERD, is present in less than half of patients with LPR.[21] An alarming example of the significance of atypical reflux symptoms came from Reavis and colleagues,[34] who reported that cough itself was the symptom most highly associated with the development of esophageal adenocarcinoma, greater than heartburn or other more familiar typical reflux symptoms.

Patients with LPR are not the same as those with GERD; LPR patients tend to have daytime, upright reflux, in contrast to those with the more familiar GERD.[35] On average, the habitus of patients with GERD reveals a higher body mass index (BMI) than normals,[36,37] which is also higher than those of patients with LPR. Halum and colleagues[38] demonstrated this in a large retrospective study in which patients with LPR had a relatively normal BMI compared with the BMI of subjects with GERD on esophageal pH probe testing in the same clinic.

With regard to the clinical history of patients with cough, Everett and Morice[39] made several potentially interesting observations in an uncontrolled 2007 publication. Within their group of 47 patients with confirmed esophageal reflux and cough, the most common cough characteristics were cough on phonation, cough in the morning when getting up out of bed, and cough around the time of eating. Throat clearing, hoarseness, dysphagia, and globus also were related but less so. Heartburn, so often noted to be present in a minority of patients with LPR, was present in 63% of their patients with reflux and cough. This study was limited, however, in that the authors did not assess if the same findings were present in patients with cough caused by other diseases. Cough is also one of the items on Belafsky's Reflux Symptom Index,[40] reflecting its clinical weight in making the provisional or working diagnosis of LPR (**Table 2**).

Office laryngoscopic evaluation for reflux and its impact on the upper airway unfortunately has been a source of great controversy in the field over the past 10 to 15 years. When performed and interpreted carefully, laryngoscopy provides helpful clinical information in cases of suspected LPR. In contrast, if LPR is diagnosed casually or without attention to specific laryngeal findings, the patient is not served. The key examination findings appear to be vocal fold edema and erythema, as well as medial arytenoid erythema (**Fig 2**).[41,42] Trauma from coughing, however, can mimic these changes. Vaezi and colleagues[43] published an important observational study dispelling the notion that generic posterior laryngitis is a useful sign in diagnosing LPR. Videolaryngoscopic examination of 100 healthy volunteers revealed that nearly 80% of subjects had at least one reflux-attributable finding on laryngoscopy. This study has been misinterpreted to mean that laryngoscopy in general is not reliable or valuable; indeed, their finding that the presence of posterior laryngitis or pachydermia is quite common is an important one but should not be misconstrued that laryngoscopy as a whole is not valuable.

As has been noted throughout this article, multichannel intraluminal impedance testing is important for detailing and distinguishing acidic and nonacidic reflux events in patients with suspected reflux-associated cough. Several interesting studies are worth mentioning here. Sifrim and colleagues[44] explored the relationship between acid reflux and cough by investigating 22 subjects with manometry, impedance, and pH monitoring. In a symptom association probability analysis, the authors looked at the connection between cough and acid, weak-acid, and weak-alkaline reflux events. First, most cough events occurred independent of reflux; of the 31% of coughs that occurred within 2 minutes of a reflux episode, 65% were associated with acidic reflux, 29% with weakly acidic reflux, and another 6% with alkaline events. This importance of the concept of symptom association is a recurring theme in reflux testing.

Table 2
Reflux symptom index (RSI)

Within the Last Month, How Did the Following Problems Affect You:	0 = No Problem 5 = Severe Problem					
Hoarseness or a problem with your voice	0	1	2	3	4	5
Clearing your throat	0	1	2	3	4	5
Excess throat mucous or postnasal drip	0	1	2	3	4	5
Difficulty swallowing food, liquid, or pills	0	1	2	3	4	5
Coughing after you ate or after lying down	0	1	2	3	4	5
Breathing difficulties or choking episodes	0	1	2	3	4	5
Troublesome or annoying cough	0	1	2	3	4	5
Sensations of something sticking in your throat or a lump in your throat	0	1	2	3	4	5
Heartburn, chest pain, indigestion, or stomach acid coming up	0	1	2	3	4	5

Adapted from Belafsky PC, Postma GN, Koufman JA. Validity and reliability of the reflux symptom index (RSI). J Voice 2002;16(2):274–77; with permission.

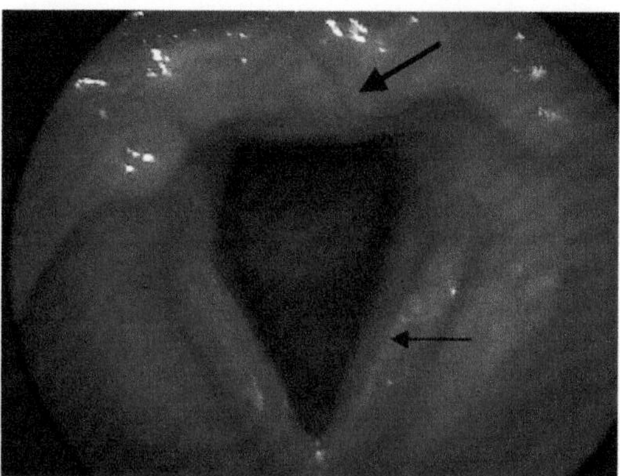

Fig. 2. Several characteristic laryngoscopic findings of a patient with LPR. Note the vocal fold edema and erythema causing a linear dimpling along the length of the vocal fold (*thin arrow,* pseudosulcus vocalis). Also note edema and erythema in the interarytenoid area, as well as the heaped-up postcricoid mucosa (*thick arrow*).

Castell and colleagues[45] recently reported on 42 female patients studied with multichannel intraluminal impedance and pH esophageal monitoring; in this way, acidic and nonacidic reflux events could be distinguished from each other, and their temporal relationship to patient symptoms could be assessed. Interestingly, the perception of acid reflux events was much more brisk, detected within the first 2 minutes following pH drop. Nonacid events detected by the impedance monitor were not felt by the patient as quickly. It is not known what impact this has on patient history and the assessment of their complaint, but it does add to the argument that while the mechanisms of these injuries may be related, they likely are distinct.

TREATMENT

The successful treatment of reflux disorders, resulting in cough or other derangements of the upper aerodigestive tract, depends on more than just expert history, physical examination, and diagnostic testing. The importance of patient counseling about food selection, laryngeal hygiene, and patient education regarding pharmacotherapy cannot be overemphasized. In this author's experience, it is a common event to see patients in clinic who have been taking PPIs for many years without apparent benefit; in these very same patients, mild interrogation reveals a 4 to 6 cups of coffee a day regime, an obsession with mints, or other deleterious habits that, unlike tobacco and alcohol intake, are not always a regular part of the clinical history. These important obstacles to symptom resolution must be identified and discussed if the patient is to improve. In Hanson's early chronic laryngitis study, lifestyle changes alone resulted in improvement in half of the cases.[46] Another major responsibility of the practitioner dealing with reflux is to assure proper drug usage. Altman's study revealed that diet counseling was performed only in about 25% of clinic visits in reflux patients; tobacco cessation and stress management discussions occurred only occasionally (4% of visits).[5]

In a recent study, Chheda and Postma[47] found that patient compliance with correct timing of PPI ingestion (ie, 15 to 45 minutes before eating) was fairly low; only 54% of patients in their study group took their PPIs in an optimal manner. The authors noted that the rate of compliance for PPIs is not significantly different than compliance rates for other drugs taken on a long-term basis. Interestingly, the rate of compliance was higher when the prescription was coming from an otolaryngologist (62%) compared with a nonotolaryngologist (40%). It is not known if this represents better education from the otolaryngology clinic experience or if this represents the impact of specialty consultation—perhaps the otolaryngologist was the second or third physician to review and insist on proper PPI usage in a given case.

The behavioral management of cough may be beneficial in complex or refractory cases. Murry and colleagues[48] have reported on respiratory retraining for patients with suspected reflux and cough in conjunction with paradoxic vocal fold dysfunction. In their initial report of five patients with symptoms refractory to 6 months of twice-daily PPI treatment, the subjects improved in their self-report of cough severity and on pulmonary function testing and laryngoscopic findings. It is not clear, of course, as to what degree each intervention had on any given patient's symptoms. This pilot was later extended to include 20 subjects, with equally striking results.[49]

Ultimately, drug therapy with PPIs continues to be the mainstay of treatment for acid reflux-associated cough. A high symptom-association probability is likely significant in predicting symptomatic improvement from drug therapy. In a recent study, Hersch and colleagues[50] followed 53 subjects undergoing pH probe testing (not impedance testing) for chronic cough; in this cohort, 55% had abnormal studies. In scrutinizing the high-degree response patients, only female sex and high symptom association probability scores were independent predictors of durable improvement. The highest response group (85%) had high symptom association, acid exposure time, and initial symptom index.

Overall, the impact of medical therapy reflux-associated cough is positive but incomplete; a recent meta-analysis by Chang and colleagues[51] from Australia concluded that the "use of a proton pump inhibitor to treat cough associated with GERD has some effect in some adults." Their review incorporated 11 papers; while the impact of treatment was positive, the effect was not universal, and the authors concluded that the actual magnitude of effect was uncertain. It is not known if the explanation of this is ultimately related to mistaken diagnosis, nonacidic injury, or patient noncompliance with therapy.

ALGINATE

An emerging alternative (or supplement) to the treatment of acid reflux is the use of alginate for managing nonacidic reflux. Alginate, available as Gaviscon in the United States and in higher concentrations as Gaviscon Advance in Europe, potentially holds great promise as an ingested material. The alginate is believed to form a raft or physical barrier to reflux, resting on top of the stomach contents and reducing the backflow of these contents above the LES. In a study of 49 subjects, McGlashan and colleagues[52] randomized patients with the clinical diagnosis of LPR based on the reflux symptom index[40] and the reflux findings score[53] to either liquid alginate suspension or nothing. Although there was some improvement in the untreated group, there was statistically significant improvement in the reflux symptom index (RSI) and reflux finding score (RFS) with treatment in the alginate group compared with controls. Although the individual components of the RFS were noted also to have improved for the most part, the cough component of the RSI was not detailed further in the report.

COMPLICATIONS RELATED TO PPI THERAPY

As a whole, the PPIs are a very safe class of drug, with a 20-year track record of remarkably broad acceptance. There are, however, very real concerns with their use, particularly in the area of cough and other LPR symptoms, because of the often long duration of use required for patients. The concerns come down to two basic areas: bacterial infection and mineral loss in bones. Garcia and Gulmez[9,10] reported on the development of bacterial gastroenteritis and bacterial pneumonitis in patients on PPI therapy. This is indeed a great concern, particularly when the drugs are used casually and without careful informed consent of the patient. It should be noted, particularly with regard to the discussion of pneumonitis that the confounding variable of coexistent upper airway disease may have skewed these numbers. It is known from large population studies that this can include disorders such as asthma, bronchitis, pulmonary fibrosis, or other diseases associated with reflux.[27] For better or worse, these complications have not occurred enough or have not been noticed enough within the otolaryngology community to have affected practice patterns.

The risk of hip fracture, on the other hand, has come to the forefront of every discussion regarding long-term PPI therapy.[7] The achlorhydria created by PPI treatment is believed to interfere with calcium absorption; furthermore, the PPIs may inhibit osteoclastic proton pumps. In a case–control study of 13,556 patients with hip fractures in the United Kingdom, the odds ratio of developing a fracture was 1.44 for patients on 1 year of therapy; the risk increased to 2.65 times with longer, higher-dose therapy such as often used in otolaryngology practice. There was a positive correlation between duration of PPI therapy and hip fracture, further emphasizing the association. Nevertheless, use of calcium citrate rather than calcium carbonate supplementation may be considered in patients taking long-term PPIs, because the citrate moiety does not require an acidic environment for absorption.

Other concerns include the development of benign gastrin adenomas, as well as the potential for altered drug metabolism of other medications (such as clopidogrel) processed through the liver.[8] Therefore, the risks of PPIs are real and need to be discussed with patients; all attempts must be made to reduce and discontinue therapy as soon as possible once symptom resolution has been achieved (or, conversely, is found to not be achievable).

PROKINETIC THERAPY

With the loss of cisapride from the US market in 2000, advocates of prokinetic therapy in the treatment of gastro-esophageal reflux have had to rely on other agents such as metoclopramide, bethanechol, erythromycin, and baclofen to achieve therapeutic improvement in their patients. In a study published in 2003, Poe and Kallay[54] reported on 214 cough patients who had been screened for primary pulmonary diseases. Of these 214 patients, 56 were believed to have GERD-related cough. Twenty-four of the 56 patients responded to PPI therapy alone. Eighteen of the remaining patients improved with addition of metoclopramide or cisapride. In over 90% of patients, cough was significantly reduced or eliminated with this medical regime. Metoclopramide and domperidone are dopaminergic antagonists that also have been used as prokinetic agents for gastrointestinal dysmotility; however, domperidone is not available for prescription in the United States. Several studies anecdotally demonstrated the usefulness of these agents in combination with PPIs for treating GERD-associated cough, in unblinded uncontrolled studies, but with fairly remarkable results. Overall, cough or hoarseness improved between 70% and 100% in these studies[55–59] In the absence of a real substitute for cisapride, however, the use of prokinetic agents for reflux-associated cough is limited by unavailability of domperidone in the United States or potential adverse effects of metoclopramide. Consideration also can be given for the use of bethanechol (as long as the patient does not have coexisting asthma) or erythromycin. Additionally, based upon recent reports, consideration also can be given for prescribing the gamma-aminobutyric acid$_B$ agonist baclofen. In a double-blind pilot study by Grossi and colleagues,[60] 21 patients with GERD were randomized to receive placebo or baclofen 10 mg four times daily. They found that the baclofen group had a reduced number of transient lower esophageal sphincter relaxations (TLOSR), as well as increased basal lower esophageal sphincter tone compared with baseline manometric pressure.

SURGERY

It is widely believed that the outcomes of surgical therapy for reflux are greater in typical reflux symptomatology than in LPR-type symptoms such as cough and hoarseness. Despite this, there is a real role for surgical management of these patients. Kaufman and colleagues[61] from the University of Washington reported on long-term surgical results in these patients in 2006. In their study, 128 patients were contacted at a mean time of 53 months following laparoscopic antireflux surgery; while heartburn and regurgitation improved in over 90% of patients, cough and hoarseness improved in only 65% to 75% of cases. Individual patient results were similar for these symptoms regardless of the presence or absence of heartburn. It should be noted that as many as one third of patients were taking some antireflux medication at follow-up. When the authors reviewed clinical data, pharyngeal probe testing was, a priori, a predictor of good outcome for these patients.

In a prospective surgical study, Ranson and colleagues[62] presented a large series of cases from a community hospital setting looking at a range of typical and atypical symptoms and the impact of laparoscopic antireflux surgery on them. Long-term data were available on 84 patients. As in other studies, the best symptom improvement occurred in heartburn and regurgitation. Of the atypical symptoms, cough and sore throat had the highest likelihood of benefiting from surgery.

In patients who are not medical responders, surgery also may be considered; along these lines, Tutuian and colleagues[63] studied patients with chronic cough despite acid suppression. Although this was done in a retrospective manner, the study is illuminating for focusing on this small but challenging group of cough patients. In their review of 50 subjects who had undergone impedance testing while on PPIs, 13 had notably positive symptom indexes for impedance-detected cough events. Of these 13 patients, 6 underwent antireflux surgery with complete symptom resolution. The authors advocate impedance testing on medications for patients with persistent cough to help select medical nonresponders for surgical treatment.

Although there is no universally agreed upon clinical pathway for evaluating and treating patients with GERD and LPR related to chronic cough, it is helpful to respect evidence-based clinical practice guidelines such as those from the American College of Chest Physicians (ACCP).[64] Generally,

> *"...when patients fit the clinical profile that has a high likelihood of predicting that GERD is the cause of cough, antireflux medical therapy should be empirically instituted. [A discussion of this profile can be found in the article entitled "Cough: a worldwide problem."] While some patients improve with minimal medical therapy, others require more intensive regimens. When empiric treatment fails, it cannot be assumed that GERD has been ruled out as a cause of chronic cough. Rather, an objective investigation for GERD is then recommended because the empiric therapy may not have been intensive enough or medical therapy may have failed. Surgery may be efficacious when intensive medical therapy has failed*

in selected patients who have undergone an extensive objective GERD evaluation."

The use of 24-hour esophageal pH and impedance monitoring, staging consequences of the disease with esophagoscopy, performing manometry with esophageal motility studies, and evaluating other root causes for GERD and LPR also should be considered when empiric therapy has failed.

SUMMARY

Reflux disease has great deleterious effects on the upper aerodigestive tract. It can cause micro- and macroscopic changes to the larynx and contributes to cough by direct irritation and by enhancing cough sensitivity to other irritants. Careful clinical history and laryngoscopic examination supplemented by reflux testing in the form of impedance testing to assure a chance of detecting nonacidic and acidic reflux events are critical in many patients. The mainstay of treatment continues to be dietary and other lifestyle interventions and drug therapy. Although PPI therapy is effective in most patients, especially those with acid reflux disease, prokinetic therapy is probably very important in those with combined acid and nonacid disease, and in those with pure nonacid disease. It is likely that failure to improve can be caused by behavioral, laryngeal hygiene, and drug compliance issues. Antireflux surgery can yield long-lasting positive outcomes in carefully selected patients despite the lower efficacy of treatment for primary upper aerodigestive tract symptoms (cough, hoarseness, sore throat) compared with heartburn and regurgitation.

REFERENCES

1. Ribeiro M, De Castro Pereira CA, Nery LE, et al. A prospective longitudinal study of clinical characteristics, laboratory findings, diagnostic spectrum, and outcomes of specific therapy in adult patients with chronic cough in a general respiratory clinic. Int J Clin Pract 2006;60(7):799–805.
2. Loehrl TA, Smith TL, Darling RJ, et al. Autonomic dysfunction, vasomotor rhinitis, and extraesophageal manifestations of gastroesophageal reflux. Otolaryngol Head Neck Surg 2002;126(4):382–7.
3. Nebel OT, Fornes MF, Castell DO. Symptomatic gastroesophageal reflux: incidence and precipitating factors. Am J Dig Dis 1976;21(11):953–6.
4. Locke GR 3rd, Talley NJ, Fett SL, et al. Prevalence and clinical spectrum of gastroesophageal reflux: a population-based study in Olmsted County, Minnesota. Gastroenterology 1997;112(5):1448–56.
5. Altman KW, Stephens RM, Lyttle CS, et al. Changing impact of gastroesophageal reflux in medical and otolaryngology practice. Laryngoscope 2005;115(7):1145–53.
6. Moayyedi P, Cranney A. Hip fracture and proton pump inhibitor therapy: balancing the evidence for benefit and harm. Am J Gastroenterol 2008;103(10):2428–31.
7. Yang YX, Lewis JD, Epstein S, et al. Long-term proton pump inhibitor therapy and risk of hip fracture. JAMA 2006;296(24):2947–53.
8. Altman KW, Radosevich JA. Unexpected consequences of proton pump inhibitor use. Otolaryngol Head Neck Surg 2009;141(5):564–6.
9. García Rodríguez LA, Ruigómez A, Panés J. Use of acid-suppressing drugs and the risk of bacterial gastroenteritis. Clin Gastroenterol Hepatol 2007;5:1418–23.

10. Gulmez SE, Holm A, Frederiksen H, et al. Use of proton pump inhibitors and the risk of community-acquired pneumonia: a population-based case-control study. Arch Intern Med 2007;167:950–5.
11. Fyke FE, Code CF, Schlegel JF. The gastroesophageal sphincter in healthy human beings. Gastroenterologia 1956;86:135–50.
12. Gawrieh S, Shaker R. Peripheral mechanisms affecting the lower esophageal sphincter tone. Gastroenterol Clin North Am 2002;31:S21–33.
13. Mittal RK, Balaban DH. The esophagogastric junction. N Engl J Med 1997;336: 924–32.
14. Dent J, Dodds WJ, Sekiguchi T, et al. Interdigestive phasic contractions of the human lower esophageal sphincter. Gastroenterology 1983;84:453–60.
15. Altschuler SM, Boyle JT, Nixon TE, et al. Simultaneous reflex inhibition of lower esophageal sphincter and crural diaphragm in cats. Am J Phys 1985;249: G586–91.
16. Adhami T, Goldblum JR, Richter JE, et al. The role of gastric and duodenal agents in laryngeal injury: an experimental canine model. Am J Gastroenterol 2004;99: 2098–106.
17. Sasaki CT, Marotta J, Hundal J, et al. Bile-induced laryngitis: is there a basis in evidence? Ann Otol Rhinol Laryngol 2005;114:192–7.
18. Johnston N, Dettmar PW, Bishwokarma B, et al. Activity/stability of human pepsin: implications for reflux attributed laryngeal disease. Laryngoscope 2007;117: 1036–9.
19. Gill GA, Johnston N, Buda A, et al. Laryngeal epithelial defenses against laryngopharyngeal reflux: investigations of E-cadherin, carbonic anhydrase isoenzyme III, and pepsin. Ann Otol Rhinol Laryngol 2005;114(12):913–21.
20. Johnston N, Wells CW, Blumin JH, et al. Receptor-mediated uptake of pepsin by laryngeal epithelial cells. Ann Otol Rhinol Laryngol 2007;116:934–8.
21. Koufman JA. The otolaryngologic manifestations of gastroesophageal reflux disease (GERD): a clinical investigation of 225 patients using ambulatory 24-hour pH monitoring and an experimental investigation of the role of acid and pepsin in the development of laryngeal injury. Laryngoscope 1991;101: 1–78.
22. Patterson N, Mainie I, Rafferty G, et al. Nonacid reflux episodes reaching the pharynx are important factors associated with cough. J Clin Gastroenterol 2009;43(5):414–9.
23. Kuhn J, Toohill RJ, Ulualp SO, et al. Pharyngeal acid reflux events in patients with vocal cord nodules. Laryngoscope 1998;108:1146–9.
24. Ylitalo R, Ramel S. Extraesophageal reflux in patients with contact granuloma: a prospective controlled study. Ann Otol Rhinol Laryngol 2002;111:441–6.
25. Hickson C, Simpson CB, Falcon R. Laryngeal pseudosulcus as a predictor of laryngopharyngeal reflux. Laryngoscope 2001;111(10):1742–5.
26. Belafsky PC, Postma GN, Koufman JA. The association between laryngeal pseudosulcus and laryngopharyngeal reflux. Otolaryngol Head Neck Surg 2002; 126(6):649–52.
27. el-Serag HB, Sonnenberg A. Comorbid occurrence of laryngeal or pulmonary disease with esophagitis in United States military veterans. Gastroenterology 1997;113(3):755–60.
28. Shaker R, Dodds WJ, Ren J, et al. Esophagoglottal closure reflex: a mechanism of airway protection. Gastroenterology 1992;102(3):857–61.
29. Lang IM, Haworth ST, Medda BK, et al. Airway responses to esophageal acidification. Am J Physiol Regul Integr Comp Physiol 2008;294(1):R211–9.

30. Javorkova N, Varechova S, Pecova R, et al. Acidification of the oesophagus acutely increases the cough sensitivity in patients with gastro-oesophageal reflux and chronic cough. Neurogastroenterol Motil 2008;20(2):119–24.
31. Morrison M, Rammage L, Emami AJ. The irritable larynx syndrome. J Voice 1999; 13(3):447–55.
32. Ferrari M, Benini L, Brotto E, et al. Omeprazole reduces the response to capsaicin but not to methacholine in asthmatic patients with proximal reflux. Scand J Gastroenterol 2007;42(3):299–307.
33. Ziora D, Jarosz W, Dzielicki J, et al. Citric acid cough threshold in patients with gastroesophageal reflux disease rises after laparoscopic fundoplication. Chest 2005;128(4):2458–64.
34. Reavis KM, Morris CD, Gopal DV, et al. Laryngopharyngeal reflux symptoms better predict the presence of esophageal adenocarcinoma than typical gastroesophageal reflux symptoms. Ann Surg 2004;239(6):849–56 [discussion: 856–8].
35. Sato K, Umeno H, Chitose S, et al. Patterns of laryngopharyngeal and gastroesophageal reflux. J Laryngol Otol 2009;123(Suppl 31):42–7.
36. Stein DJ, El-Serag HB, Kuczynski J, et al. The association of body mass index with Barrett's oesophagus. Aliment Pharmacol Ther 2005;22(10):1005–10.
37. Smith KJ, O'Brien SM, Smithers BM, et al. Interactions among smoking, obesity, and symptoms of acid reflux in Barrett's esophagus. CancerEpidemiol Biomarkers Prev 2005;14:2481–6.
38. Halum SL, Postma GN, Johnston C, et al. Patients with isolated laryngopharyngeal reflux are not obese. Laryngoscope 2005;115(6):1042–5.
39. Everett CF, Morice AH. Clinical history in gastroesophageal cough. Respir Med 2007;101(2):345–8.
40. Belafsky PC, Postma GN, Koufman JA. Validity and reliability of the reflux symptom index (RSI). J Voice 2002;16(2):274–7.
41. Hanson DG, Jiang J, Chi W. Quantitative color analysis of laryngeal erythema in chronic posterior laryngitis. J Voice 1998;12(1):78–83.
42. Park W, Hicks DM, Khandwala F, et al. Laryngopharyngeal reflux: prospective cohort study evaluating optimal dose of proton pump inhibitor therapy and pretherapy predictors of response. Laryngoscope 2005;115(7):1230–8.
43. Hicks DM, Ours TM, Abelson TI, et al. The prevalence of hypopharynx findings associated with gastroesophageal reflux in normal volunteers. J Voice 2002; 16(4):564–79.
44. Sifrim D, Dupont L, Blondeau K, et al. Weakly acidic reflux in patients with chronic unexplained cough during 24 hour pressure, pH, and impedance monitoring. Gut 2005;54(4):449–54.
45. Agrawal A, Roberts J, Sharma N, et al. Symptoms with acid and nonacid reflux may be produced by different mechanisms. Dis Esophagus 2009;22(5):467–70.
46. Hanson DG, Kamel PL, Kahrilas PJ. Outcomes of antireflux therapy for the treatment of chronic laryngitis. Ann Otol Rhinol Laryngol 1995;104(7):550–5.
47. Chheda NN, Postma GN. Patient compliance with proton pump inhibitor therapy in an otolaryngology practice. Ann Otol Rhinol Laryngol 2008;117(9):670–2.
48. Murry T, Tabaee A, Aviv JE. Respiratory retraining of refractory cough and laryngopharyngeal reflux in patients with paradoxical vocal fold movement disorder. Laryngoscope 2004;114(8):1341–5.
49. Murry T, Tabaee A, Owczarzak V, et al. Respiratory retraining therapy and management of laryngopharyngeal reflux in the treatment of patients with cough and paradoxical vocal fold movement disorder. Ann Otol Rhinol Laryngol 2006; 115(10):754–8.

50. Hersh MJ, Sayuk GS, Gyawali CP. Long-term therapeutic outcome of patients undergoing ambulatory ph monitoring for chronic unexplained cough. J Clin Gastroenterol 2009.
51. Chang AB, Lasserson TJ, Kiljander TO, et al. Systematic review and meta-analysis of randomised controlled trials of gastro-oesophageal reflux interventions for chronic cough associated with gastro-oesophageal reflux. BMJ 2006; 332(7532):11–7.
52. McGlashan JA, Johnstone LM, Sykes J, et al. The value of a liquid alginate suspension (Gaviscon Advance) in the management of laryngopharyngeal reflux. Eur Arch Otorhinolaryngol 2009;266(2):243–51.
53. Belafsky PC, Postma GN, Koufman JA. The validity and reliability of the reflux finding score (RFS). Laryngoscope 2001;111(8):1313–7.
54. Poe RH, Kallay MC. Chronic cough and gastroesophageal reflux disease: experience with specific therapy for diagnosis and treatment. Chest 2003;123(3): 679–84.
55. Irwin R, Zawacki JK, Curley FJ, et al. Chronic cough as the sole presenting manifestation of gastroesophageal reflux. Am Rev Respir Dis 1989;140:294–300.
56. Irwin R, Curley FJ, French CL. Chronic cough: the spectrum and frequency of causes, key components of the diagnostic evaluation, and outcome of specific therapy. Am Rev Respir Dis 1990;141:640–7.
57. Fitzgerald J, Allen CJ, Craven MA, et al. Chronic cough and gastroesophageal reflux. Can Med Assoc J 1989;140:520–4.
58. Dordal M, Baltazar MA, Roca I, et al. Nocturnal spasmodic cough in the infant: evolution after antireflux treatment. Allerg Immunol (Paris) 1994;26:53–8.
59. DuPont C, Molkhou P, Petrovic N, et al. Treatment using motilium of gastroesophageal reflux associated with respiratory manifestations in children. Ann Pediatr 1989;36:148–50.
60. v Grossi L, Spezzaferro M, Sacco LF, et al. Effect of baclofen on oesophageal motility and transient lower oesophageal sphincter relaxations in GORD patients: a 48-h manometric study. Neurogastroenterol Motil 2008;20(7):760–6.
61. Kaufman JA, Houghland JE, Quiroga E, et al. Long-term outcomes of laparoscopic antireflux surgery for gastroesophageal reflux disease (GERD)-related airway disorder. Surg Endosc 2006;20(12):1824–30.
62. Ranson ME, Danielson A, Maxwell JG, et al. Prospective study of laparoscopic nissen fundoplication in a community hospital and its effect on typical, atypical, and nonspecific gastrointestinal symptoms. JSLS 2007;11(1):66–71.
63. Tutuian R, Mainie I, Agrawal A, et al. Nonacid reflux in patients with chronic cough on acid-suppressive therapy. Chest 2006;130(2):386–91.
64. Irwin RS. Chronic cough due to gastroesophageal reflux disease. Chest 2006; 129:80S–94S.

Rhinogenic Laryngitis, Cough, and the Unified Airway

John H. Krouse, MD, PhD[a,*], Kenneth W. Altman, MD, PhD[b]

KEYWORDS

- Respiratory inflammatory processes • Cough
- Laryngeal pathophysiology • Mucus

Extensive epidemiologic and physiologic data gathered in the past decade suggest that the respiratory tract, from the eustachian tube and the paranasal sinuses through to the distal bronchioles, functions as a unified, organized, and interrelated unit. Both local inflammatory processes and the systemic propagation of inflammation through trafficking of inflammatory mediators promote a system-wide response in the respiratory mucosa through which pathology in one portion of this system can stimulate and influence pathophysiological changes at a site distal to the initial site of inflammation. The model developed to study and explain these observations has been termed the *unified airway model* and has been recently described:

> *The presence and severity of disease processes within the upper and lower airways are linked closely, and exacerbations of disease in one component of the airway are likely to encourage worsening of airway disease diffusely.*[1]

Several proposed mechanisms have been offered to provide a physiologic framework for understanding the unified airway response. In the early and mid–twentieth century, one primary hypothesis involved a putative nasobronchial reflex, in which neurogenic communication occurred reflexively between the nose and the bronchial apparatus. While early studies appeared to offer some support for this hypothesis,[2,3] attempts to replicate these findings failed and interest in a nasobronchial reflex waned. A second hypothesis involved the proposed protective mechanism that the nose offered in supporting normal pulmonary function. An observation that occluding the nose in patients with exercise-induced bronchospasm could worsen pulmonary

[a] Department of Otolaryngology–Head and Neck Surgery, Temple University School of Medicine, 3440 North Broad Street, Kresge West 102, Philadelphia, PA 19106, USA
[b] Department of Otolaryngology-Head and Neck Surgery, Mount Sinai School of Medicine, Annenberg 10th Floor, One Gustave Levy Place, Box 1189, New York, NY 10029, USA
* Corresponding author.
E-mail address: jkrouse@temple.edu (J.H. Krouse).

Otolaryngol Clin N Am 43 (2010) 111–121
doi:10.1016/j.otc.2009.11.005
0030-6665/10/$ – see front matter

function was offered in support of this mechanism.[4] Again, similar studies have not replicated these effects, and this mechanism has also fallen into disfavor.

More recently, a model of shared inflammation has become of primary interest as a mechanism to account for many observations seen in unified airway disease. Histologically and functionally, the respiratory mucosa throughout the upper and lower respiratory tracts consists of a uniform pseudostratified columnar epithelium that demonstrates similar responses to stimulation with various agents. Many chronic inflammatory conditions of the respiratory tract, including allergic rhinitis, chronic rhinosinusitis, and asthma, share the system-wide expression of Th2 cytokines, such as interleukin (IL)-4, IL-5, and IL-13, as well as the proliferation and influx of cellular mediators, such as eosinophils. Elegant studies conducted by Braunstahl[5,6] have shown that stimulation with antigen at one respiratory site can result in expression of these inflammatory cytokines at a location distant from the site of stimulation. These findings suggest that there is "inflammatory crosstalk" that occurs throughout the respiratory tract, and that inflammatory processes can therefore progress from one portion of the system to another without difficulty. The activation of Th2 lymphocytes in the nose can lead to the differentiation and activation of immune cells from precursors in the nasal mucosa and bone marrow, leading to recruitment of these newly generated cells throughout the respiratory system.[7] This model of shared respiratory inflammation appears to provide a useful mechanism in understanding processes that occur in the unified airway, and provides a platform to direct future research studies in the area.

LARYNGEAL INVOLVEMENT IN THE UNIFIED AIRWAY

While there has been extensive discussion of how the upper and lower airways interact in acute and chronic illness, the role of the larynx has not been widely described and is currently not well understood. While clinicians have frequently considered the role of allergic rhinitis and asthma in their patients with laryngitis, dysphonia, and cough, systematic study in this area has been uncommon. The larynx possesses a unique anatomic role. It is situated between the upper and lower airways and is therefore a conduit for both upstream and downstream trafficking of mucus and mucopurulent secretions. Effects on the larynx that lead to symptoms of cough and dysphonia could therefore occur either through (1) direct effects of airway inflammation in the laryngeal structures, (2) manifestations of the trafficking of materials through this anatomic region, or (3) the development of secondary edema (particularly in the interarytenoid area as well as the vocal process of the arytenoids) as a result of the cough.

At the cellular level, two leukocyte populations are present and can participate in acute and chronic laryngeal inflammation: (1) mast cells and (2) eosinophils. Mast cells act as the primary cellular mediators of the acute allergic response. When exposed to an antigen in a previously sensitized individual, mast cells degranulate and release histamine and other vasoactive compounds rapidly into the local tissues. While mast cells are abundant in the mucosa of the epiglottis and immediate subglottis, they are not present in the mucosa of the true glottis and vocal folds.[8] Pathophysiologically, these mast cell populations occur in those regions of the larynx that are most responsive to acute anaphylactic reactions: the supraglottis and subglottis. Edema of the vocal folds in the setting of anaphylaxis is less common and pronounced, and cellular infiltration of the larynx in anaphylaxis is often characterized by the presence of eosinophils at postmortem.[9]

In chronic laryngeal inflammation, however, the most common presenting symptoms include dysphonia, transient throat clearing, and cough.[10] In fact, nonproductive coughing episodes are often described as a primary complaint of patients with chronic allergic laryngitis.[11] Diffuse laryngeal inflammation can be appreciated in acute laryngitis, especially in the epiglottis and immediate subglottis. In chronic laryngitis, however, inflammatory changes appear to be confined to the vocal folds, with minimal erythema and no compromise on the airway.[12,13] In addition, animal models show the presence of eosinophils in the laryngeal mucosa among sensitized rats after exposure.[14]

A small body of clinical research has discussed the effects of allergic influences on the larynx. Chadwick[15] suggested that laryngeal dysfunction and symptom expression are influenced by both inflammatory and biomechanical laryngeal disturbances in allergic patients. These factors act synergistically to create chronic changes in the larynx and adjacent airway, and produce the range of symptoms commonly experienced by these patients, including dysphonia, throat clearing, and cough. In another paper, Corey and colleagues[16] described two forms of allergic laryngitis: (1) acute, (anaphylactic) and (2) chronic. The acute, anaphylactic response represents an acute angioedema, in which there is rapid edema of the lips, tongue, pharynx, and larynx in response to exposure to a sensitized antigen. This type of acute response can also be accompanied by systemic symptoms, such as urticaria, dyspnea, and tachycardia, and can rapidly proceed to become life threatening. Acute asphyxia is the primary cause of death among these individuals. In contrast, chronic laryngeal allergy presents with a different symptom complex and a much less aggressive course. Symptoms include hoarseness, throat clearing, globus sensation, and cough, and are often seen coseasonally in patients with allergic rhinitis. Physical examination of these patients demonstrates mild vocal fold edema, increased presence of mucus in the endolarynx, mild to moderate erythema of the arytenoid mucosa, and thick mucus strands that can bridge the vocal folds.[16,17]

Several researchers have examined the interaction between physiologic and behavioral factors in the pathogenesis of symptoms among patients with presumed laryngeal allergy. Cohn and colleagues,[18] for example, have suggested that symptoms of allergic rhinitis, such as pharyngeal dryness and postnasal drainage, lead to mucosal irritation in the larynx and pharynx, which then provokes a sense of itching or tickling in the throat and leads to such behaviors as throat clearing and coughing. Abusive behaviors can then injure the vocal folds, leading to mucosal tears, hemorrhage, and Reinke edema. This cycle of inflammatory and biomechanical influences can result in a downward spiral among patients with respiratory allergy, and can lead to chronic changes in laryngeal anatomy and function.

Direct stimulation of the larynx with antigen in sensitized individuals has also been shown to provoke observable adverse effects in the larynx and pharynx. In a series of experiments from our voice laboratory at Wayne State University Department of Otolaryngology–Head and Neck Surgery, Temple University School of Medicine, subjects demonstrated to be allergic to the house dust mite *Dermatophagoides pteronyssinus* by skin testing underwent direct inhalational challenge of the larynx with aerosolized antigen in increasing concentrations.[19,20] With increasing exposure, subjects demonstrated not only the presence of increased mucus in the larynx, but also coughing and throat clearing with dyspnea (**Fig. 1**). It was unclear whether this mucus was generated within the larynx itself or was transported to the larynx from the lungs during cough. In sensitized subjects, there was also a rapid decline in pulmonary function, suggesting immediate-onset bronchospasm with antigen challenge. These findings support the observation that increased mucus in the larynx and cough are two prominent and reproducible findings among patients with allergic laryngeal symptoms. In addition, the same laboratory has

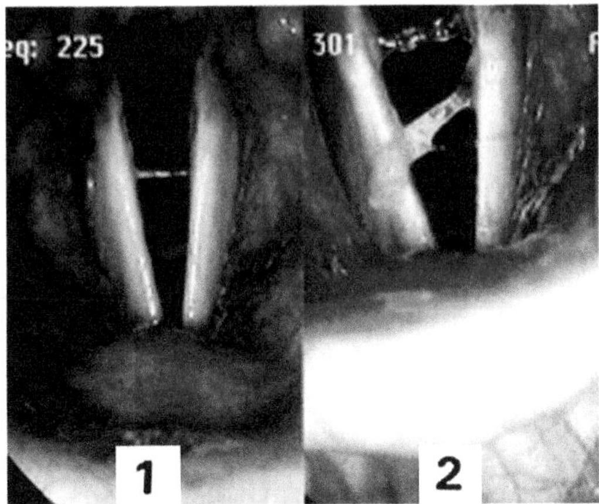

Fig. 1. Videostroboscopic image of a dust mite–allergic subject (1) before and (2) following direct provocation of the larynx with inhalation of dust mite antigen. Note the significant increase in mucus following challenge. (*From* Dworkin JP, Stachler RJ. Management of the patient with laryngitis. In: Krouse JH, Derebery MJ, Chadwick SJ, editors. Managing the allergic patient. Philadelphia: Elsevier; 2007. p. 261; with permission.)

demonstrated that allergic individuals may perceive subtle voice changes even in the absence of more significant symptoms, such as cough.[21]

Other researchers have confirmed the roles of increased mucus production and upstream and downstream mucus trafficking in patients with chronic laryngeal allergy. In observing a large number of patients from a professional voice practice, these researchers noted the common coexistence of irregular glottic edema, excessive sticky mucus secretions in the endolarynx, and dysphonia among symptomatic patients with allergic rhinitis.[22] Some of these patients had symptoms of reflux, although many did not. In addition, about 25% of patients in this study demonstrated abnormalities in pulmonary function testing, again confirming that both upper and lower airway influences were present in many individuals. The study confirms the complex interaction that can occur in these allergic patients with dysphonia and cough.

MUCUS, NEUROLOGIC REFLEXES, AND NEUROGENIC INFLAMMATION

The many roles of mucus are important in both health and disease. Mucus is continuous from the nasal vestibule to the distal alveoli, and serves multiple functions including:

- Humidification of inspired air, which lowers oxygen tension for circulatory exchange and reduces dehydration of the mucosa
- Warming of the inspired air to provide temperature equilibration in the lungs
- Mechanical protection of the underlying mucosa, clearance of foreign particles (including bacterial, viral, and fungal elements), and preservation of ciliary function
- Communication between the upper and lower respiratory tracts to signal a protective response to caustic material and disease.

In addition, mucus gene expression is modified in response to different disease states, as well as exposure to infection, caustic inhalants, and particulate/irritant material.[23]

Although the sinonasal-bronchial reflex has fallen out of favor as a predominant mechanism unifying the upper and lower airways, there is anecdotal evidence of neural reflexes in the airway based on clinical observation. These observations include:

- The tendency of a patient to cough when a flexible endoscope is first placed into the nares, and laryngeal "guarding" (adduction) when the scope is advanced into the pharynx
- Perceived shortness of breath with new-onset nasal obstruction or placement of bilateral nasal packing
- The smooth muscle constriction present in bronchial hyperreactivity (and in response to upper respiratory stimulation of the unified airway) is under both local as well as neurologic control
- Neurologic reflexes present in cough involve vagal nuclei that have broad influence within the respiratory as well as digestive tracts.[24]

The autonomic nervous system has been implicated in reflexive behavior associated with nonallergic/vasomotor rhinitis, allergic rhinitis, and gastroesophogeal reflux disease associated with bronchial hyperreactivity. In the example of vasomotor rhinitis, Loehrl and colleagues[25] demonstrated a hypoactive sympathetic nervous system relative to the parasympathetic nervous system compared with controls. Furthermore, disruption of the cervical sympathetic supply to the nose has been shown to result in chronic inflammation and nasal eosinophilia on the affected side, providing support for the interaction of the autonomic nervous system and the inflammatory response.[26,27] Also, Lodi and colleagues[28] demonstrated significant autonomic dysfunction in patients with gastroesophogeal reflux disease and asthma.

The inflammatory process is now known to involve submucosal mediators, such as substance P, and other mediators that modulate sensory nerve excitability.[29,30] This nerve excitability is responsible for instigating a cough response,[31–33] and also potentially plays a central role in impaired laryngeal sensory feedback, which is common in many voice disorders. Although the concept of "neurogenic inflammation" is still controversial, it makes sense that neurogenic mediators are present and that these mediators link (1) surveillance (by the mucus, inflammatory mediators, and resulting altered mucus gene expression), (2) sensory nerve sensitivity modulation, and (3) a systemic nervous system response.[24] However, the clinical importance of these links has yet to be determined.

DIAGNOSIS OF CHRONIC RHINOGENIC LARYNGITIS

For the purposes of this discussion, chronic rhinogenic laryngitis is defined as inflammation of the larynx resulting in related symptoms and signs that last for at least 2 weeks.[17] The term *rhinogenic laryngitis* is not fully satisfactory, since inflammation of the larynx can occur from both upstream and downstream influences, but will frame the problem accurately for the otolaryngologist treating these types of patients. It may be also be argued that the term *rhinogenic laryngitis* refers to upper respiratory disease involving or influencing the larynx, without the concurrence of lower respiratory disease as part of the unified airway. The term *rhinogenic laryngitis* also indicates a distinction from *reflux laryngitis* or *laryngopharyngeal reflux*, the latter postulated to be the most common (and often empirically diagnosed) cause of chronic laryngitis.

Symptoms of rhinogenic laryngitis include odynophagia, globus sensation, hoarseness, and cough, and are often accompanied by abusive vocal behaviors, such as straining and throat clearing. The degree of symptomatology can be mild or severe and, in many patients, can be longstanding. Since the differential diagnosis of laryngeal pathologies includes malignant neoplasms, a full head and neck examination with indirect or endoscopic visualization of the larynx is essential for all individuals whose symptoms do not rapidly and fully resolve with treatment.

History of the patient with suspected rhinogenic laryngitis must include those factors traditionally evaluated in any patient with laryngeal dysfunction. Any history of gastroesophageal reflux disease or its treatment is important and may be contributory to the patient's symptoms. In addition, a history of smoking, alcohol use, and vocal abuse is important, as is a past history of laryngeal trauma or surgery. The presence of previous or concurrent respiratory diseases, such as allergic rhinitis, recurrent acute or chronic rhinosinusitis, and asthma, would also raise the suspicion that an inflammatory process may be involved in the patient's laryngeal symptoms. In addition, a full history of pharmacotherapy, both active and prior, will help to evaluate any current medications that may be having an adverse effect on the larynx, as well as to suggest contributory influences, such as rhinitis or asthma.

Evaluation of the patient's allergies should involve a full history as it relates to upper and lower airway inflammatory processes. Family history of allergic rhinitis or asthma raises the likelihood that a patient will also have allergic disease. Age of onset of respiratory symptoms is also important, as childhood onset suggests a higher likelihood of allergic disease. Exposure history and any triggering factors known to the patient can elicit allergen-specific information useful in diagnosis and treatment planning. The presence of asthma increases the likelihood of rhinitis dramatically, as patients with asthma have concurrent rhinitis in 80% or more of cases.[34] Any history of skin testing or of immunotherapy is relevant and suggests that allergies may play an important role in the patient's laryngeal symptoms as well.

The physical examination of the patient with suspected rhinogenic laryngitis should involve a full head and neck examination, as well as a laryngeal examination, auscultation of the chest, and possibly spirometry for pulmonary function assessment. In patients with rhinitis, changes in the color of the nasal mucosa and in the character of the nasal mucus are common. In allergic rhinitis, the nasal mucosa often appears pale and boggy, with increased clear, sticky, mucoid secretions present in the nasal cavity. By contrast, there is in patients with nonallergic rhinitis often more of a hyperemic appearance to the mucosa. It must be remembered that mixed allergic-nonallergic rhinitis is common, and not all patients with allergic rhinitis demonstrate the classic pale appearance of the nasal mucosa. In addition, the presence of purulence in the nasal cavity, or of purulent discharge on nasal endoscopic examination, suggests acute or chronic rhinosinusitis. The tympanic membranes should also be visualized for signs of effusion or retraction, and the face should be observed for signs of any periorbital venous pooling that would also suggest allergic rhinitis.

Visualization of the larynx is important, and fiber-optic examinations in the office provide the best means to fully evaluate the larynx, either with or without stroboscopic assistance. In the allergic larynx, the primary finding will be thick, tenacious mucus within the endolarynx, often bridging the vocal folds in tenacious bands. In addition, erythema or paleness can commonly be seen in the posterior larynx, although this finding is frequent in reflux laryngitis as well. Changes, such as vocal fold edema, can be appreciated, as can small vocal nodules, but these findings are likely secondary to the abusive behavioral effects that often accompany the increased sense of mucus and irritation that can occur in rhinogenic laryngitis. If the laryngeal examination is performed with a transoral Hopkins rod laryngoscope, then nasal and nasopharyngeal contributions to laryngeal inflammation may be missed. **Fig. 2** shows an example of nasopharyngeal and posterior pharyngeal "cobblestoning" of

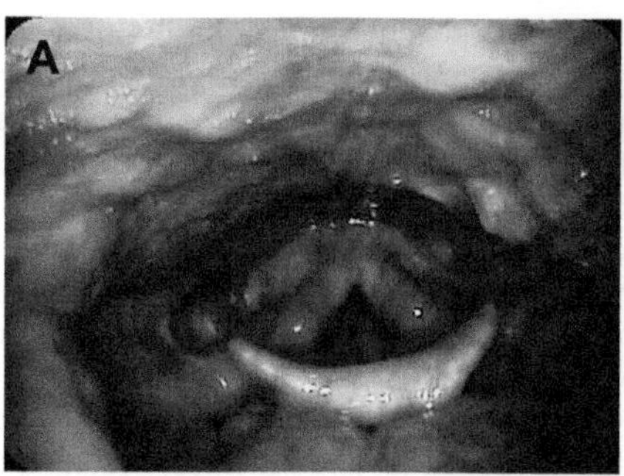

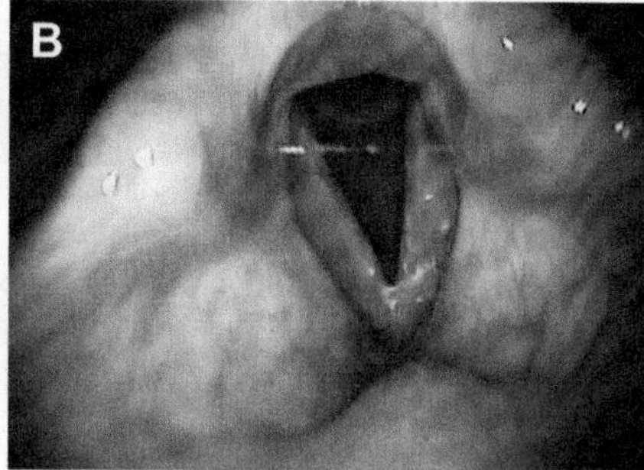

Fig. 2. (*A*) Flexible distal-chip evaluation showing nasopharyngeal and posterior oropharyngeal cobblestoning of the mucosa. (*B*) Stroboscopic image of the vocal folds showing dense airway mucus typical of rhinogenic laryngitis.

the mucosa, as well as dense airway mucus consistent with rhinologic sources contributing to laryngeal symptoms and findings.

Despite these findings, it is often difficult to distinguish between rhinogenic laryngitis and laryngopharyngeal reflux laryngitis solely by physical examination and initial response to empiric use of medication. There is a significant risk of "symptomatic confusion" by both the patient and primary physician regarding the sensation of "postnasal drip." Therefore, objective testing plays an important role when the patient fails to make expected progress with first-line therapy. This testing may include formal allergy testing, computed tomography scan of the sinuses, and/or 24-hour esophageal pH and impedance probe monitoring.

Finally, evaluation of the lungs is important, given the coexistence of asthma among many patients with upper respiratory disease. Auscultation of the chest can determine wheezing in patients with asthma, although this is a late sign and is suggestive of more severe disease. Spirometry can also be useful to detect less severe degrees of asthma, although patients with mild asthma can have relatively preserved levels of pulmonary function between periods of exacerbation. In cases where a diagnosis of asthma is more critical among these patients, methacholine challenge can be used to determine the degree of bronchial hyperresponsiveness and mild bronchoconstriction.

According to Naito and colleagues,[11] three criteria can be used to suggest a diagnosis of allergic laryngitis, and may be generally extended to the diagnosis of rhinogenic laryngitis:

- History of allergic disease, preferably confirmed by skin or in vitro testing
- Pharyngolaryngeal itching, globus sensation, and/or dry cough for more than 3 weeks
- Local laryngeal edema, with paleness of the arytenoid mucosa.

These clinical findings can be supported by biopsies demonstrating eosinophilia or mast cell infiltration in mucosal samples from the larynx, although this procedure is not necessary in framing a presumptive diagnosis. In addition, response to antiallergy or anti-inflammatory medications would support the diagnosis.

MODEL FOR CHRONIC RHINOGENIC LARYNGITIS

It is clear that the respiratory tract functions as an integrated, unified airway unit, and that influences in one portion of this system can result in changes in other, more distant sites. It is also clear that the larynx functions as an integral component of this unified airway, and that common influences from both the upper and lower respiratory tracts can lead to changes in the larynx and the production of laryngeal symptoms, including hoarseness, throat clearing, and cough. These laryngeal symptoms can be generated by both inflammatory and behavioral factors, and the interaction of these influences can lead to a downward spiral with increasing laryngeal dysfunction and resistance to treatment. In cases of chronic laryngitis, direct mucosal effects can occur through persistent allergic stimulation and mediator release, and mucus production in both the upper and lower respiratory systems can result in the trafficking of mucus both upstream and downstream. The increase in thick, sticky mucus in the larynx will result in compensatory behaviors, both volitional and reflexive, resulting in dysphonia and cough.

A specific model for this synergistic process has been proposed by Dworkin and Stachler[17] for inhalant allergen exposure. A modified version of this is shown in **Fig. 3**. This model may be extended to include indolent sinusitis, as well as secondary effects from respiratory irritants, and involves three primary components present in cases of chronic rhinogenic laryngitis:

1. Inflammatory effects occur at all levels of the respiratory tract, leading to mediator release and increased edema and mucus production in the nose, sinuses, pharynx, and lungs.
2. This increased mucus is transported throughout the respiratory tract, both upstream and downstream, and results in increased mucus as the level of the larynx.

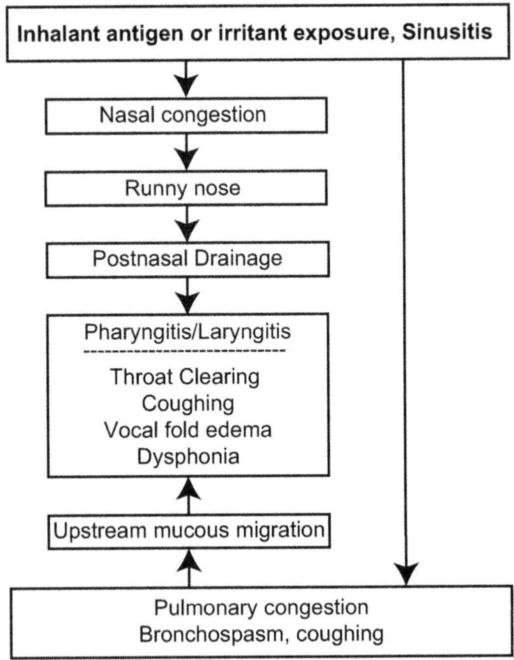

Fig. 3. Flow diagram. Downstream and upstream inflammatory reactions may induce laryngeal changes and symptoms. (*Modified from* Dworkin JP, Stachler RJ. Management of the patient with laryngitis. In: Krouse JH, Derebery MJ, Chadwick SJ, editors. Managing the allergic patient. Philadelphia: Elsevier; 2007. p. 262; with permission.)

3. Increased mucus and irritation in the larynx and pharynx lead to compensatory behaviors, including throat clearing and coughing, which result in anatomic and histologic changes to the laryngeal mucosa, with observable, discrete laryngeal pathologies, such as vocal fold edema and mucosal irregularities.

It is these final symptoms and behaviors that often motivate the patient to seek treatment.

SUMMARY

The increasing recognition of concurrent and synergistic inflammatory processes in respiratory pathophysiology and their effects on the larynx suggests that an evaluation of patients with laryngeal symptoms, such as hoarseness, throat clearing, and cough, should involve an assessment of acute and chronic processes in the upper and lower airways. Direct effects of allergic inflammation in the nose, paranasal sinuses, and lungs; trafficking of mucus and mucopurulent secretions upstream and downstream in both allergic and infectious processes; and secondary compensatory behaviors, such as throat clearing, can all contribute to the development and persistence of chronic laryngeal changes and ongoing patient symptoms. When evaluating a patient with complaints of dysphonia and cough, the otolaryngologist must consider the potential impact of these coexisting conditions, apply appropriate diagnostic methods to assess these potential conditions, and recommend treatment strategies designed to address the comprehensive and interactive nature of processes in the unified airway.

REFERENCES

1. Krouse JH. The unified airway—conceptual framework. Otolaryngol Clin North Am 2008;41:257–66.
2. Sluder G. Asthma as a nasal reflex. JAMA 1919;73:589–91.
3. Kaufman J, Chen JC, Wright GW. The effect of trigeminal resection on reflex bronchoconstriction after nasal and nasopharyngeal irritation in man. Am Rev Respir Dis 1970;101:768–9.
4. Shturman-Ellstein R, Zeballos RJ, Buckley JM, et al. The beneficial effect of nasal breathing on exercise-induced bronchoconstriction. Am Rev Respir Dis 1978; 118:65–73.
5. Braunstahl GJ, Kleinjan A, Overbeek SE, et al. Segmental bronchial provocation induces nasal inflammation in allergic rhinitis patients. Am J Respir Crit Care Med 2000;161:2051–7.
6. Braunstahl GJ, Overbeek SE, Kleinjan A, et al. Nasal allergy provocation induces adhesion molecule expression and tissue eosinophilia in upper and lower airways. J Allergy Clin Immunol 2001;107:469–76.
7. Steinke JW, Borish L. The role of allergy in chronic rhinosinusitis. Immunol Allergy Clin North Am 2004;24:45–57.
8. Domeij S, Dahlqvist A, Erikkson A, et al. Similar distribution of mast cells and substance P and calcitonin gene-related peptide-immunoreactive nerve fibers in the adult human larynx. Ann Otol Rhinol Laryngol 1996;105:825–31.
9. Pumphrey RHS, Roberts ISD. Postmortem findings after fatal anaphylactic reactions. J Clin Pathol 2000;53:273–6.
10. Alimov AL. The clinical symptomatology in the diagnosis of allergy in acute and chronic laryngitis. Vestn Otorinolaringol 1968;30:71–5.

11. Naito K, Baba R, Ishii G, et al. Laryngeal allergy: a commentary. Eur Arch Otorhinolaryngol 1999;256:455–7.
12. Williams RI. Allergic laryngitis. Ann Otol Rhinol Laryngol 1972;81:558–64.
13. Pang LQ. Allergy of the larynx, trachea, and bronchial tree: symposium on allergy and otolaryngology. Otolaryngol Clin North Am 1974;7:719–34.
14. Naito K, Iwata S, Yokoyama N. Laryngeal symptoms to patients exposed to Japanese cedar pollen: allergic reactions and environmental pollution. Eur Arch Otorhinolaryngol 1999;256:209–11.
15. Chadwick SJ. Allergy and the contemporary laryngologist. Otolaryngol Clin North Am 2003;36:957–88.
16. Corey JP, Gungor A, Karnell M. Allergy for the laryngologist. Otolaryngol Clin North Am 1998;31:189–205.
17. Dworkin JP, Stachler RJ. Management of the patient with laryngitis. In: Krouse JH, Derebery MJ, Chadwick SJ, editors. Managing the allergic patient. Philadelphia: Elsevier; 2007. p. 233–72.
18. Cohn JR, Sataloff RT, Branton C. Responsive asthma-related voice dysfunction to allergen immunotherapy: a case report of confirmation by methacholine challenge. J Voice 2001;15:558–60.
19. Reidy PM, Dworkin JP, Krouse JH. Laryngeal effects of antigen stimulation challenge with perennial allergen Dermatophagoides pteronyssinus. Otolaryngol Head Neck Surg 2003;128:455–62.
20. Dworkin JP, Reidy PM, Stachler RJ, et al. Effects of sequential Dermatophagoides pteronyssinus antigen stimulation on anatomy and physiology of the larynx. Ear Nose Throat J 2009;88:793–9.
21. Krouse JH, Dworkin JP, Carron MA, et al. Baseline laryngeal effects among individuals with dust mite allergy. Otolaryngol Head Neck Surg 2008;138:149–51.
22. Jackson-Menaldi CA, Dzul AI, Holland RW. Allergies and vocal fold edema: a preliminary report. J Voice 1999;13:113–22.
23. Rogers DF, Barnes PJ. Treatment of airway mucus hypersecretion. Annu Mediaev 2006;38:116–25.
24. Altman KW, Simpson CB, Amin MR, et al. Cough and paradoxical vocal fold motion. Otolaryngol Head Neck Surg 2002;127:501–11.
25. Loehrl TA, Smith TL, Darling RJ, et al. Autonomic dysfunction, vasomotor rhinitis, and extraesophageal manifestations of gastroesophageal reflux. Laryngoscope 2002;112:1762–5.
26. Fowler EP. Unilateral vasomotor rhinitis due to interference with the cervical sympathetic system. Arch Otolaryngol 1943;37:710–2.
27. Millonig AF, Harris HE, Gardner JW. Effect of autonomic denervation on nasal mucosa: interruption of sympathetic and parasympathetic fibers. Arch Otolaryngol 1950;52:359–68.
28. Lodi U, Harding SM, Coghian HC, et al. Autonomic regulation in asthmatics with gastroesophageal reflux. Chest 1997;111:65–70.
29. Barnes PJ. Neurogenic inflammation in the airways. Respir Physiol 2001;125:145–54.
30. Undem BJ, Lee M-G. Basic mechanisms of cough: current understanding and remaining questions. Lung 2008;186(Suppl 1):S10–6.
31. McLeod RL, Correll CC, Jia Y, et al. TRPV1 antagonists as potential antitussive agents. Lung 2008;186(Suppl 1):S59–65.

32. Brenn D, Richter F, Schaible HG. Sensitization of unmyelinated sensory fibers of the joint nerve to mechanical stimuli by interleukin-6 in the rat: an inflammatory mechanism of joint pain. Arthritis Rheum 2007;56(1):351–9.
33. Hu C, Wedde-Beer K, Auais A, et al. Nerve growth factor and nerve growth factor receptors in respiratory syncytial virus-infected lungs. Am J Physiol Lung Cell Mol Physiol 2002;283(2):L494–502.
34. Corren J. Allergic rhinitis and asthma: how important is the link? J Allergy Clin Immunol 1997;99:S781–6.

Cough Due to Asthma, Cough-Variant Asthma and Non-Asthmatic Eosinophilic Bronchitis

Dhan Desai, MBBS, MRCP, Chris Brightling, MBBS, MRCP, PhD*

KEYWORDS

• Cough • Asthma • Nonasthmatic eosinophilic bronchitis
• Sputum • Exhaled nitric oxide

Chronic cough is defined as a cough lasting for more than 8 weeks with no clinical or radiological evidence of lung disease; it usually results in referral for specialist assessment. An anatomic diagnostic protocol has been constructed in several studies, and this protocol helps identify the causal process in most of these patients.[1–6] Asthma accounts for about one in four cases of cough. Sputum induction was one the first validated noninvasive techniques to assess airway inflammation and led to the identification of nonasthmatic eosinophilic bronchitis. This condition manifests like asthma with sputum eosinophilia and accounts for 10% of cases of chronic cough, but unlike asthma, there is no airway dysfunction.[7] This article summarizes the current understanding of the similarities and differences between asthma and nonasthmatic eosinophilic bronchitis in terms of the immunopathogenesis, natural history and clinical management. The main features and differences between the asthma, cough variant asthma, and nonasthmatic eosinophilic bronchitis are as shown in **Table 1**.

DEFINITION, DIAGNOSIS, AND PREVALENCE

Asthma is the leading cause for chronic cough, accounting for 24% to 29% cases, and these percentages were fairly similar in multiple prospective studies of adult nonsmokers.[1–6] Classic asthma presents most commonly with cough, wheeze, and

---

Funding from Wellcome Senior Clinical Fellowship (CB).
Department of Infection, Inflammation, and Immunity, University of Leicester, Institute for Lung Health, Glenfield Hospital, Groby Road, LE3 9QP, UK
* Corresponding author.
E-mail address: ceb17@le.ac.uk (C.E. Brightling).

Otolaryngol Clin N Am 43 (2010) 123–130
doi:10.1016/j.otc.2009.11.006 oto.theclinics.com
0030-6665/10/$ – see front matter

Table 1
Clinical and pathologic features of eosinophilic bronchitis compared with classical asthma and cough variant asthma

	Eosinophilic Bronchitis	Classical Asthma	Cough Variant Asthma
Symptoms	Cough, often upper airway symptoms	Breathlessness, cough, wheeze	Isolated cough
Presence of atopy	↔	↑	↑
Airway hyper-responsiveness	-	+	+
Response to bronchodilator	-	+	+
Cough reflex hypersensitivity	↑	↔	↑ or ↔
Sputum eosinophil count	↑	↑ or ↔	↑ or ↔
Mast cells within airway smooth muscle bundles	-	+	+
Response to corticosteroids	Good	Good in presence of sputum eosinophilia	Good in presence of sputum eosinophilia

dyspnea and chest tightness. Cough variant asthma, as the title suggests, presents with cough in isolation.[8] Asthmatic patients may have normal physical examination and spirometry; hence when a cause for cough is being sought, bronchial challenge testing may reveal the presence of reactive airways disease. Antiasthma treatment in the form of bronchodilators, inhaled corticosteroids, or a short course of oral prednisolone (usually 0.5 mg/kg for 2 weeks), may resolve the cough, which confirms the diagnosis.

Nonasthmatic eosinophilic bronchitis is defined as a chronic cough in patients with no symptoms or objective evidence of variable airflow obstruction, normal airway hyper-responsiveness (provocative concentration of methacholine producing a 20% decrease in forced expiratory volume in 1 minute (FEV_1), PC_{20} greater than 16 mg/mL), and sputum eosinophilia.[1] An accepted upper cut-off level of greater than 3% nonsquamous sputum eosinophils is used as indicative of eosinophilic bronchitis, as this is outside the 90th percentile for normal patients (1.1%).[9] This level of sputum eosinophilia has been associated with a corticosteroid response in asthma and chronic obstructive pulmonary disease (COPD).[10,11]

Importantly, another cause of chronic cough has been described, particularly in Japanese populations, that is characterized by the presence of eosinophilic airway inflammation and atopy, without airway hyper-responsiveness known as atopic cough.[12,13] This condition is very similar to nonasthmatic eosinophilic bronchitis, except that the latter includes patients with and without atopy. It is therefore likely that atopic cough represents a subgroup of nonasthmatic eosinophilic bronchitis rather than a distinct condition, although further comparative studies are required.

The information gained by measuring airway inflammation only recently has been more widely recognized. Herein lies the problem with establishing the true prevalence of nonasthmatic eosinophilic bronchitis, as most reports of the causes of chronic cough did not include these investigations. In the few studies where airway inflammation was measured, however, it accounted for 10 to 30% of cases of chronic cough. In a 2-year prospective study of chronic cough at a specialist center, 91 patients were identified among an initial 856 referrals. A sputum induction was performed on carefully selected patients, those in whom the diagnosis was unclear despite examination and initial testing. This led to the identification of 12 (13.2%) patients who had nonasthmatic eosinophilic bronchitis, representing about 30% of patients who underwent sputum induction.[1]

EXHALED NITRIC OXIDE AS A SURROGATE FOR SPUTUM EOSINOPHILIA

Sputum induction and analysis require technical support and training, which have limited their widespread application. A simpler, cheaper near-patient biomarker of eosinophilic inflammation is therefore attractive. Exhaled nitric oxide (eNO) levels are increased in asthma, cough variant asthma, and nonasthmatic eosinophilic bronchitis,[14–16] and expression of inducible nitric oxide synthase is up-regulated in the epithelium of asthmatics.[17] Both of these features respond to corticosteroid therapy. The correlation between eNO and sputum eosinophilia is good in corticosteroid-naïve patients, but this relationship is weaker once patients are treated.[16] In asthma following treatment with anti-interleukin (IL)-5, the sputum eosinophil count is markedly attenuated without affecting eNO, suggesting that this relationship represents an epiphenomenon rather than a causal association.[18] The application of eNO to guide corticosteroid therapy in asthma has been disappointing[19–21] compared with success with sputum eosinophil counts[22,23] and therefore questions its role in monitoring patients and titrating their therapy. This, however, does not detract from its potential as a biomarker for eosinophilic inflammation during the workup of patients as part of the diagnostic investigations. Indeed, Hayn and colleagues[24] reported that eNO had good positive and negative predictive values for response to corticosteroids in chronic cough with a sensitivity and specificity above 85%. Similarly, eNO has a strong negative predictive value for a sputum eosinophilia in nonasthmatic eosinophilic bronchitis[25] and for cough variant asthma.[26] It therefore probably has clinical utility as part of the initial evaluation for chronic cough before the use of corticosteroid therapy for the exclusion of cough variant asthma and nonasthmatic eosinophilic bronchitis. Therefore, although sputum induction and processing would be desirable in the routine assessment of chronic cough, eNO does provide valuable information in cases where analysis of sputum is not possible.

PATHOGENESIS

The etiology remains unknown, but both asthma and nonasthmatic eosinophilic bronchitis can be associated with exposure to inhaled aeroallergen or an occupational sensitizer.[27,28] These conditions share many immunopathological features including a similar degree of sputum,[15,29] bronchoalveolar lavage,[15,30] and biopsy eosinophilia, and a similar degree of reticular basement membrane thickening.[15,31] Similarly, there are increased sputum concentrations of cysteinyl–leukotrienes and eosinophilic cationic protein.[29] IL-5 and granulocyte macrophage colony stimulating factor gene expression are increased in bronchoalveolar lavage in both asthma and nonasthmatic eosinophilic bronchitis.[30] The role of vascular endothelial growth factor (VEGF) is unclear, as one study found VEGF levels similar in both asthma and nonasthmatic eosinophilic bronchitis,[32] while another study showed higher sputum VEGF concentration in the asthma group.[33] This is implicated in causing airway narrowing by increasing vascular permeability and subsequently mucosal edema.

In asthma, mast cell numbers in airway smooth muscle were increased, but not in nonasthmatic eosinophilic bronchitis,[31] and the number of airway smooth muscle mast cells was correlated inversely with airway hyperresponsiveness.[31,32] Histamine and prostaglandinD2 sputum concentrations are increased in non-asthmatic eosinophilic bronchitis. This supports the view that mast cells are localized and activated in more superficial airway epithelium in nonasthmatic eosinophilic bronchitis, whereas in asthma they lie deeper in close association with the airway smooth muscle.[31] IL-13 expression is increased in asthma in bronchial submucosa, sputum, and peripheral blood T-cells.[34–37]

The airway narrowing that characterizes asthma is not seen in nonasthmatic eosinophilic bronchitis. It is a consequence of airway remodeling, which is active in both conditions but only results in disordered airway geometry in the former.[38] Thus, although there is an overlap in the immunopathogenesis of both conditions, the pathways of airway inflammation are likely to ultimately lead to the differences in clinical expression between asthma and nonasthmatic eosinophilic bronchitis. In summary, airway hyper-responsiveness in asthma is caused in part by the localization of activated mast cells to airway smooth muscle bundle, as evidenced by increased IL-13 expression and airway narrowing, whereas cough is mediated in part by infiltration into the superficial airway by eosinophils and mast cells. These key differences in the immunopathology of asthma and nonasthmatic eosinophilic bronchitis and their clinical consequences are illustrated in **Fig. 1**.

DISEASE PROGRESSION

Few studies have examined the natural history of nonasthmatic eosinophilic bronchitis because of the lack of large case series. A 10-year follow-up evaluation of 12 patients

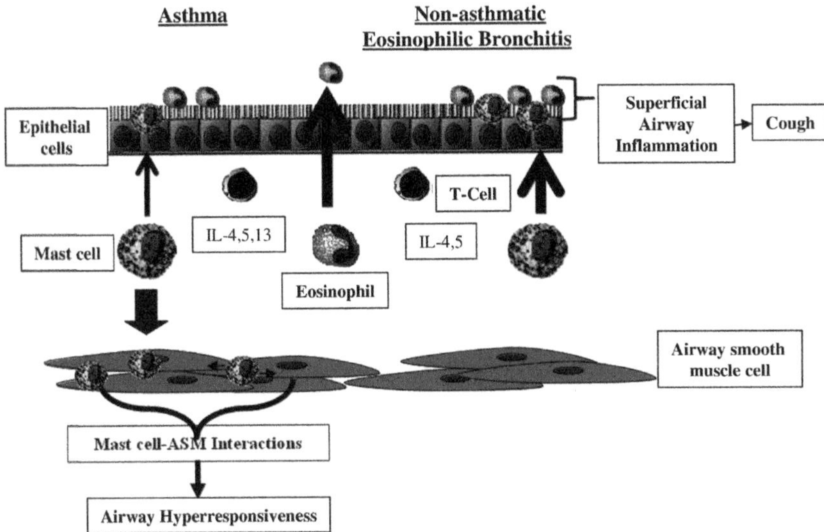

Fig. 1. Inflammatory cell localization in the airway wall and its functional consequences. Mast cell localization to the airway smooth muscle bundle is a feature of asthma and has been implicated in the development of airway hyper-responsiveness. Inflammatory cell localization to the superficial airway is a feature of asthma and nonasthmatic eosinophilic bronchitis and may be important in chronic cough.

with nonasthmatic eosinophilic bronchitis suggests that this condition is generally benign and self-limiting.[39] A larger series of patients has been reported recently, suggesting that this condition is rarely self-limiting.[28] The data were available from 32 patients with nonasthmatic eosinophilic bronchitis who were followed for more than 1 year. Only one patient had complete resolution of symptoms, with no sputum eosinophilia while not receiving any steroid therapy. Twenty one (66%) had persistent symptoms or ongoing airway inflammation. Three (9%) patients developed asthma with typical symptoms and airway hyper-responsiveness. Five (16%) developed fixed airflow obstruction.

There may be a causal association between nonasthmatic eosinophilic bronchitis and COPD. Sputum eosinophilia has been observed in up to 40% of patients with COPD, with no history of asthma and with no evidence of airway hyper-responsiveness.[10,40] A case has been reported of a patient who over a 2-year period developed persistent airflow obstruction.[41] The patient's cough improved with inhaled corticosteroids, but the sputum eosinophilia continued.

The natural history of cough variant asthma is not entirely clear, mainly because of lack of sufficient data. In a 4-year retrospective study of 42 patients, 7 went into remission, and 13 developed classical asthma.[42] Thus, in some cases, it appears as a precursor of classic asthma, and whether patients develop fixed airflow obstruction is uncertain.

TREATMENT

Where the onset appears to be related to an inhaled aeroallergen, occupational exposure, or identifiable trigger, avoidance strategy initially is recommended. Anti- inflammatory treatment is mainly in the form of corticosteroids.

Current recommendations for asthma and cough variant asthma are to use inhaled therapy with bronchodilators and corticosteroids first,[43] with leukotriene receptor antagonists added as the next step. Small trials have demonstrated that theophylline and zafirlukast are also useful. Difficult cases may need treatment with systemic corticosteroids, usually oral prednisolone, but these are to be used only as an exception because of the unfavorable adverse effect profile of systemic corticosteroid usage. Monitoring both clinical response and airway inflammation is recommended in this last group of patients to guide intensity of corticosteroid therapy. Patients with chronic cough without evidence of airway eosinophilia do not respond to corticosteroid therapy, and attempts should be made to reduce or withdraw this.[44]

Inhaled corticosteroid therapy for nonasthmatic eosinophilic bronchitis is associated with symptomatic improvement and a significant fall in sputum eosinophilia.[45,46] Oral corticosteroids rarely are required. Treatment duration is guided by symptomatic response and monitoring airway inflammation. Management decisions can be difficult to make if these parameters are discordant. In one study, capsaicin cough sensitivity, which was increased moderately before treatment,[46] improved toward normal after treatment with budesonide (400 μg inhaled twice daily) for 4 weeks, and there was a significant positive correlation between the treatment-induced change in cough sensitivity and sputum eosinophil count. These findings suggest that heightened cough sensitivity contributes to the cough in nonasthmatic eosinophilic bronchitis and that eosinophilic airway inflammation is causally associated with the increased cough sensitivity. However, importantly in a group of severe asthmatics, anti-IL-5 therapy had profound effects upon the frequency of severe exacerbations without an impact upon cough.[18] This questions a causal relationship between eosinophilic inflammation in asthma and cough and perhaps raises the potential importance of other mechanisms such as mast cell interactions with superficial nerves. Antileukotriene and antihistaminic therapy have not yet been tried in nonasthmatic eosinophilic bronchitis, but the increase of these mediators in sputum samples suggests that they may have efficacy. Atopic cough, in addition, appears to respond to antihistaminic therapy.[13]

SUMMARY

Asthma and nonasthmatic eosinophilic bronchitis are common causes of chronic cough that in general respond well to corticosteroid therapy. Sputum induction has provided a reliable tool to measure airway inflammation and can be applied to the management of chronic cough, but in a setting where this test is unavailable, eNO may help to guide the use of corticosteroids. In addition to its value in the management of nonasthmatic eosinophilic bronchitis, the study of this condition also has shed light on the potential relationship between airway inflammation and dysfunction. Specifically, mast cell location to the airway smooth muscle bundle is a key determinant of the development of airway hyper-responsiveness, whereas location of inflammatory cells in the epithelium may be important in cough. There is a need to improve the understanding of the causes of these conditions, their natural history, and the role of other current and emerging therapies.

REFERENCES

1. Brightling CE, Ward R, Goh KL, et al. Eosinophilic bronchitis is an important cause of chronic cough. Am J Respir Crit Care Med 1999;160:406–10.
2. Carney IK, Gibson PG, Murree-Allen K, et al. A systematic evaluation of mechanisms in chronic cough. Am J Respir Crit Care Med 1997;156:211–6.
3. Ayik SO, Basoglu OK, Erdinc M, et al. Eosinophilic bronchitis as a cause of chronic cough. Respir Med 2003;97:695–701.
4. Irwin RS, Corrao WM, Pratter MR. Chronic persistent cough in the adult: the spectrum and frequency of causes and successful outcome of specific therapy. Am Rev Respir Dis 1981;123:413–7.
5. Irwin RS, Curley FJ, French CL. Chronic cough. The spectrum and frequency of causes, key components of the diagnostic evaluation, and outcome of specific therapy. Am Rev Respir Dis 1990;141:640–7.
6. McGarvey LP, Heaney LG, Lawson JT, et al. Evaluation and outcome of patients with chronic nonproductive cough using a comprehensive diagnostic protocol. Thorax 1998;53:738–43.
7. Gibson PG, Dolovich J, Denburg J, et al. Chronic cough: eosinophilic bronchitis without asthma. Lancet 1989;1:1346–8.
8. Corrao WM, Braman SS, Irwin RS. Chronic cough as the sole presenting manifestation of bronchial asthma. N Engl J Med 1979;300(12):633–7.
9. Belda J, Leigh R, Parameswaran K, et al. Induced sputum cell counts in healthy adults. Am J Respir Crit Care Med 2000;161:475–8.
10. Pizzichini E, Pizzichini MM, Gibson P, et al. Sputum eosinophilia predicts benefit from prednisone in smokers with chronic obstructive bronchitis. Am J Respir Crit Care Med 1998;158:1511–7.
11. Pavord ID, Brightling CE, Woltmann G, et al. Noneosinophilic corticosteroid unresponsive asthma. Lancet 1999;353:2213–4.
12. Fujimura M, Ogawa H, Nishizawa Y, et al. Comparison of atopic cough with cough variant asthma: is atopic cough a precursor of asthma? Thorax 2003;58:14–8.

13. Fujimura M, Ogawa H, Yasui M, et al. Eosinophilic tracheobronchitis and airway cough hypersensitivity in chronic nonproductive cough. Clin Exp Allergy 2000; 30:41–7.
14. Berlyne GS, Parameswaran K, Kamada D, et al. A comparison of exhaled nitric oxide and induced sputum as markers of airway inflammation. J Allergy Clin Immunol 2000;106:638–44.
15. Brightling CE, Symon FA, Birring SS, et al. Comparison of the immunopatholgy of eosinophilic bronchitis and asthma. Thorax 2003;58:528–32.
16. Smith AD, Cowan JO, Filsell S, et al. Diagnosing asthma: comparisons between exhaled nitric oxide measurements and conventional tests. Am J Respir Crit Care Med 2004;169(4):473–8.
17. Redington AE, Meng QH, Springall DR, et al. Increased expression of inducible nitric oxide synthase and cyclo-oxygenase-2 in the airway epithelium of asthmatic subjects and regulation by corticosteroid treatment. Thorax 2001; 56(5):351–7.
18. Haldar P, Brightling CE, Hargadon B, et al. Mepolizumab and exacerbations of refractory eosinophilic asthma. N Engl J Med 2009;360(10):973–84.
19. Smith AD, Cowan J, Brasset KP, et al. Use of exhaled nitric oxide measurements to guide treatment in chronic asthma. N Engl J Med 2005;352(21):2163–73.
20. Shaw DE, Berry MA, Thomas M, et al. The use of exhaled nitric oxide to guide asthma management: a randomised controlled trial. Am J Respir Crit Care Med 2007;176(3):231–7.
21. Pijnenburg MW, Bakker EM, Hop WC, et al. Titrating steroids on exhaled nitric oxide in children with asthma: a randomized controlled trial. Am J Respir Crit Care Med 2005;172:831–6.
22. Green RH, Brightling CE, McKenna S, et al. Reduced asthma exacerbations with management strategy directed at normalising the sputum eosinophil count. Lancet 2002;360:1715–21.
23. Jayaram L, Pizzichini MM, Cook RJ, et al. Determining asthma treatment by monitoring sputum cell counts: effect on exacerbations. Eur Respir J 2006;27(3): 483–94.
24. Hayn PY, Morgenthaler TI, Lim KG. Use of nitric oxide in predicting response to inhaled corticosteroids for chronic cough. Mayo Clin Proc 2007;82:1350–5.
25. Oh MJ, Lee JY, Lee B, et al. Exhaled nitric oxide measurement is useful for the exclusion of nonasthmatic eosinophilic bronchitis in patients with chronic cough. Chest 2008;14:990–5.
26. Chatkin JM, Ansarin K, Silkoff PE, et al. Exhaled nitric oxide as a noninvasive assessment of chronic cough. Am J Respir Crit Care Med 1999;159(6):1810–3.
27. Lemiere C, Efthimiadis A, Hargreave FE. Occupational eosinophilic bronchitis without asthma: an unknown occupational airway disease. J Allergy Clin Immunol 1997;100:852–3.
28. Berry MA, Hargadon B, McKenna S, et al. Observational study of the natural history of eosinophilic bronchitis. Clin Exp Allergy 2005;35(5):598–601.
29. Brightling CE, Ward R, Woltmann G, et al. Induced sputum inflammatory mediator concentrations in eosinophilic bronchitis and asthma. Am J Respir Crit Care Med 2000;162:878–82.
30. Gibson PG, Zlatic K, Scott J, et al. Chronic cough resembles asthma with IL-5 and granulocyte-macrophage colony-stimulating factor gene expression in bronchoalveolar cells. J Allergy Clin Immunol 1998;101:320–6.
31. Brightling CE, Bradding P, Symon FA, et al. Mast cell infiltration of airway smooth muscle in asthma. N Engl J Med 2002;346:1699–705.

32. Siddiqui S, Mistry V, Doe C, et al. Airway hyperresponsiveness is dissociated from airway wall structural remodelling. J Allergy Clin Immunol 2008;122(2):335–41.
33. Kanazawa H, Nomura S, Yoshikawa J. Role of microvascular permeability on physiologic differences in asthma and eosinophilic bronchitis. Am J Respir Crit Care Med 2004;169:1125–30.
34. Saha SK, Berry MA, Parker D, et al. Increased sputum and bronchial biopsy IL-13 expression in severe asthma. J Allergy Clin Immunol 2008;121(3):685–91.
35. Siddiqui S, Cruse G, McKenna S, et al. IL-13 expression by blood T cells and not eosinophils is increased in asthma compared to non-asthmatic eosinophilic bronchitis. BMC Pulm Med 2009;9:34.
36. Berry MA, Parker D, Neale N, et al. Sputum and bronchial submucosal IL-13 expression in asthma and eosinophilic bronchitis. J Allergy Clin Immunol 2004; 114(5):1106–9.
37. Park SW, Jangm HK, An MH, et al. Interleukin-13 and interleukin-5 in induced sputum and eosinophilic bronchitis: comparison with asthma. Chest 2005; 128(4):1921–7.
38. Siddiqui S, Gupta S, Cruse G, et al. Airway wall geometry in asthma and nonasthmatic eosinophilic bronchitis. Allergy 2009;64(6):951–8.
39. Hancox RJ, Leigh R, Kelly MM, et al. Eosinophilic bronchitis. Lancet 2001; 358(9287):1104.
40. Brightling CE, Monteiro W, Ward R, et al. Sputum eosinophilia and short-term response to prednisolone in chronic obstructive pulmonary disease: a randomised controlled trial. Lancet 2000;356:1480–5.
41. Brightling CE, Woltmann G, Wardlaw AJ, et al. Development of irreversible airflow obstruction in a patient with eosinophilic bronchitis without asthma. Eur Respir J 1999;14:1228–30.
42. Matsumoto H, Niimi A, Takemura M, et al. Prognosis of cough variant asthma: a retrospective analysis. J Asthma 2006;43(2):131–5.
43. Dicpinigaitis PV. Chronic cough due to asthma: ACCP evidence-based clinical practice guidelines. Chest 2006;129(Suppl 1):75S–9S.
44. Pizzichini MM, Pizzichini E, Parameswaran K, et al. Nonasthmatic chronic cough: no effect of treatment with an inhaled corticosteroid in patients without sputum eosinophilia. Can Respir J 1999;6:323–30.
45. Gibson PG, Hargreave FE, Girgis-Gabardo A, et al. Chronic cough with eosinophilic bronchitis: examination for variable airflow obstruction and response to corticosteroid. Clin Exp Allergy 1995;25:127–32.
46. Brightling CE, Ward R, Wardlaw AJ, et al. Airway inflammation, airway responsiveness, and cough before and after inhaled budesonide in patients with eosinophilic bronchitis. Eur Respir J 2000;15:682–6.

The Spectrum of Nonasthmatic Inflammatory Airway Diseases in Adults

Sidney S. Braman, MD[a,b,*], Muhanned Abu-Hijleh, MD[a,b]

KEYWORDS

• Chronic productive cough • Mucopurulent sputum
• Chronic bronchitis • Bronchiectasis • Bronchiolitis

Mucus secretion and cough provide a normal first-line defense against inhaled gases, particles, and microorganisms. Normally, approximately 50 mL of sputum is produced each day by the airway mucus-secreting tissue, the goblet cells in the epithelium, and submucosal seromucus glands. The viscoelasticity of the mucus is conferred by glycoproteins, called mucins, whose components are encoded by specific mucin (MUC) genes. The mucus is eliminated by the action of mucociliary clearance to the hypopharynx, where it is swallowed and rarely noticed. When the burden of gases, particles, or microorganisms that are inhaled becomes excessive, for example, as seen in cigarette smokers, those with noxious occupational exposures, or those with an influenza infection, it results in inflammatory and immune responses in the airways. One consequence is an overproduction of mucus. This may overwhelm mucociliary clearance mechanisms and cause chronic productive cough. The expectorated mucus is usually clear or white (mucoid) unless there is a high bacterial load in the respiratory secretions that causes the mucus to have a yellow or green color (purulent). The production of green sputum is a surrogate marker for intense bronchial inflammation and the presence of bacterial pathogens in increasing concentrations.[1] A change of sputum from mucoid to purulent reflects an increased number of neutrophils containing the green pigment myeloperoxidase. Syndromes associated with chronic productive cough discussed in this article include chronic bronchitis, bronchiectasis, and infectious and

[a] Department of Medicine, Division of Pulmonary and Critical Care Medicine, Warren Alpert Medical School of Brown University, Rhode Island Hospital, 593 Eddy Street, Providence, RI 02903, USA

[b] Division of Pulmonary, Sleep and Critical Care Medicine, Department of Medicine, Warren Alpert Medical School of Brown University, Rhode Island Hospital, 593 Eddy Street, Providence, RI 02903, USA

* Corresponding author. Division of Pulmonary, Sleep and Critical Care Medicine, Department of Medicine, Warren Alpert Medical School of Brown University, Rhode Island Hospital, 593 Eddy Street, Providence, RI 02903.

E-mail address: Sidney_braman@brown.edu (S.S. Braman).

Otolaryngol Clin N Am 43 (2010) 131–146
doi:10.1016/j.otc.2009.11.007
0030-6665/10/$ – see front matter. Published by Elsevier Inc.

noninfectious bronchiolitis (**Box 1**). Bacterial bronchitis and unsuspected bacterial suppurative airway disease are discussed elsewhere in this issue.

CHRONIC BRONCHITIS

Most smokers produce excessive amounts of sputum each day, as much as 100 mL/d more than normal. This results in cough and sputum production. The term, *chronic bronchitis*, has been used to describe this cough phlegm syndrome since the early nineteenth century, and in the mid–twentieth century, the British Medical Research Council definition became widely accepted: "a disease of the bronchi that is manifested by cough and sputum expectoration occurring on most days for at least 3 months of the year and for at least 2 consecutive years when other pulmonary or cardiac causes for the chronic productive cough are excluded."[2] Many, but not all, patients with chronic bronchitis develop expiratory flow limitation. Spirometry testing shows that reduced expiratory flow and measures, such as the forced expiratory volume in the first second of expiration (FEV_1), have been used to identify and stage the degree of airflow obstruction.[3] Often in smokers with chronic bronchitis, destruction of alveolar walls (emphysema) also develops and this contributes to airflow limitation. The presence of chronic bronchitis without airflow obstruction has been referred to as *simple chronic bronchitis* and when accompanied by airflow obstruction the term, *chronic obstructive bronchitis*, or, more commonly, *chronic obstructive pulmonary disease (COPD)*, is used.

The excess mucus production in patients with chronic bronchitis occurs as a result of an increase in the size and number of the submucosal glands and an increase in the number of goblet cells on the surface epithelium. Mucous gland enlargement and hyperplasia of the goblet cells[4] are, therefore, the pathologic hallmarks of chronic bronchitis and the amount of the gland correlates with the amount of intraluminal mucus.[5] Goblet cells are normally absent in the small airways, and their presence there (often referred to as mucous metaplasia) is important to the development of COPD. The increase in mucus is linked specifically with an increase in MUC5B in the bronchiolar lumen.[6] There is also upregulation of MUC5AC in the airway epithelium of patients with COPD and chronic cough compared to smokers without COPD and

Box 1
Definitions

Chronic bronchitis is a disease of the bronchi characterized by abnormal inflammatory response to noxious particles and gases (primarily cigarette smoking) and progressive airflow limitation. Its is usually manifested by cough and chronic sputum expectoration occurring on most days for at least 3 months of the year and for at least 2 consecutive years, when other pulmonary or cardiac causes for the chronic productive cough are excluded.

Bronchiectasis is an airway disorder associated with chronic cough and production of mucopurulent sputum related to chronic inflammation and infection. This eventually leads to bronchial wall damage, dilation, and permanent destruction. The pathologic features include intense inflammation, thickening, and constrictions of the airway wall, and resulting tortuosity, dilatation, ectasia, and eventual destruction of the distal bronchi and bronchioles.

Bronchiolitis encompasses a spectrum of infectious/postinfectious, inflammatory, and idiopathic syndromes that can affect the small airways less than or equal to 2 mm in diameter. This process can lead to variable degrees of injury to the bronchiolar epithelium and reversible or irreversible structural damage. Bronchiolitis can be the only manifestation of various clinical syndromes or may be a part of a spectrum of histopathologic and radiographic findings that may also involve the large airways and lung parenchyma.

nonsmokers.[6] In the larger airways of patients with chronic bronchitis, there is a reduction in the serous acini of the submucosal glands. This depresses local defenses to bacterial adherence, because these glands are known to produce microbial deterrents, such as lactoferrin, antiproteases, and lysozyme. Other epithelial alterations that are seen in patients with chronic bronchitis are a reduction in the number and length of the cilia and squamous metaplasia. The mucociliary abnormalities of chronic bronchitis cause the formation of a continuous sheet or blanket of mucus lining the airways instead of the discreet deposits of mucus seen in normal airways. Pooling of the secretions also may occur. This provides an additional source of bacterial growth and is likely important in the establishment of a chronic colonization in the tracheobronchial tree. These bacteria cause a release of toxins that can further damage the cilia and epithelial cells. Bacterial exoproducts are known to stimulate mucus production, slow ciliary beating, impair immune effector cell function, and destroy local immunoglobulins. This vicious cycle[7] is especially seen in current smokers acompared with former smokers.

The cause of cough in patients with chronic bronchitis is multifactorial. Airway inflammation and excessive bronchial secretions are likely to activate the afferent limb of the cough reflex.[8] There is evidence that the cough receptors are heightened in patients with chronic bronchitis as it has been demonstrated that capsaicin-induced cough is increased.[9] When airflow obstruction is present, it often leads to an ineffective cough as a result of decreased expiratory flow, which, coupled with impaired mucociliary clearance, results in the further retention of secretions and a vicious cycle of chronic recurrent coughing.[10,11] Even in the absence of airflow obstruction and with a short smoking history, impaired mucociliary clearance has been shown in young smokers. This occurs because of abnormal clearance in the small airways. Patients with advanced disease and evidence of airway obstruction have mucus retention in the small peripheral airways and larger central airways.[12,13] This cycle is worsened during episodes of acute viral and bacterial infections that are common in patients with chronic bronchitis, referred to as an acute exacerbation of COPD.[14]

Smoking and Chronic Bronchitis

The association of chronic cough and excessive mucus production with cigarette smoking has been established for decades. The pioneering work of Comstock and colleagues[15] in middle-aged smokers showed that cigarette smokers had considerably more cough and phlegm than nonsmokers and that pipe and cigar smokers had intermediate levels of these symptoms. Those who quit smoking showed considerable improvement in these symptoms. Two decades later, the longitudinal Scottish Heart Health Study[16] showed that current cigarette smokers had rates of chronic cough and chronic phlegm four to five times those of never-smokers and symptoms were more prevalent in men than in women (32.3% versus 6.5% for men and 24% versus 5.5% for women for chronic cough; 31% versus 8.3% for men and 21% versus 5.5% for women for chronic phlegm). The higher symptom rates in men were found in smokers, exsmokers, and never-smokers. There were substantially lower rates of chronic cough and chronic phlegm within a year of stopping smoking. Even 10 years after stopping, rates of symptoms among exsmokers remained a little above those of never-smokers. These studies emphasize the importance of smoking cessation in relieving cough and sputum production with chronic bronchitis. A widely held belief is that smoking cessation will lead to an increase in cough but this has proved unlikely among relatively healthy smokers who stop smoking and should not be a barrier to maintaining abstinence for most smokers.[17]

More recently a 30-year Finnish study on the cumulative incidence of chronic bronchitis in middle-aged men was reported.[18] The cumulative incidence of chronic bronchitis and COPD was 42% and 32%, respectively, in continuous smokers and 22% and 12% in nonsmokers. The symptoms of chronic bronchitis began at a median age of 55 years in smokers and in never-smokers at the age of 60 years. In this study the presence of chronic bronchitis resulted in a 13 mL per year excess in the longitudinal decline in pulmonary function and a higher mortality rate. The study was done in a rural environment, hence many were farmers. Occupational exposure to organic dusts, such as grain dust, may explain these findings in nonsmokers.

Thus, there is a strong association between smoking and cough and mucus production and there is evidence that excessive mucus production has a negative effect on the decline in pulmonary function with aging. In prospective studies of a middle-aged population, a rapid decline of FEV_1 has also been associated with the presence of severe airflow obstruction (FEV_1/forced vital capacity <70% and FEV_1 <50% predicted), age 50 or older, female gender, and black race.[19] The presence of chronic productive cough in a smoker should raise suspicion of underlying COPD and should prompt vigorous smoking cessation measures and lung function testing.

Acute Exacerbation of Chronic Bronchitis (Chronic Obstructive Pulmonary Disease)

In 2000, an international panel of chest physicians proposed a definition for an acute exacerbation of chronic bronchitis in patients with COPD that is widely accepted: "a sustained worsening of the patient's condition, from the stable state and beyond normal day-to-day variations, that is acute in onset and necessitates a change in treatment in patients with underlying COPD."[20] Three subtypes (types 1, 2, and 3) have been identified that helped direct therapy. They were based on the occurrence of all or some of three specific symptoms: increased shortness of breath, increased cough and sputum volume, and increased sputum purulence.[21] The presence of all three symptoms (type 1) implies a greater severity of disease and calls for treatment with antibiotics.[21] Nonspecific systemic symptoms, such as fatigue, malaise, and fever, may be present and evidence of a systemic inflammatory response during a COPD exacerbation can be demonstrated by elevated blood levels of IL-6, tumor necrosis factor α, and C-reactive protein.[14]

Causes of Chronic Obstructive Pulmonary Disease Exacerbations

Viral and bacterial infections are the main causative agents associated with COPD exacerbations and there is also epidemiologic evidence that high levels of air pollution with SO_2, NO_2, ozone, and airborne particulates may play a contributory role. The use of polymerase chain reaction technology has led to a greater recognition of the importance of respiratory viruses in the pathogenesis of exacerbations. At least 30% to 50% of all exacerbations are associated with a respiratory virus[22] and this is especially seen in the winter months when these infections are more prevalent in the general community. In one prospective community study, rhinovirus was detected in 58% of virus-induced exacerbations and 23% of all COPD exacerbations.[23] Other viruses that have been detected are the coronovirus, influenza virus, parainfluenza virus adenovirus, and respiratory syncytial virus.[22] Bacteria are also an important cause of COPD exacerbations but viruses are associated with more severe exacerbations and recovery is more prolonged.[14] Pathogenic bacteria can be found in approximately 50% of exacerbations and the acquisition of a new strain of bacterial pathogen is associated with a twofold risk of a new exacerbation.[24] Typical bacteria associated with a COPD exacerbation are *Haemophilus influenzae, Moraxella catarrhalis*, and *Streptococcus pneumoniae*. Empiric therapy is usually given to cover these organisms as the sputum is not routinely cultured. There is evidence that multidrug-resistant bacteria, most commonly nonfermenting gram-negative bacilli, such as *Pseudomonas aeruginosa, Acinetobacter baummani* and *Stenotrophomonas maltophilia*, are becoming increasingly common with severe exacerbations. For severe exacerbations or those refractory to first-line treatment, a sputum culture and sensitivity may prove useful.[25] Also, many patients hospitalized with an acute exacerbation of COPD have concomitant viral and bacterial infections. Such patients tend to have greater severity of illness and longer lengths of hospital stay. A severe exacerbation of COPD can lead to hypoxemic and hypercarbic respiratory failure that requires an ICU level of care and carries a high mortality. Patients with a higher frequency of exacerbations, in general, have a more profound deterioration in overall health status and a greater decline in lung function over time.

There are few clinical clues that may be helpful to distinguish viral-induced from bacterial-induced exacerbations of COPD. It is usually difficult to make this distinction. Patients with cold symptoms (nasal congestion, rhinorrhea, sore throat) and fever are more likely to have viruses detected from nasal aspirates. Sputum purulence as a result of increased numbers of white blood cells can be seen with viral or bacterial infection but the presence of green purulent sputum is especially predictive of a high bacterial load.[26]

Treatment of an Acute Exacerbation of Chronic Obstructive Pulmonary Disease

Bronchodilator therapy has a role in the prevention and treatment of COPD exacerbations and is recommended for stable chronic bronchitis and for an acute exacerbation.[27] Short-acting inhaled β-agonists, such as albuterol, and anticholinergics, such as ipratropium, are effective in improving symptoms and lung function in patients with an exacerbation. They are often given together but there is no evidence that the combination is more effective than a single agent. Oral corticosteroids (such as prednisone [40–60 mg]) have been shown to reduce hospitalizations and relapses after emergency department visits and for patients who require hospitalization; systemic corticosteroids improve symptoms more quickly and reduce hospital length of stay compared with placebo.[28] Long-acting inhaled β-agonists, such as formoterol and salmeterol, and anticholinergics, such as tiotropium, reduce exacerbation rates in patients with COPD. The combination treatment with a long-acting β-agonist and inhaled corticosteroid reduces exacerbation rates greater than the individual components alone.[29] The use of antibiotics for treatment of an acute exacerbation of chronic bronchitis is recommended as it shortens the course of the illness. There is, however, some uncertainty about their use because of conflicting clinical trial results. Antibiotics are most effective in patients with purulent sputum and in those with a greater severity of illness (those with the three cardinal symptoms of increased cough, increased sputum volume, and increased dyspnea) and in those with more severe airflow obstruction at baseline. The choice of antibiotics should be based on local bacterial resistance patterns[3] and first-line drugs include macrolides, cephalosporins, doxycycline, and amoxicillin. For treatment failures and those who are hospitalized, other agents, such as fluoroquinolones and amoxicillin/clavulanate, are required. The use of antibiotics (macrolides) for prophylaxis in patients with frequent (three or more per year) exacerbations is effective[30] and further clinical trials are necessary to confirm the risks ands benefits. Mucolytic agents and expectorants have not proved useful in the prevention or treatment of exacerbations of chronic bronchitis.[27]

BRONCHIECTASIS

Bronchiectasis is another cough phlegm syndrome caused by chronic inflammation and infection of the airways. Like chronic bronchitis, bronchiectasis is associated with chronic cough, production of mucopurulent sputum, and, when there is extensive lung involvement, shortness of breath. Unlike chronic bronchitis, the inflammation and infection seen with bronchiectasis causes the bronchial walls to become damaged and dilated, and this results in permanent destruction of bronchi. The pathologic features include intense inflammation, thickening, and constrictions of the airway wall and resulting tortuosity, dilatation, ectasia, and eventual destruction of the distal bronchi and bronchioles. Earlier changes include squamous metaplasia, desquamation of the lining epithelium, and extensive areas of necrotizing ulceration. The mucus found in the airways contains large numbers of neutrophils, and metalloproteinases and collagenases released by these cells are thought to play an important role in the destructive process of bronchiectasis. As the disease progresses, fibrosis of bronchial or bronchiolar walls occurs and peribronchiolar fibrosis also develops, leading to varying degrees of subtotal or total obliteration of bronchiolar lumens. The bronchi may become so dilated (up to four times their size) that on cut surfaces of pathologic specimens they appear as cysts filled with mucopurulent secretions. Clearance of mucus and bacteria by normal mucociliary mechanisms from bronchiectatic areas is impaired and a vicious cycle of repeated or prolonged bronchial infections, suppuration, and destruction ensues. This is the cause of the cough phlegm syndrome, the chronic infection with frequent exacerbations, the progressive decline of lung function and quality of life, and, for some, eventual mortality.

Clinical Features of Bronchiectasis

The physical findings of bronchiectasis are nonspecific and may include localized or diffuse crackles or wheezes and coarse rhonchi caused by retained airway secretions. The routine chest roentgenogram may be unable to detect the abnormalities or may underestimate the degree of bronchiectasis. High-resolution CT scan (HRCT) has become the standard method of diagnosis. A common classification of bronchiectasis is based on the anatomic variations demonstrated by HRCT; the terms, *cylindrical, varicose*, and *cystic (saccular) bronchiectasis*, have been used to describe the extent of bronchial distortion and destruction (**Fig. 1**). More extensive involvement of the lungs and the presence of the cystic changes predict a much poorer prognosis. The natural history of this disease is usually associated with recurrent exacerbations of bronchial infection and decline of lung function. In later stages of the disease, progressive dyspnea, poor quality of life, cachexia, and cor pulmonale may occur and hemoptysis may complicate the course of the illness as a result of new and enlarged bronchial circulation to the areas of destroyed lung. In milder forms of the disease, patients may be relatively asymptomatic and may not demonstrate bacteria in their sputum, unless an acute infection (exacerbation) occurs. The organisms that usually infect patients with bronchiectasis are similar to those associated with chronic bronchitis: *H influenzae, M catarrhalis*, and *S pneumoniae*. Nonenteric gram-negative bacteria and *Staphylococcus aureus* are also commonly seen, however, and colonization and infection with *P aeruginosa* are frequently found in more advanced stages. Patients with *P aeruginosa* are more likely to have a more accelerated decline of lung function and more frequent exacerbations. Nontuberculous mycobacteria, *Nocardia*, and *Aspergillus* also may be cultured from the sputum of patients with bronchiectasis and their presence may represent airway colonization in a compromised airway or active infection. Anerobic bacteria are less frequently isolated from bronchiectatic airways.

Causes of Bronchiectasis

The causes and predisposing factors for bronchiectasis are usually categorized as (1) local bronchiectasis, caused by a local bronchial obstruction, poor airway clearance,

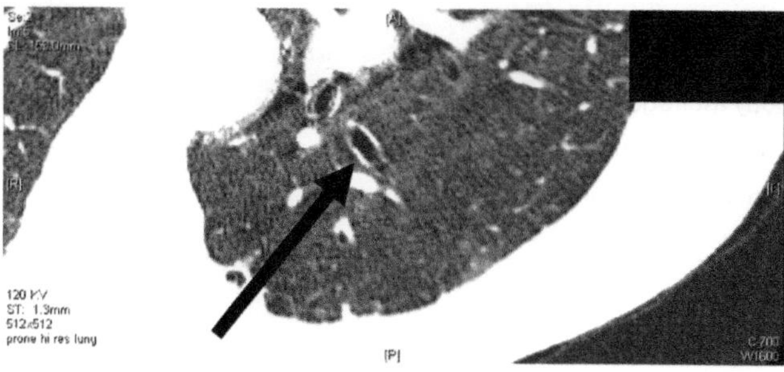

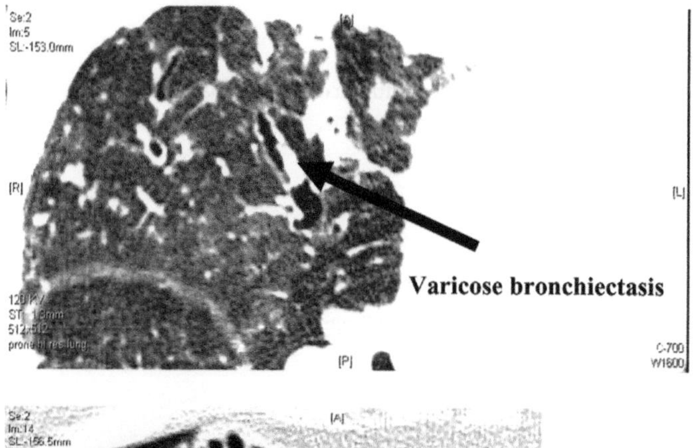

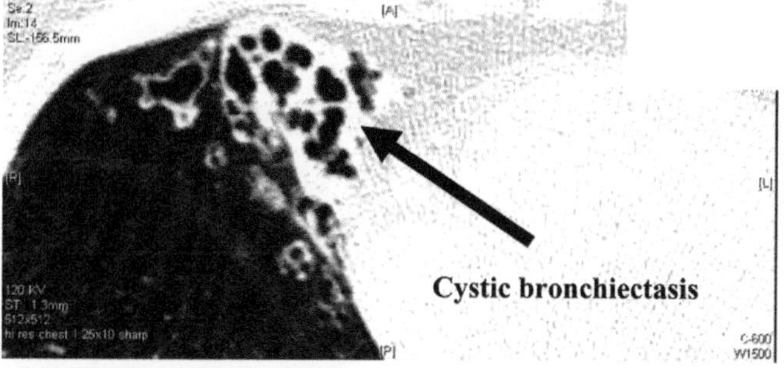

Fig. 1. HRCT classification of bronchiectasis: cylindrical bronchiectasis—thickening of the airway wall and airway enlargement (mild); varicose bronchiectasis—tortuosity of the airway with evidence of bronchial stricture and ectasia (more severe); and cystic bronchiectasis—lung destruction with thick walled cysts and peribronchial fibrosis (most severe).

and distal infection or by a primary local infection, such as pneumonia, that does not completely resolve, or (2) diffuse bronchiectasis, associated with a systemic disease or immune deficiency that causes diffuse airway abnormalities, which impair mucociliary clearance and lead to chronic infection and the cycle of wall distortion and destruction. These causes are listed in **Box 2**. A review of these causes with an overview of this topic has recently been published.[31]

Treatment of Bronchiectasis

The goals of therapy for bronchiectasis are to mobilize airway secretions, reduce inflammation, and treat and prevent infection. The ideal management of

Box 2
Conditions associated with diffuse and local bronchiectasis

Focal disease

Airway obstruction

- Foreign body aspiration
- Bronchial stricture (right middle lobe syndrome)
- Endobronchial mass (carcinoma, adenoma)

Postinfection

- Bacterial
- Viral
- Mycobacterial (tuberculosis and nontuberculous mycobacteria)

Diffuse disease

Postinfection

- Measles, pertussis
- Mycobacterial (tuberculosis and nontuberculous mycobacteria)

Congenital syndromes

- CF
- Primary ciliary dyskinesia
- Young's syndrome
- Tracheobronchomegaly
- Cartilage deficiency (Williams-Campbell syndrome)
- Marfan syndrome
- α_1-Antitrypsin deficiency
- Yellow nail syndrome

Immunodeficiency states

- Primary immunoglobulin deficiency (IgG, IgA)
- HIV/AIDS
- Chronic lymphatic leukemia
- Chemotherapy immune depression
- Immune modulation post transplantation

Immune-mediated diseases

- Allergic bronchopulmonary aspergillosis
- Rheumatoid arthritis
- Relapsing polychondritis
- Sjögren's syndrome
- Inflammatory bowel disease

Gastroesophageal reflux disease

Chronic aspiration

- Esophageal dysmotolity
- Dysphagia
- Chronic illicit drug abuse

Idiopathic

bronchiectasis has been offered in an evidenced-based review.[32] Bronchodilators, short- and long-acting, are commonly used because physiologic testing often shows airflow obstruction. Although this is reasonable, there are no randomized studies that show their benefit. The mucolytic drug, recombinant human DNase, has proved effective (improved lung function and reduced exacerbation rates) in bronchiectasis associated with cystic fibrosis (CF). This agent is not effective, however, in non-CF bronchiectasis. Dry powder mannitol and hypertonic saline inhalation show promise for therapy for bronchiectasis as both improve tracheobronchial clearance in a variety of conditions complicated by chronic productive cough. Long-term, randomized, controlled studies with these agents are needed to determine their usefulness in patients with non-CF bronchiectasis. Mechanical aides such as chest physiotherapy, postural drainage, airway oscillatory devices, high-frequency assisted airway clearance, and mechanically assisted cough have been advocated to assist patients in removing airway secretions. Although many patients report improvement with these modalities, their efficacy is not proved in non-CF bronchiectasis.

Inhaled corticosteroids have been used in patients with non-CF bronchiectasis and short-term studies (4 to 6 weeks) show little improvement of lung function and productive cough. A 1-year trial with inhaled fluticasone (500 μg twice a day) showed improvement in 24-hour sputum volume in the entire group of bronchiectasis patients studied, and in those with *P aurugenosa* infection, an improvement in 24-hour sputum volume and exacerbations frequency was seen.[33] There is insufficient data to recommend the routine use of inhaled corticosteroids in patients with bronchiectasis, however.[34] The potential risk of increased respiratory infections associated with the use of inhaled corticosteroids is a particular concern in this patient population. Other anti-inflammatory approaches, such as systemic corticosteroids and ibuprofen, also cannot be recommended, especially because of safety concerns with long-term use. Chronic macrolide therapy has shown benefit in patients with bronchiectasis, including reducing sputum volume, decreasing exacerbation rates, and improving lung function.[35,36] It is not clear whether or not the antimicrobial benefits or anti-inflammatory actions of macrolide therapy cause this improvement. The benefits of maintenance antibiotics, with macrolides or other antimicrobial agents, are uncertain and the overall benefits and long-term risks will have to be assessed in future studies before firm recommendations can be made. The role of inhaled antibiotics (tobramycin) has also been found effective for CF bronchiectasis, but trials in non-CF bronchiectasis with tobramycin, gentamycin, and colistin are less encouraging.[37–40] Future trials are needed to determine the risks and benefits of this therapy.

Patients with bronchiectasis may experience an exacerbation of symptoms similar to those seen with an exacerbation of chronic bronchitis. Because of the high bacterial load and high likelihood of highly virulent organisms, antibiotics are the mainstay of treatment for an exacerbation. The selection of an antibiotic depends on the organisms that may be infecting the patient. It has been recommended that sputum cultures be taken frequently and antibiotic sensitivity patterns monitored closely. In patients who have had recent antibiotic exposure, resistance to these antimicrobials should be suspected. Because of the heterogeneity of patients and the small number of therapeutic trials to guide antibiotic choices, care of the patient must be individualized.[31] Surgery might be considered for local disease that is highly symptomatic. Also, resection may become an urgent consideration for massive hemoptysis caused by bleeding from a bronchiectatic area of the lung.

BRONCHIOLITIS IN ADULTS

Bronchiolitis encompasses a spectrum of pathologic inflammatory processes that affect the small airways (2 mm or less in diameter), and cough is one of the common symptoms of this disorder. The inflammation can involve any cell line (eosinophils, lymphocytes, macrophages, and neutrophils) and can lead to variable degrees of injury to the bronchiolar epithelium. The resulting structural distortion can be reversible or irreversible (bronchiolectasis and fibrosis).[41] Bronchiolitis can be the only manifestation of various clinical syndromes or may be a part of a spectrum of histopathologic and radiographic findings that may also involve the large airways and lung parenchyma. The epidemiology of bronchiolitis has not been well established, although it seems generally uncommon. The spectrum of disorders causing bronchiolitis includes a variety of infections/postinfectious syndromes and inflammatory and idiopathic disorders.

Etiology of Bronchiolitis in Adults

Box 3 lists the common causes of bronchiolitis. Infectious and postinfectious clinical syndromes are common causes associated with bronchiolitis in adults. The interaction between acute infection, immune response, structural changes, and subsequent chronic colonization or chronic active infection of the small airways can lead to a variety of chronic symptoms, including a nonproductive or productive cough. Viral syndromes associated with bronchiolitis are more common in children. Specific causes include adenoviruses, respiratory syncytial virus, influenza, and parainfluenza viruses, among others. HIV can result in bronchiolitis, primarily related to the HIV infection or as a result of an inflammatory immune response. Secondary infections related to immune suppression can also cause bronchiolitis in HIV patients. Other immune-compromised patients, such as those receiving immune suppression after organ transplantation, patients with common variable immune deficiency, and patients on chemotherapy for malignancy, are at risk to develop viral bronchiolitis.

The clinical presentation of infectious bronchiolitis syndrome caused by *Mycoplasma pneumoniae* in adults is similar to the clinical presentation of pneumonia caused by this organism.[42] The role of chronic *M pneumoniae* infection in patients with chronic cough remains controversial.[43] Similarly, chronic cough due to infection

Box 3
An overview of the causes of bronchiolitis

Infections and postinfectious: bacterial and viral pathogens

Hypersensitivity pneumonitis: organic and nonorganic antigens

Inhalational injury: toxic and irritant gas or fumes inhalation, including smoking and occupational exposures

Systemic inflammatory disease: connective tissue disease

Medications

Organ transplantation: lung, heart-lung, and bone marrow

Inflammatory bowel disease

Idiopathic bronchiolitis: cryptogenic organizing pneumonia (COP), cryptogenic constrictive bronchiolitis, and diffuse panbronchiolitis (DPB)

Other causes: radiation injury, vasculitis, primary biliary cirrhosis, paraneoplastic syndromes, bronchiolitis associated with other interstitial lung disease (ILD), and large airway disease with *Chlamydia pneumoniae* as a result of chronic bronchiolitis or bronchitis has been suggested.[44,45] The evidence for such a chronic infection using serologic studies and cultures remains inconclusive. Typical and atypical mycobacterial infections can also cause bronchiolitis with or without bronchiectasis and may result in chronic cough. Bronchiolitis has also been associated with infections caused by the streptococcus, nocardia, legionella, and *Pneumocystis jirovecci* organisms. It is thought that the sequence of the initial acute infection, the postinfectious inflammatory response, and subsequent bacterial colonization may lead to chronic cough in patients with infectious bronchiolitis.

The inhalation of organic or nonorganic material can cause hypersensitivity pneumonitis and manifest as bronchiolitis, with or without involvement of the larger airways and lung parenchyma. More than 300 syndromes related to specific occupational and other environmental exposures are well described in the literature (eg, bird fancier's disease related to exposure to specific bird antigens). Direct injury of the small airways related to inhalation of toxins or aspiration can also lead to bronchiolitis. Respiratory bronchiolitis–ILD related to smoking and other irritants is an example of direct inhalational injury that can cause inflammatory bronchiolitis. Respiratory bronchiolitis–ILD likely begins with inflammation in the small airways and extends to the air spaces and interstitium. The inflammation can be chronic and associated with nonspecific symptoms, including cough. Bronchiolitis has also been associated with several systemic inflammatory diseases, including systemic lupus erythematosus, rheumatoid arthritis, Sjögren's syndrome, and dermatomyositis/polymyositis complex. It has also been reported to occur with primary biliary cirrhosis and paraneoplastic disorders. Some medications can cause bronchiolitis (eg, amiodarone, sulfasalazine, cephalosporins, and penicillamine).[46,47] Bronchiolitis obliterans with progressive airflow obstruction can be a manifestation of bone marrow, lung, and heart-lung transplantation with chronic dry or productive cough. Bronchiolitis can also be a manifestation of radiation injury, vasculitis, and interstitial lung disease.

Inflammatory bowel disease, including ulcerative colitis and Crohn's disease, can affect the central airways, small airways, and lung parenchyma with a pattern of inflammation similar to involvement of the large intestine. Toxicity related to medications used in the treatment of this disease and infection related to immune suppression can also involve the respiratory system.[48] The spectrum of pathology involving the small airways in patients with inflammatory bowel disease includes lymphocytic bronchiolitis and necrotizing and granulomatous bronchiolitis. Chronic cough and sputum production are common manifestations. The pulmonary symptoms seem to correlate with the activity of the disease in the large intestine and generally do not respond to surgical resection of the involved bowel. There is an inconsistent response to inhaled and systemic steroids, but a trial with these agents is reasonable.

Idiopathic bronchiolitis syndromes, including COP, cryptogenic constrictive bronchiolitis, and DPB are diagnosed in an appropriate clinical setting when there is no obvious underlying infectious or systemic inflammatory processes that are known to cause bronchiolitis. COP has predominant features of pneumonia with chronic relapsing symptoms, including persistent productive cough. This disorder is associated with proliferative bronchiolitis that involves the small airways, alveolar ducts, and alveolar spaces (see histopathologic features of bronchiolitis, discussed later). Cryptogenic constrictive bronchiolitis is associated with progressive airflow obstruction in the absence of an obvious cause, including inhalational injury or other predisposing factors. Although an occasional patient in the United States may have the condition, DPB is primarily found in Japan, Korea, and China. An interaction between genetic predisposition and environmental factors is probably instrumental in the development of this specific small airway disease. Treatment with macrolide antibiotics is associated with improved symptoms and survival in patients with this disease and is likely related to the anti-inflammatory effects of macrolides. Treatment of associated infections is important in all idiopathic small airway disorders.

The Histopathology of Bronchiolitis

Bronchiolitis can be associated with constriction of the small airways (constrictive bronchiolitis with or without complete obliteration of the lumen) or proliferation of fibrous tissue within the airway lumen (proliferative bronchiolitis). Other forms include follicular bronchiolitis with hyperplasia of the bronchus-associated lymphoid tissue, seen with connective tissue disorders and immune deficiency states, chronic bronchitis with fibrosis (airway-centered interstitial fibrosis), and DPB. Mixed patterns are common and there is considerable overlap seen with these syndromes.[49] Distinguishing between these different histopathologic patterns and the recognition of a predominant pattern, however, is important in determining prognosis and therapy. Proliferative patterns are generally more responsive to treatment and reversible when compared to constrictive bronchiolitis. Fortunately constrictive bronchiolitis is rare, as it is more progressive and less responsive to treatment. Thoracoscopic or open lung biopsy is the gold standard for obtaining adequate tissue and determining the pattern of inflammation of the bronchiolitis. Bronchoscopy with or without transbronchial biopsies is a reasonable initial step to rule out infection and may be adequate in the appropriate clinical setting. At times, pathologic confirmation may not be necessary, for example in patients with typical clinical presentation (eg, hypersensitivity pneumonitis with obvious exposure history) and typical radiographic findings.

Clinical, Radiographic, and Physiologic Evaluation of Bronchiolitis

Patients with bronchiolitis can present with different clinical syndromes that include productive or dry cough, dyspnea, night sweats, weight loss, fatigue, wheezing, and chest tightness. A comprehensive history that includes all past medical conditions, medications, occupational history, and potential environmental exposures is the cornerstone of the evaluating patients with bronchiolitis. Physical findings include wheezing, inspiratory crackles, and manifestations of systemic disorders, including skin, joints, and eye manifestations. Radiographic studies and physiologic evaluation by pulmonary function tests are the reasonable next steps in evaluating these patients.

A chest radiograph may demonstrate nonspecific hyperinflation, an interstitial pattern, air-space disease, or normal lung parenchyma. HRCT is the most sensitive test for evaluating patients with suspected bronchiolitis. Features of bronchiolitis on HRCT are variable. They include dilation of the small airways (bronchiolectasis), thickening of the airways (small and larger airways), bronchiectasis, ground glass attenuation, mosaic pattern on expiratory films suggestive of air trapping, centrilobular nodules, and tree-in-bud opacities (branching opacities).[50] Features associated with interstitial lung disease or other diseases can also be recognized on HRCT when bronchiolitis is associated with such conditions. Unfortunately, a normal HRCT scan does not completely rule out bronchiolitis as the resolution of the CT scan is limited to airways approximately 2 mm in diameter. In such instances it may be helpful to obtain inspiratory and expiratory films when considering bronchiolitis (especially constrictive bronchiolitis), as the appearance of the mosaic pattern on expiration can be a useful finding.

Lung function tests, including spirometry, lung volumes, and diffusion capacity, are helpful to further characterize the pattern of bronchiolitis and the severity of the disease and to follow the response to treatment. Constrictive bronchiolitis is generally associated with airflow obstruction, whereas proliferative bronchiolitis is usually associated with a restrictive pattern. Mixed patterns of restriction and obstruction are also possible and the diffusion capacity is generally impaired in both conditions. Lung function may be normal during the early stages of bronchiolitis. The difference between lung volumes obtained using body plethysmography (measuring the total thoracic gas content) and helium dilution techniques (measuring the volume of thoracic gas communicating with the mouth through the small and large airways) may help characterize the severity of obstruction and follow the response to treatment. The more the difference between the two techniques, the worse the degree of obstruction.

Management of Bronchiolitis

Prior to initiating specific treatment, physicians should secure a diagnosis of the clinical syndrome associated with bronchiolitis, taking into consideration the clinical presentation, radiographic studies, physiologic evaluation, potential bronchoscopy, and thoracoscopic (or open) lung biopsy. The histopathologic pattern of bronchiolitis and severity of the disease should be characterized. The treatment of bronchiolitis depends on the cause, underlying disorder, and severity. The focus of treatment should be on the underlying disease in patients with bronchiolitis secondary to known illness (eg, connective tissue disorders). Avoidance of exposures in patients with suspected bronchiolitis related to hypersensitivity pneumonitis or exposure to toxins/irritants is essential. Discontinuation of any medications suspected of causing bronchiolitis is also essential. Treatment with antimicrobial agents is the cornerstone of treatment of patients with suspected or confirmed infectious bronchiolitis. Patients may require prolonged courses of oral or intravenous antibiotics or other antimicrobial agents.

Systemic steroids are usually effective in proliferative bronchiolitis and cases related to hypersensitivity pneumonitis or toxic/irritant exposures with improvement in symptoms and reversibility of radiographic and pulmonary function abnormalities.[51] The response of constrictive bronchiolitis to systemic steroids is variable and generally less impressive with progressive disease and significant pulmonary limitations. Other immune-modifying agents, including azathioprine, cyclophosphamide, and anti–tumor necrosis factor α could be considered in patients not responding to systemic steroids. Augmentation of immune suppression is the treatment of choice for bronchiolitis associated with organ transplantation. Long-term treatment with macrolide antibiotics is effective in improving the symptoms and survival in patients with DPB due to the anti-inflammatory effects.[52] Low-dose long-term macrolide treatment could be considered for other patterns of bronchiolitis, especially constrictive bronchiolitis, as the response to steroids is generally poor, and in patients with proliferative bronchiolitis not responding to systemic steroids. Treatment with inhaled steroids could be considered in patients with mild disease. Inhaled bronchodilators and specific symptomatic treatment of cough are also reasonable.

REFERENCES

1. Gompertz S, O'Brien C, Bayley DL, et al. Changes in bronchial inflammation during acute exacerbations of chronic bronchitis. Eur Respir J 2001;17:1112–9.
2. Oswald N, Harold J, Martin W. Clinical pattern of chronic bronchitis. Lancet 1953; 265:639–43.
3. Celli BR, MacNee W, Agusti A, et al. Standards for the diagnosis and treatment of patients with COPD: a summary of the ATS/ERS position paper. Eur Respir J 2004;23:932–46.

4. Oswald N, Harold J, Martin W, et al. Mucin expression in peripheral airways of patients with chronic obstructive lung disease. Histopathology 2004;45:477–8.
5. Saetta M, Turato G, Baraldo S. Goblet cell hyperplasia and epithelial inflammation in peripheral airways of smokers with both symptoms of chronic bronchitis and chronic airflow limitation. Am J Respir Crit Care Med 2000;161:1016–21.
6. Aikawa T, Shimura S, Sasaki H, et al. Morphometric analysis of intraluminal mucus in airways in chronic obstructive pulmonary disease. Am Rev Respir Dis 1989; 140:477–82.
7. Sethi S. Bacterial infection and the pathogenesis of COPD. Chest 2000;117: 380S–5S.
8. Higgenbottam T. Chronic cough and the cough reflex in common lung diseases. Pulm Pharmacol Ther 2002;15:241–7.
9. Doherty M, Mister R, Pearson M, et al. Capsaicin responsiveness and cough in asthma and chronic obstructive pulmonary disease. Thorax 2000;55:643–9.
10. Houtmeters E, Gosselink R, Gayan-Ramirez G, et al. Regulation of mucociliary clearance in health and disease. Eur Respir J 1999;13:949–50.
11. Foster W. Mucociliary transport and cough in humans. Pulm Pharmacol Ther 2002;15:277–82.
12. Smaldone G, Foster W, O'Riordan T, et al. Regional impairment in mucociliary clearance in chronic obstructive pulmonary disease. Chest 1993;103:1390–6.
13. Foster W, Longenbach E, Bergofsky E. Disassociation of mucociliary function in central and peripheral airways in asymptomatic smokers. Am Rev Respir Dis 1985;132:633–7.
14. Celli BR, Barnes PJ. Exacerbations of chronic obstructive pulmonary disease. Eur Respir J 2007;29:1224–38.
15. Comstock GW, Brownlow WJ, Stone RW, et al. Cigarette smoking and changes in respiratory findings. Arch Environ Health 1970;21:50–7.
16. Brown CA, Crombie, Smith WC, et al. The impact of quitting smoking on symptoms of chronic bronchitis: results of the Scottish Heart Health Study. Thorax 1991;46:112–6.
17. Warner DO, Colligan RC, Hurt RD, et al. Cough following initiation of smoking abstinence. Nicotine Tob Res 2007;9:1207–12.
18. Pelkonen M, Notkola IL, Nissinen A, et al. Thirty year cumulative incidence of chronic bronchitis and COPD in relation to 30 year pulmonary function and 40 year mortality: a follow-up in middle-aged rural men. Chest 2006;130:1129–37.
19. Mannino DM, Reichert MM, Davis KJ. Lung function decline and outcomes in an adult population. Am J Respir Crit Care Med 2006;173:985–90.
20. Rodriguez-Roisin R. Toward a consensus definition for COPD exacerbations. Chest 2000;117:398S–401S.
21. Anthonisen NR, Manfreda J, Warren CP, et al. Antibiotic therapy in exacerbations of chronic obstructive pulmonary disease. Ann Intern Med 1987;106:196–204.
22. Varkey JB, Varkey B. Viral infections in patients with chronic obstructive pulmonary disease. Curr Opin Pulm Med 2008;14:89–94.
23. Seemungal T, Harper-Owen R, Bhowmik A, et al. Respiratory viruses, symptoms, and inflammatory markers in acute exacerbations and stable chronic obstructive pulmonary disease. Thorax 2002;57:759–64.
24. Sethi S, Evans N, Grant BJ, et al. New strains of bacteria and exacerbations of chronic obstructive pulmonary disease. N Engl J Med 2002;347:465–71.
25. Nseir S, Di Pompeo C, Cavestri B, et al. Multiple drug resistant bacteria in patients with acute severe exacerbation of chronic obstructive pulmonary disease: prevalence, risk factors and outcome. Crit Care Med 2006;34:2959–66.

26. Balter MS, La Forge J, Low DE, et al. Canadian guidelines for the acute exacerbation of chronic bronchitis. Can Respir J 2003;10(Suppl B):3B–32B.
27. Braman S. Chronic cough due to chronic bronchitis: ACCP evidence-based clinical practice guidelines. Chest 2006;129:104S–15S.
28. Niewoehner DE. The role of systemic corticosteroids in acute exacerbation of chronic obstructive pulmonary disease. Am J Respir Med 2002;1:243–8.
29. Calverley PM, Anderson JA, Celli B, et al. Salmeterol and fluticasone propionate and survival in chronic obstructive pulmonary disease. N Engl J Med 2007;356: 775–89.
30. Seemungal TA, Wilkinson TM, Hurst JR, et al. Long-term erythromycin therapy is associated with decreased chronic obstructive lung disease exacerbations. Am J Respir Crit Care Med 2008;178:1139–47.
31. O'Donnell AE. Bronchiectasis. Chest 2008;134:815–23.
32. Rosen M. Chronic cough due to bronchiectasis: ACCP evidence-based clinical practice guidelines. Chest 2006;129:122S–31S.
33. Tsang KW, Tan KC, Ho PL, et al. Inhaled fluticasone in bronchiectasis: a 12 month study. Thorax 2005;60:239–43.
34. Kapur N, Bell S, Kolbe J, et al. Inhaled steroids for bronchiectasis. Cochrane Database Syst Rev 2009;(1):CD000996.
35. Tsang KW, Ho PI, Chan KN, et al. A pilot study of low-dose erythromycin in bronchiectasis. Eur Respir J 1999;13:361–4.
36. Cymbala AA, Edmonds AC, Bauer MA, et al. The disease modifying effects of twice-weekly oral azithromycin in patients with bronchiectasis. Treat Respir Med 2005;4:117–22.
37. Barker KF, Couch L, Fiel SB, et al. Tobramycin solution for inhalation reduces sputum *Pseudomonas aeruginosa* density in bronchiectasis. Am J Respir Crit Care Med 2000;162:481–5.
38. Scheinberg P, Shore E. A pilot study of the safety and efficacy of tobramycin solution for inhalation in patients with severe bronchiectasis. Chest 2005;127: 1420–6.
39. Lin HC, Cheng HF, Wang CH, et al. Inhaled gentamicin reduces airway neutrophil activity and mucus secretion in bronchiectasis. Am J Respir Crit Care Med 1997; 155:2024–9.
40. Steinfort DP, Steinfort C. Effect of long-term nebulized colistin on lung function and quality of life in patients with chronic bronchial sepsis. Intern Med J 2007; 37:495–8.
41. Brown KK. Chronic cough due to nonbronchiectatic suppurative airway disease (bronchiolitis): ACCP evidence-based clinical practice guidelines. Chest 2006; 129(Suppl 1):132S–7S.
42. Cha SI, Shin KM, Kim M, et al. *Mycoplasma pneumoniae* bronchiolitis in adults: clinicoradiologic features and clinical course. Scand J Infect Dis 2009;3:1–5.
43. Birkebaek NH, Jensen JS, Seefeldt T, et al. *Chlamydia pneumoniae* infection in adults with chronic cough compared with healthy blood donors. Eur Respir J 2000;16(1):108–11.
44. Hammerschlag MR, Chirgwin K, Roblin PM, et al. Persistent infection with *Chlamydia pneumoniae* following acute respiratory illness. Clin Infect Dis 1992;14: 178–82.
45. Andersen P. Pathogenesis of lower respiratory tract infections due to *Chlamydia, Mycoplasma, Legionella* and viruses. Thorax 1998;53(4):302–7.
46. Ryu JH, Myers JL, Swensen SJ. Bronchiolar disorders. Am J Respir Crit Care Med 2003;168:1277–92.

47. Ryu JH. Classification and approach to bronchiolar diseases. Curr Opin Pulm Med 2006;12:145–51.
48. Camus P, Colby TV. The lung in inflammatory bowel disease. Eur Respir J 2000; 15:5–10.
49. Visscher DW, Myers JL. Bronchiolitis: the pathologist's perspective. Proc Am Thorac Soc 2006;3(1):41–7.
50. Pipavath SJ, Lynch DA, Cool C, et al. Radiologic and pathologic features of bronchiolitis. AJR Am J Roentgenol 2005;185:354.
51. King TE Jr. Bronchiolitis. Clin Chest Med 1993;14:607.
52. Nagai H, Shishido H, Yoneda R, et al. Long-term low dose administration of erythromycin to patients with diffuse panbronchiolitis. Respiration 1991;58:145.

Pharmacologic Management of Cough

Donald C. Bolser, PhD

KEYWORDS

• Cough • Antitussive • Cough suppressant • Dystussia
• Atussia • Dysphagia

This review provides an update on advances in the pharmacology of coughing and antitussives. There are a number of informative reviews on recent work in the area of antitussives.[1–7] These reviews note the limited amount of new information that has become available on the effects of these drugs in humans in the last several years. Furthermore, in double-blind placebo controlled trials in humans with chronic or acute cough, no new drugs been shown to be effective as antitussive agents.[2–6] This review focuses on some new information on antitussives. The review is expanded to include the potential therapeutic impact of enhancement of cough in patients who suffer from dystussia,[8] or impaired cough.

ANTITUSSIVES

My previous review,[9] as well as an earlier one by other investigators,[10] noted that, in recent studies, commonly prescribed antitussives, such as codeine and dextromethorphan, had limited or no efficacy relative to placebo in humans with chronic cough. As such, these drugs were not recommended for suppression of cough. Since that time, a comprehensive study of the effect of codeine on chronic cough in patients with chronic obstructive pulmonary disease (COPD) has been published.[11] This report confirmed a lack of efficacy of codeine to suppress cough in this patient group. However, Morice and coworkers[12] have shown a 40% decrease in cough scores in patients treated with an oral formulation of a low (5 mg) dose of morphine. This dosing regime was well tolerated by their patients. Doubling this dose of morphine resulted in a higher frequency of side effects, such as sedation. The use of morphine as an antitussive is likely to be limited by widespread caution regarding the side effect liability of the drug,[5] regardless of how well tolerated this opioid is in any particular study.

This work was supported by R33 HL089104 from the National Institutes of Health.
Department of Physiological Sciences, College of Veterinary Medicine, University of Florida, Gainesville, FL 32610-0144, USA
E-mail address: bolser@vetmed.ufl.edu

Otolaryngol Clin N Am 43 (2010) 147–155
doi:10.1016/j.otc.2009.11.008 oto.theclinics.com
0030-6665/10/$ – see front matter

The results of this study raise three additional important points:

1. It is possible to observe significant antitussive effects of an orally active opioid in humans with chronic cough. The lack of efficacy of codeine (up to 60 mg by mouth) in recent studies[11,13] may be related to specific issues with the molecule itself rather than to μ-opioid agonists in general. Indeed, the cough suppressant effects of codeine are not blocked by naloxone in the cat,[14] suggesting that this drug has actions at nonopioid receptors.
2. Although Morice and colleagues[12] showed activity of morphine to suppress cough scores in humans with chronic cough, the drug did not alter the sensitivity of these patients to an inhaled irritant (citric acid). Another study[15] with dextromethorphan in smokers showed significant effects of this drug relative to placebo on cough sensitivity to inhaled citric acid, but there was no difference between active and placebo groups for subjective measures of coughing. These findings call to question the relevance of irritant aerosol challenge in the evaluation of the activity of putative cough suppressants in humans.
3. Antitussive drugs rarely prevent humans from coughing with an antitussive drug. This point should be considered in light of the widely held misconception that new cough suppressants should not be developed because they will eliminate the ability to protect the airway with the cough reflex.

Recent cough research should expand our knowledge of the genesis of this airway protective behavior in humans. Several recent studies have focused in particular on the effects of antitussives on sensory, motor, and mechanical aspects of cough. The production of cough can be associated with significant sensations, termed *urge to cough*.[13,16] In dose-response studies with inhaled irritants,[13] these sensations occur in advance of the actual behavior and directly increase in intensity with the number of coughs and dose of irritant. Cough (and presumably the urge to cough) can be suppressed voluntarily,[17,18] suggesting that there are endogenous neurochemicals in the human that can mediate this effect. Eccles and coworkers[17] showed that voluntary cough suppression is not opioid-mediated in humans. The presence of these sensations associated with the production of coughing indicates that this behavior is not simply an involuntary reflex phenomenon involving only brainstem mechanisms in the human. To be sure, vigorous chronic cough cannot be eliminated solely through voluntary means. However, pharmacologic approaches that address sensory issues involved in the production of cough may yield novel cough suppressants. This argument is subject to the caveat that no information yet exists that demonstrates suppression by antitussives of the urge to cough in humans with chronic cough. In normal subjects, codeine (30 and 60 mg) did not alter cough sensitivity, electromyograms of abdominal muscles, airflows, or sensations associated with capsaicin-induced cough.[13] The role of urge to cough in the action of antitussive drugs in humans awaits specific studies that use effective cough suppressants.

In smokers, nicotine has been thought to have a cough-promoting effect through its excitatory effects on pulmonary afferents.[19–21] However, recent findings in smokers suggest that nicotine actually has a cough-suppressant effect.[22] Smokers who refrained from smoking for 12 hours had greater levels of anxiety and higher cough responses and urge-to-cough ratings in response to inhalation of capsaicin than those in age-matched nonsmokers. When the smokers were administered nicotine gum during abstinence from smoking, anxiety levels, cough responses, and urge-to-cough ratings were not different from those in the placebo or the nonsmoking group.[22] The investigators concluded that nicotine modulated the central neural state of the smokers, which reduced anxiety, sensations, and cough responses. Regardless of mechanism, nicotine replacement normalized an elevated cough response and acted as a cough suppressant.[22] These results are consistent with other findings showing that spontaneous coughing increases in the subacute period following cessation of smoking.[23] This putative cough suppressant effect of nicotine may account for the ability of smokers to inhale cigarette smoke repeatedly each day without violent coughing. Nicotine penetrates the nervous system readily and the probability of a central action of this drug on the cough reflex in these subjects must be considered high.

In my previous review of this topic,[9] I concluded that mucolytic agents were not recommended to suppress cough in patients with chronic bronchitis. These drugs may have other benefits, such as increased cough clearance and improvement of other symptoms. I further recommended only one anticholinergic agent, ipratropium bromide, for cough suppression.[9] Although new information related to some of these recommendations has appeared in the last several years, it does not appear that sufficient evidence has accumulated to warrant a change in these recommendations. New information has been published on several drugs with mucolytic or anticholinergic activity that have an antitussive effect in patients groups with chronic or acute cough.

N-acetylcysteine was administered in a double-blind clinical trial to patients who had been exposed to sulfur-mustard gas.[24] This drug significantly improved cough, dyspnea, and several components of pulmonary function in these patients. Both the treatment and placebo groups received fluticasone and salmeterol, raising the possibility that N-acetylcysteine had a synergistic effect with these drugs. The investigators suggested that the antioxidant effects of this drug were responsible for its therapeutic effects.[24]

Another antioxidant agent and putative mucolytic agent, erdosteine, when combined with amoxicillin, has recently been shown to be significantly more effective in reducing cough in children with acute lower respiratory illness than this antibiotic and placebo.[25] This was a randomized double-blinded and placebo-controlled study and the combination of erdosteine and amoxicillin reduced visual analog scores for cough by approximately 90% compared with 76% for amoxicillin plus placebo.[25] Note the large placebo effect, which is typical for studies in which cough is an end point. Erdosteine also significantly decreased interleukin 8 (IL-8) in sputum of current smokers with COPD,[26] which is consistent with an anti-inflammatory effect.

These observations are consistent with the potential use of these drugs in combination therapies for the relief of cough in selected patient populations. Mucolytic drugs have not been effective as antitussive agents when used as monotherapies.[9] The extent to which these drugs will be useful for the suppression of cough on a widespread basis is unknown and awaits larger scale clinical trials.

A small-scale double-blind placebo-controlled study was conducted on the effect of the anticholinergic agent tiotropium on cough due to acute upper airway viral infection.[27] Tiotropium significantly inhibited cough sensitivity to capsaicin after the first dose and out to 7 days relative to placebo.[27] The treatment group also had significantly improved spirometry, but this effect was not correlated with cough sensitivity changes, suggesting that bronchodilatation was not responsible for the effect on cough sensitivity. The cough-suppressant activity of tiotropium in this study contrasts with the findings of Casaburi and colleagues,[28] who showed no effect of this drug on cough in patients with COPD. As noted above, Morice and colleagues[12] showed that cough due to inhaled irritants is not an accurate predictor of the activity of antitussive drugs in patients with airway disease. The extent to which tiotropium will suppress spontaneous coughing in patients with acute upper airway viral illness is unknown (**Table 1**).

Table 1
Influence of selected agents on cough

Drug	Mechanism	Outcome
Codeine	Opioid	No effect on cough due to COPD
Morphine	Opioid	40% decrease in cough in patients with chronic cough refractory to specific therapy; well tolerated but long-term use potentially limited by side effects
Dextromethorphan	Nonopioid	Slight but significant decrease in cough due to upper airway disorders; no effect on smoker's cough
N-acetylcysteine	Possible antioxidant effect	Significant cough alleviation in patients with chemical injury to lungs
Erdosteine	Possible antioxidant effect	Potentiates cough suppressant effect of antibiotics during airway infection
Tiotropium	Unknown	Decreased capsaicin sensitivity; no effect on cough due to COPD

Enhancement of Cough

Awareness of the significance of dystussia is increasing. While chronic cough is associated with significant morbidity and quality-of-life issues,[6] dystussia is life threatening.[29,30] Dystussia and atussia[8] represent a breakdown in endogenous mechanisms for airway protection. Airway protection, which is the prevention and/or correction of aspiration (**Table 2**), is accomplished through the expression of a constellation of different behaviors, which include coughing, swallowing, expiration reflex, laryngeal adduction, and apnea. During the pharyngeal phase of swallowing, aspiration is prevented by closure of the vocal folds, changes in breathing, elevation of the larynx, and movement of the epiglottis to protect the laryngeal orifice.[31] In awake humans, swallowing preferentially occurs during the expiratory phase of breathing, usually resulting in a prolonged expiration and resetting of the breathing cycle.[32] The expiration reflex prevents aspiration by changing breathing pattern and producing a ballisticlike expiratory airflow to "blow" adherent material away from the vocal folds.[33] If aspiration occurs, coughing corrects this problem by producing high-velocity airflows that create shear forces to dislodge and eject material from the airway.[34]

In neurologic disease, airway protective mechanisms are frequently impaired, leading to increased risk of pulmonary infection. In patients with acute stroke or Parkinson disease, those with dysphagia and aspiration also have profound dystussia.[8,35] Furthermore, the risk of aspiration due to dysphagia can be predicted by several

Table 2
Important terms in airway protection

Term	Definition
Airway protection	Prevention and/or correction of aspiration
Dystussia	Impaired cough
Atussia	Inability to cough
Silent aspiration	Aspiration with atussia

mechanical features of voluntary cough in stroke patients.[29,30] These impairments of swallowing and coughing contribute to a high risk of aspiration,[29] which "seeds" the subglottic airways with pathogen-laden material,[36] resulting in a high prevalence of aspiration pneumonia. Mortality rates of aspiration pneumonia can approach 40%.[29] High rates of aspiration also occur in patients following anterior cervical spinal surgery (over 40%), in elderly patients in long-term care facilities, those with gastrointestinal problems, and those with other neurologic disorders, such as Parkinson disease.[29] Relationships have been objectively quantified between disordered swallowing and dystussia in patients with Parkinson disease.[37]

Aspiration can occur with atussia and is termed *silent aspiration*.[29] Patients with silent aspiration have a 13-fold increased risk of developing pneumonia.[38] By definition, patients with atussia and dysphagia have a high risk of developing pneumonia and this group exemplifies the consequences of impaired airway protection.

Atussia can occur with normal swallowing in patients with cervical spinal injuries, leading to the development of pulmonary complications.[39] Pneumonia is one of the leading causes of death in this patient group.[39] Although intubation and mechanical ventilation represent strong contributors to the risk of pulmonary infection in patients with cervical spinal injuries, it is widely accepted that impaired cough is a significant risk factor.[39]

As many as 30% of healthy elderly subjects may aspirate at least once during a sequential swallowing paradigm, indicating that aspiration can occur even in the absence of pathology.[40] Spontaneous coughing in normal subjects may well be a response to these minor aspiration events.

Detection of Dystussia and Atussia

Assessment of disordered cough is usually performed in context with an effort to predict competency of airway protective mechanisms in patients with neurologic disease. These assessments are most frequently based on subjective measures, such as cough sounds with or without a water-drinking challenge, and/or appearance of cough strength or quality during either voluntary or induced cough maneuvers.[30,41] These bedside tests can have highly variable sensitivities and specificities when compared with videofluoroscopy in predicting risk of aspiration.[30,42] Cough sounds in particular may have some utility in differentiating between patient groups with chronic cough and/or suppression of this behavior by antitussive drugs.[43,44] However, this approach is only useful in concert with advanced objective analytic methodologies, which can include computational analysis.[43,44] Subjective assessments represent an effort to simplify the measurement of a complex and multiphasic motor act produced by coordinated activation of a host of upper-airway and chest-wall muscles.[34] Atussia in response to cough-promoting stimuli probably lends itself to precise measurement by subjective observation. However, approaches that validate subjective assessments of dystussia by comparison to objective measures of cough mechanics are most likely to yield tests that have high sensitivities and specificities. Objective measures of cough mechanics have been shown to have high sensitivity and specificity in predicting risk of aspiration in patients with neurologic disease.[30,35]

Voluntary cough can only be used in patients who are awake and capable of following verbal commands. Previous reports that have objectively analyzed voluntary cough in patients with neurologic disease have employed instrumentation that acquired, filtered, and recorded cough airflow signals with high fidelity.[30,35,37,45] Although these recordings can be made at bedside, the instrumentation can be expensive. Presumably, less expensive handheld spirometers can be employed to acquire and process these signals, but this assumption has yet to be validated.

Features of the cough airflow waveform that have been shown to be most useful in the evaluation of dystussia are peak expiratory airflow, expulsive flow rise-time, and cough volume acceleration, which is the product of peak expiratory airflow and expulsive flow rise-time.[30,35,37] The duration of the compression phase may a be useful measure of dystussia in some patient groups,[37,45] but not in others.[35] The duration of the compression phase during cough is difficult to measure by subjective observation, which highlights the importance of objective measurements of cough airflows in patients in which dystussia is suspected. Other methods for eliciting cough, such as challenge with irritant aerosols,[46] may also have significant value in identifying patients at risk of aspiration. As with voluntary cough, the ultimate value of this method will become clearer as we learn more about the predictive nature of objective and subjective measures of coughing in patients at risk of aspiration.

Treatment

There are currently no Food and Drug Administration–approved pharmacologic treatments for enhancement of coughing in patients with dystussia or atussia. Most therapeutic strategies are centered on physical therapy techniques. In patients with spinal injuries, external movement of the chest wall and/or abdomen to increase expiratory airflows has been employed with limited efficacy.[47] Electrical stimulation of expiratory muscles has not been very effective, although recent trials of intrathecal electrical stimulation have proven effective in restoring expiratory airflow sufficient to simulate coughing.[48,49] As this is an invasive method, it is likely to be most appropriate for tetraplegic patients.

Other nonpharmacological approaches may have promise in restoring impaired cough. In patients with Parkinson disease who have dysphagia and dystussia, expiratory muscle strength training has proven effective in improving peak expiratory airflows and rise-times during voluntary cough.[45] In patients with dysphagia, it is common to employ behavioral methodologies to improve swallow function, and these approaches can have significant therapeutic effects.[29] It is unknown if these methods also can improve coughing, which would represent a "cross-behavioral" therapeutic effect.

It is well known that coughing can be elicited by inhalation of irritant chemicals, such as acidic solutions and capsaicin, as well as of nebulized distilled water.[50] The production of cough in response to inhalation of an acidic aerosol has been used to assess risk of pneumonia in patients with acute stroke.[46] In this study, cough was assessed by subjective measures. Sixteen percent of the patients with abnormal cough exhibited atussia in response to inhalation of acidic solutions.[46] However, Yamanda and colleagues[51] showed that elderly patients with a history of aspiration pneumonia have a reduced cough sensitivity to inhaled citric acid. Furthermore, these investigators showed that the urge to cough of these patients was reduced at low-dosage ranges of citric acid.[51] Although this study was conducted in a small number of patients, it does raise the possibility that both sensory and motor components of coughing may be impaired for months after aspiration pneumonia. The extent to which inhalation of irritant chemicals could be used as a therapeutic modality to enhance cough in patients with dystussia and/or atussia is unknown. Presumably, these widely used tests for cough sensitivity could be employed repeatedly in patient groups at risk of aspiration and dystussia to enhance sensory feedback specific to airway protection. This approach would be analogous to "forced use" of paretic limbs in rehabilitation strategies for stroke patients.[52] Alternatively, responsive patients with dystussia could be challenged with inhaled irritants at standard intervals to promote coughing.

SUMMARY

Low-dose oral morphine can inhibit chronic cough, but the use of this opioid as an antitussive agent may be limited by its side effect profile. Several studies have questioned the value of inhaled irritants in understanding pathologic cough and its response to antitussives. A new measure of coughing, urge to cough, has recently been identified and may become useful in understanding the mechanisms of cough production and suppression in the awake human. In selected patient populations, some proposed mucolytic drugs may be useful as adjunct therapies to suppress cough.

Dystussia is the impairment of cough and represents a life-threatening problem in patients with neurologic disease. There is a strong association between dystussia and dysphagia, and patients with both have a high risk for aspiration. There is a significant unmet need for more information regarding the diagnosis and treatment of dystussia and the mechanisms that underlie this breakdown in airway protection in patients with neurologic diseases.

ACKNOWLEDGMENTS

I thank Teresa Pitts for her valuable feedback on the manuscript.

REFERENCES

1. Canning BJ. Central regulation of the cough reflex: therapeutic implications. Pulm Pharmacol Ther 2009;22(2):75–81.
2. Dicpinigaitis PV. Currently available antitussives. Pulm Pharmacol Ther 2009; 22(2):148–51.
3. Chung KF. Chronic cough: future directions in chronic cough: mechanisms and antitussives. Chron Respir Dis 2007;4(3):159–65.
4. Chung KF. Effective antitussives for the cough patient: an unmet need. Pulm Pharmacol Ther 2007;20(4):438–45.
5. Chung KF. Currently available cough suppressants for chronic cough. Lung 2008; 186(Suppl 1):S82–7.
6. Chung KF. Clinical cough VI: the need for new therapies for cough: disease-specific and symptom-related antitussives. Handb Exp Pharmacol 2009;187: 343–68.
7. Pavord ID, Chung KF. Management of chronic cough. Lancet 2008;371(9621): 1375–84.
8. Chung KF, Bolser D, Davenport P, et al. Semantics and types of cough. Pulm Pharmacol Ther 2009;22(2):139–42.
9. Bolser DC. Cough suppressant and pharmacologic protussive therapy: ACCP evidence-based clinical practice guidelines. Chest 2006;129(1 Suppl): 238S–49S.
10. Irwin RS, Boulet LP, Cloutier MM, et al. Managing cough as a defense mechanism and as a symptom. A consensus panel report of the American College of Chest Physicians. Chest 1998;114(2 Suppl Managing):133S–81S.
11. Smith J, Owen E, Earis J, et al. Effect of codeine on objective measurement of cough in chronic obstructive pulmonary disease. J Allergy Clin Immunol 2006; 117(4):831–5.
12. Morice AH, Menon MS, Mulrennan SA, et al. Opiate therapy in chronic cough. Am J Respir Crit Care Med 2007;175(4):312–5.

13. Davenport PW, Bolser DC, Vickroy T, et al. The effect of codeine on the urge-to-cough response to inhaled capsaicin. Pulm Pharmacol Ther 2007;20(4):338–46.
14. Chau TT, Carter FE, Harris LS. Antitussive effect of the optical isomers of mu, kappa and sigma opiate agonists/antagonists in the cat. J Pharmacol Exp Ther 1983;226(1):108–13.
15. Ramsay J, Wright C, Thompson R, et al. Assessment of antitussive efficacy of dextromethorphan in smoking related cough: objective vs. subjective measures. Br J Clin Pharmacol 2008;65(5):737–41.
16. Davenport PW. Clinical cough I: the urge-to-cough: a respiratory sensation. Handb Exp Pharmacol 2009;187:263–76.
17. Hutchings HA, Eccles R. The opioid agonist codeine and antagonist naltrexone do not affect voluntary suppression of capsaicin induced cough in healthy subjects. Eur Respir J 1994;7(4):715–9.
18. Hutchings HA, Eccles R, Smith AP, et al. Voluntary cough suppression as an indication of symptom severity in upper respiratory tract infections. Eur Respir J 1993;6(10):1449–54.
19. Karlsson JA, Zackrisson C, Lundberg JM. Hyperresponsiveness to tussive stimuli in cigarette smoke-exposed guinea-pigs: a role for capsaicin-sensitive, calcitonin gene-related peptide-containing nerves. Acta Physiol Scand 1991;141(4):445–54.
20. Kou YR, Frazier DT, Lee LY. The stimulatory effect of nicotine on vagal pulmonary C-fibers in dogs. Respir Physiol 1989;76(3):347–56.
21. Lee LY, Gu Q. Cough sensors. IV. Nicotinic membrane receptors on cough sensors. Handb Exp Pharmacol 2009;187:77–98.
22. Davenport PW, Vovk A, Duke RK, et al. The urge-to-cough and cough motor response modulation by the central effects of nicotine. Pulm Pharmacol Ther 2009;22(2):82–9.
23. Cummings KM, Giovino G, Jaen CR, et al. Reports of smoking withdrawal symptoms over a 21 day period of abstinence. Addict Behav 1985;10(4):373–81.
24. Ghanei M, Shohrati M, Jafari M, et al. N-acetylcysteine improves the clinical conditions of mustard gas-exposed patients with normal pulmonary function test. Basic Clin Pharmacol Toxicol 2008;103(5):428–32.
25. Balli F, Bergamini B, Calistru P, et al. Clinical effects of erdosteine in the treatment of acute respiratory tract diseases in children. Int J Clin Pharmacol Ther 2007;45(1):16–22.
26. Dal Negro RW, Visconti M, Micheletto C, et al. Changes in blood ROS, e-NO, and some pro-inflammatory mediators in bronchial secretions following erdosteine or placebo: a controlled study in current smokers with mild COPD. Pulm Pharmacol Ther 2008;21(2):304–8.
27. Dicpinigaitis PV, Spinner L, Santhyadka G, et al. Effect of tiotropium on cough reflex sensitivity in acute viral cough. Lung 2008;186(6):369–74.
28. Casaburi R, Briggs DD, Donohue JF, et al. The spirometric efficacy of once-daily dosing with tiotropium in stable COPD. Chest 2000;118:1294–302.
29. Smith Hammond CA, Goldstein LB. Cough and aspiration of food and liquids due to oral-pharyngeal dysphagia: ACCP evidence-based clinical practice guidelines. Chest 2006;129(1 Suppl):154S–68S.
30. Smith Hammond CA, Goldstein LB, Horner RD, et al. Predicting aspiration in patients with ischemic stroke: comparison of clinical signs and aerodynamic measures of voluntary cough. Chest 2009;135(3):769–77.
31. Logemann JA. Swallowing physiology and pathophysiology. Otolaryngol Clin North Am 1988;21(4):613–23.

32. Paydarfar D, Gilbert RJ, Poppel CS, et al. Respiratory phase resetting and airflow changes induced by swallowing in humans. J Physiol 1995;483(Pt 1):273–88.
33. Korpas J, Tomori Z. Cough and other respiratory reflexes. Basel; New York: S. Karger; 1979.
34. Leith DE, Butler JP, Sneddon SL, et al. Cough. Handbook of physiology. The respiratory system, V. III. Mechanics of breathing, part I. Bethesda (MD): American Physiological Society; 1986. p. 315–36.
35. Smith Hammond CA, Goldstein LB, Zajac DJ, et al. Assessment of aspiration risk in stroke patients with quantification of voluntary cough. Neurology 2001;56(4):502–6.
36. Scannapieco FA. Role of oral bacteria in respiratory infection. J Periodontol 1999; 70(7):793–802.
37. Pitts T, Bolser D, Rosenbek J, et al. Voluntary cough production and swallow dysfunction in Parkinson's disease. Dysphagia 2008;23(3):297–301.
38. Pikus L, Levine MS, Yang YX, et al. Videofluoroscopic studies of swallowing dysfunction and the relative risk of pneumonia. AJR Am J Roentgenol 2003;180(6):1613–6.
39. Schilero GJ, Spungen AM, Bauman WA, et al. Pulmonary function and spinal cord injury. Respir Physiol Neurobiol 2009;166(3):129–41.
40. Butler SG, Stuart A, Markley L, et al. Penetration and aspiration in healthy older adults as assessed during endoscopic evaluation of swallowing. Ann Otol Rhinol Laryngol 2009;118(3):190–8.
41. Smith Hammond C. Cough and aspiration of food and liquids due to oral pharyngeal dysphagia. Lung 2008;186(Suppl 1):S35–40.
42. Ramsey DJ, Smithard DG, Kalra L. Early assessments of dysphagia and aspiration risk in acute stroke patients. Stroke 2003;34(5):1252–7.
43. Pavesi L, Subburaj S, Porter-Shaw K. Application and validation of a computerized cough acquisition system for objective monitoring of acute cough: a meta-analysis. Chest 2001;120(4):1121–8.
44. Piirila P, Sovijarvi AR. Differences in acoustic and dynamic characteristics of spontaneous cough in pulmonary diseases. Chest 1989;96(1):46–53.
45. Pitts T, Bolser D, Rosenbek J, et al. Impact of expiratory muscle strength training on voluntary cough and swallow function in Parkinson disease. Chest 2009; 135(5):1301–8.
46. Addington WR, Stephens RE, Widdicombe JG, et al. Effect of stroke location on the laryngeal cough reflex and pneumonia risk. Cough 2005;1:4.
47. Jaeger RJ, Turba RM, Yarkony GM, et al. Cough in spinal cord injured patients: comparison of three methods to produce cough. Arch Phys Med Rehabil 1993; 74(12):1358–61.
48. DiMarco AF, Kowalski KE, Geertman RT, et al. Lower thoracic spinal cord stimulation to restore cough in patients with spinal cord injury: results of a National Institutes of Health–sponsored clinical trial. Part I: methodology and effectiveness of expiratory muscle activation. Arch Phys Med Rehabil 2009;90(5):717–25.
49. DiMarco AF, Kowalski KE, Geertman RT, et al. Lower thoracic spinal cord stimulation to restore cough in patients with spinal cord injury: results of a National Institutes of Health–sponsored clinical trial. Part II: clinical outcomes. Arch Phys Med Rehabil 2009;90(5):726–32.
50. Dicpinigaitis PV. Experimentally induced cough. Pulm Pharmacol Ther 2007; 20(4):319–24.
51. Yamanda S, Ebihara S, Ebihara T, et al. Impaired urge-to-cough in elderly patients with aspiration pneumonia. Cough 2008;4:11.
52. Nudo RJ, Friel KM. Cortical plasticity after stroke: implications for rehabilitation. Rev Neurol (Paris) 1999;155(9):713–7.

Assessing Efficacy of Therapy for Cough

Jaclyn A. Smith, MRCP, PhD

KEYWORDS

- Cough counts • Cough reflex • Acoustics • Clinical trials
- Quality of life

Cough consistently is reported to be the most common symptom for which patients seek medical advice[1,2] and it has substantial impacts on quality of life for sufferers.[1] As a consequence, cough represents a significant financial burden; for example, in the United Kingdom, over £100 million/year is spent on over-the-counter antitussives[2] (of questionable efficacy), and the cost to the national economy is estimated at £1 billion annually due to absenteeism from work, reduced productivity, physician consultations, and prescription costs.[3] Despite these facts, safe, effective, and acceptable antitussive agents are lacking. Although this may result partly from poor research investment in understanding of the mechanisms underlying cough and hence the identification of novel treatment targets, the lack of well-validated tools for the accurate measurement of cough in clinical trials also may have impeded progress.

The aim of any effective ant-tussive agent should be to reduce the amount of coughing experienced by the patient sufficiently for the patient to appreciate an improvement in cough severity, and regard the magnitude of the improvement as sufficient to outweigh any adverse effects or risks associated with the treatment. A recent focus group study provided some useful insights into how patients with chronic cough perceive the severity of this symptom.[4] The study concluded that the three main dimensions of cough severity were: frequency of coughing, intensity or physical discomfort associated with coughing, and disruption caused by coughing (**Fig. 1**).

Dr Smith is funded by an MRC Clinician Scientist Award. She has received remuneration for advice, and the department also has received financial support from GlaxoSmithKline, Pfizer, Schering Plough, Procter & Gamble, Vectura, and Sound Biotech. Her department additionally has received funding to support studies from the Moulton Charitable Trust and a Manchester University Stepping Stones Award.
JAS is an inventor on a patent describing a novel method for cough detection, filed by the University Hospital of South Manchester and licensed to Vitalograph Limited, United Kingdom. JAS has an industrial collaboration with Vitalograph Limited, United Kingdom to develop a commercial cough monitoring system.
Respiratory Research Group, University of Manchester, 2nd Floor Education and Research Centre, University Hospital of South Manchester, Southmoor Road, Manchester, M23 9LT, UK
E-mail address: jacky.smith@manchester.ac.uk

Otolaryngol Clin N Am 43 (2010) 157–166
doi:10.1016/j.otc.2009.11.014 oto.theclinics.com
0030-6665/10/$ – see front matter

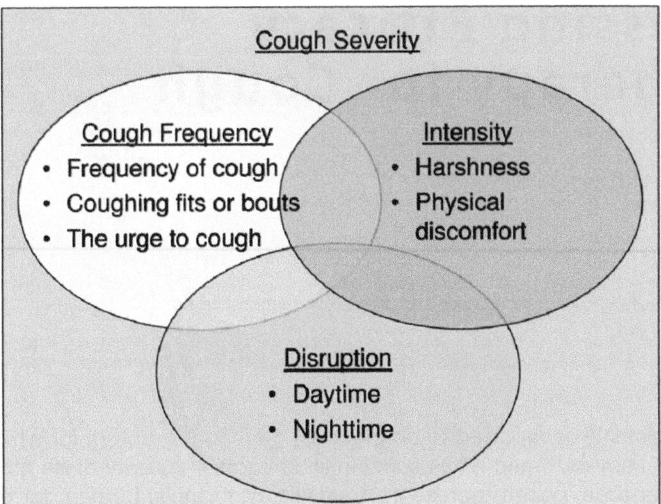

Fig. 1. Dimensions of the severity of chronic cough from the perspective of patients. (*Adapted From* Vernon M, Leidy NK, Nacson A, et al. Measuring cough severity: perspectives from the literature and from patients with chronic cough. Cough 2009;5:7; with permission.)

The most sensitive tools for capturing the efficacy of therapies for cough are likely to be those that are able to encapsulate these aspects of cough. In recent years, considerable progress has been made in the understanding of how best to measure cough, including the development of novel tools for the objective assessment of cough frequency and the assessment of the disruption and physical discomfort caused by coughing using cough-specific quality-of-life instruments. This article summarizes the current knowledge about methodologies for assessing cough therapies, the patient groups to study, and the design of clinical trials.

SUBJECTIVE ASSESSMENTS OF COUGH

In clinical practice and also in clinical trials, one of the quickest and easiest methods for documenting cough severity is to use either a numerical scoring system or visual analog scale.

Numerical Scoring Systems

Various numerical scoring systems have been used to assess the severity of cough and treatment responses.[5–8] In their simplest forms, patients merely are asked to score their cough severity from 0 to 10[5] or on Likert scales separately describing increasing frequency or severity.[8] For assessing cough in children, scales for the parents' observations are needed in addition to those for the child.[6–8] Other systems have used separate scales to describe coughing during the day and night, such as that used by Hsu and colleagues[9] (**Table 1**). This scale uses descriptors of cough frequency for scores from 0 to 2 and then supplements these with description of disruption for scores from 3 to 5, which may be confusing for patients, as infrequent coughing may still be very disruptive.

Visual Analog Scales

Visual analog scales (VAS) have been used widely for assessingmany symptoms, but particularly pain. VAS for cough assessment consists of the usual 100 mm scale often

Table 1
Numerical cough scoring system

Score	Day	Night
0	No cough during the day	No cough during the night
1	Cough for one short period	Cough on waking only
2	Cough for more than two short periods	Wake once or early because of cough
3	Frequent coughing that did not interfere with usual daytime activities	Frequent waking because of cough
4	Frequent coughing that did interfere with usual daytime activities	Frequent cough most of the night
5	Distressing cough most of the day	Distressing cough most of the night

Data from Hsu JY, Stone RA, Logan-Sinclair RB, et al. Coughing frequency in patients with persistent cough: assessment using a 24-hour ambulatory recorder. Eur Respir J 1994;7(7):1246–53.

marked at the extremes from "no cough" to "very severe"[5] or "worst cough".[6] Some patient instruction may be required to ensure the scale is used correctly. The author has found cough VAS to correlate moderately with objective cough frequency (**Fig. 2**).[6]

There are several limitations to subjective cough assessments that must be appreciated. First, the subject has to recall the severity of his or her cough over a period of time, for example scoring their cough severity on waking for the previous night or even estimating cough severity over periods of up to 2 weeks.[7] Cough events are episodic, and some subjects may have difficulty remembering their symptoms, while others may be very vigilant and score more accurately. Recall bias also may prove a problem when subjects rate the change in cough symptoms over time. Global ratings of change scales are in common use, but rely on subjects comparing their current state to their recollection of a previous state. A recent study has demonstrated that such scale ratings are correlated strongly with the subject's present state, rather than the change in state.[8] The section on cough quality-of-life measures discusses this further. Other sources of variability in such measures include the influences of the patient's mood, his or her expectations if an intervention is involved, and also the effect of physical complications of coughing. Patients who experience complications such as cough

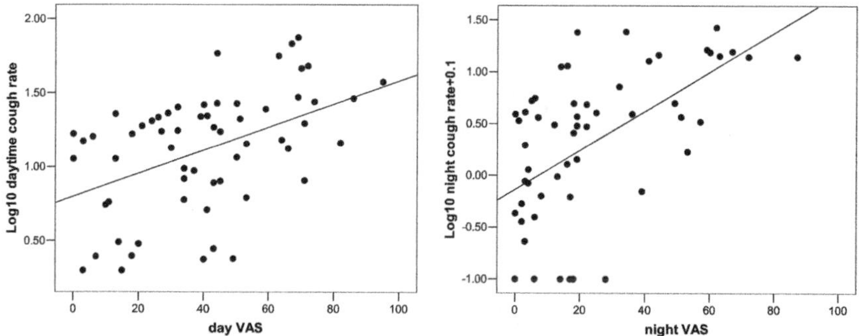

Fig. 2. Relationship between cough reflex sensitivity to citric acid and ambulatory objective cough frequency in patients with chronic cough. (*Adapted from* Decalmer SC, Webster D, Kelsall AA, et al. Chronic cough: how do cough reflex sensitivity and subjective assessments correlate with objective cough counts during ambulatory monitoring? Thorax 2007;62(4):332; with permission.)

syncope and incontinence are likely to score cough highly on any scale even if the episodes of coughing are few.

Although the previously mentioned factors limit the accuracy of subjective scores when compared with more objective cough measures, they are nonetheless important in their own right, as they do accurately reflect a patient's perception of the severity of his or her cough. It remains to be seen whether better targeting subjective assessments to address the different aspects of cough severity as suggested by Vernon and colleagues[4] may make these measures more sensitive to change with interventions for cough.

COUGH REFLEX SENSITIVITY TESTING

The inhalation of irritant substances (capsaicin, citric acid, distilled water) in increasing concentrations can be used as a measure of the sensitivity of a subject's cough reflex.[10] Capsaicin is the most commonly used agent and has been shown to be safe,[11] and it has good long- and short-term reproducibility.[12] Additionally, studies have used these challenges to demonstrate the effect of several drugs on cough reflex sensitivity.[13–16] Although in the past variability in challenge methodologies made study results difficult to compare, the recent European Respiratory Society (ERS) guidelines have aimed to standardize the equipment and challenge regimens used.[17]

The sensitivity of the cough reflex is clearly mechanistically interesting in the study of cough. For example, cough thresholds are lower in females compared with males, and citric acid and capsaicin thresholds moderately correlate with one another and, therefore, probably represent subtly different aspects of the cough reflex.[18] There is sizeable overlap in cough threshold measurements between healthy volunteers and chronic cough patients,[19] however, perhaps suggesting that these measures largely represent the airway protective reflex common to both groups, rather than the hypersensitivity that leads to profound coughing in chronic cough. This may explain why it has been found that cough reflex sensitivity correlates weakly to moderately with spontaneous cough frequency in chronic cough (**Fig. 3**),[6] asthma,[20] and chronic obstructive pulmonary disease (COPD)[21] and is, therefore, a poor surrogate for cough counting.

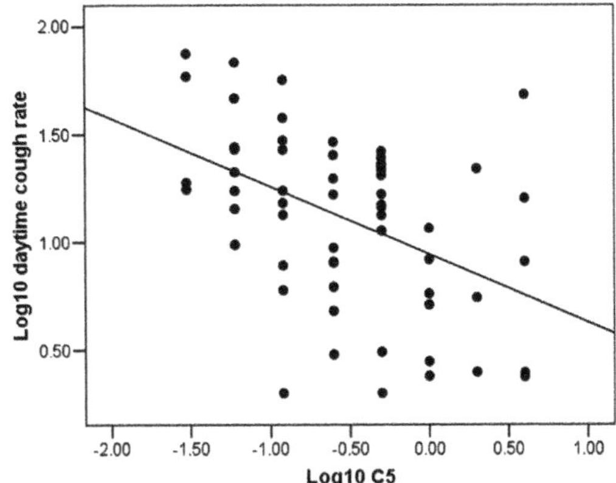

Fig. 3. Relationships between cough VAS and objective cough counts. (*Adapted from* Decalmer SC, Webster D, Kelsall AA, et al. Chronic cough: how do cough reflex sensitivity and subjective assessments correlate with objective cough counts during ambulatory monitoring? Thorax 2007;62(4):333; with permission.)

OBJECTIVE COUGH COUNTING

With the development of portable digital sound recording devices, it has become possible to make high-quality acoustic cough recordings from patients over 24-hour periods to quantify coughing. Cough is under considerable conscious control. Therefore, monitoring cough in an unobtrusive manner, while patients go about their usual activities, is far more likely to give an accurate measure of the symptom, than making assessments in laboratory conditions over shorter periods of time, where placebo effects have been found to be substantial.[22]

Cough Recording Devices

Manually counting of coughs from digital sound recordings has been validated against cough counting from audiovisual recordings and found to be more sensitive to detect cough sounds because of the better sound quality.[23] Trained cough counters are able to achieve excellent interobserver agreement for cough counting, but the main drawback is the time-consuming nature of the process. The author, however, has performed numerous clinical studies using manual cough counting,[12,20,24–28] but the time taken to complete the counting limits the size of studies and the number of measures feasible per individual. Several groups are developing automated cough detection systems, but none is fully validated for use over 24 hours. A detailed review of challenges in automated cough detection has been published elsewhere.[13]

The only currently commercially available cough monitoring systems are the Lifeshirt (Vivometrics Incorporated, Ventura, California) and the newly developed Cough-COUNT (Karmel Sonix, Haifa, Israel). The validation data available for both of these devices are limited. The Lifeshirt detects cough from a combination of sounds measured by a throat microphone and induction plethysmography to measure chest wall movement. Although the induction plethysmography is built into a tight lycra vest to allow the device to be mostly be hidden under clothing, it is far from unobtrusive. It has been shown to detect 78% of coughs in a small number of patients with COPD studied in laboratory conditions.[14] The CoughCOUNT device so far only has been validated for detecting voluntary coughing in healthy individuals; its ability to detect spontaneous coughing is not yet known.[15]

The Leicester cough monitor has been the most widely published system, but as with many other devices, validation is limited.[16] The system is not fully automated, and it is unclear to what extent the user input may influence performance. The performance of the system only has been assessed over 2 hours per subject despite 24-hour recording capabilities.[29] Comparison with cough counts performed at another center was initially encouraging, but subsequently it was revealed that the recordings had been filtered before analysis.[18] Furthermore, the system relies upon an off-the-shelf mp3 player, and no commercialization seems to be planned.

The Hull Automated Cough Counter (HACC) recognizes cough from sound recordings using neural network-based technology, and is undergoing further development.[19]

The author has been developing a cough monitoring system (Vitalojak) with a commercial company (Vitalograph Limited, Buckinghamshire, United Kingdom) based upon studies of the relationships between the physiologic changes that occur during coughing and how these relate to the cough sound produced.[20,24] To optimize cough detection, the author believes it is necessary to calibrate cough detection to an individual's cough sounds by collecting voluntary coughs from increasing lung volumes. This facilitates not only cough detection, as very low volume coughs can be discounted, but also may allow classification of coughs by estimating the starting volume from the cough sound. The author currently is working to assess whether this may be a useful surrogate for cough intensity.[30] In the meantime, the author has used a custom-built recording device for quantifying cough using manual cough counting and found weak to moderate correlations between cough counts and cough-related quality of life and subjective scores.[6,21,25,31] The addition of a parameter reflecting the intensity of coughs over a 24-hour period may independently explain further variance in these scales and provide a more comprehensive measure than simple counts.

HEALTH-RELATED QUALITY OF LIFE

Health-related quality of life refers to an individual's physical, emotional, and social well-being, and their ability to perform day-to-day tasks. The recent development of cough-specific quality-of-life tools now allows quantification of the disruption caused by coughing, and it generally is accepted that the burden of cough can be considered to fall into physical, psychological, and social domains.

Three cough quality-of-life tools are in current use, the Cough Quality of Life Questionnaire (CQLQ),[26] the Leicester Cough Questionnaire (LCQ),[7] and the Chronic Cough Impact Questionnaire (CCIQ).[27] All are easily used clinically, self-administered, and contain many similar items, suggesting consistent themes in different patient cohorts. The CQLQ and LCQ have been published most widely; both questionnaires have been developed in patients with chronic cough, validated against generic quality-of-life scales, and found to be repeatable and responsive to change. Furthermore, these questionnaires have been applied successfully in other conditions characterized by cough such as asthma, acute cough, bronchiectasis, pulmonary fibrosis, and COPD.[21,28,31,32]

The minimally important difference (MID) for a quality-of-life scale (as for any measure) is key in assessing the impact of a novel treatment for patients. The MID often is calculated by retrospectively comparing changes in the scale to a global rating of change, as performed for the LCQ.[33] Fletcher and colleagues,[8] in their publication reporting the MID for the CQLQ, found the MID was significantly underestimated using a global rating of change scale compared with a prospective measure of current quality of life applied before and after treatment, the Punum Ladder. The twofold difference in MID that was reported is likely to be due to the reliance of the global rating upon a patient's recall of his or her previous state to report a change, suggesting the higher estimate is the most accurate representation of the MID.

SELECTING PATIENT GROUPS FOR TESTING COUGH THERAPIES

When deciding the type of patients in whom an antitussive drug might be tested, there are several important considerations. Obviously, the mechanism of action of the drug, if specific to a particular condition, may dictate the population recruited; however, if a drug is expected to suppress cough generally, then some patient groups may have advantages over others. There is always a concern that cough should not be suppressed in subjects with a productive cough because of the theoretical risk of sputum stasis and infection. For the testing of novel therapies, clearly patients with significant expectoration such as bronchiectasis would not be appropriate candidates, but hopefully, further studies in the future will help to assess the extent to which coughing may be excessive in some individuals rather than appropriate for sputum clearance.

Patients presenting with chronic cough (>8 weeks duration) and a normal chest radiograph may provide a useful model for the testing of antitussive agents. These patients have relatively high cough frequencies[6] and stable symptoms that have advantages for study power/sample size and allow for crossover designed studies. Furthermore, there is some suggestion that placebo effects in this patient group are minimal, perhaps because they have low expectations of treatment success.[34] Objective cough frequency in these patients has been shown to be significantly greater in females than males and tends to increase with age, and so for parallel study designs, stratification of groups by these factors is important.[35]

Patients with acute cough (<3 weeks duration) present by far the largest patient group and therefore market for antitussive agents. Because of the short duration of illness and rapid improvement for most patients with acute cough, this condition always has been thought to be a difficult group to study requiring parallel trial designs and with difficulty discerning a treatment effect. In this author's experience, using objective cough counts, cough rates are high in acute coughing subjects, relatively stable, and highly repeatable over a 2-day period (JA Smith, unpublished data, 2009), suggesting objective cough counts may make trials in acute coughing conditions easier to perform.

Finally, some experts have advocated the use of patients with subacute cough (3 to 8 weeks duration) for testing antitussive agents. In a recent multicenter trial, testing the efficacy of a novel antitussive agent (NOP1 agonist), the identification and recruitment of such patients proved extremely difficult.[36]

CLINICAL TRIAL DESIGN

As with any clinical trial, double-blind randomized controlled trials are required to assess the effects of a novel antitussive over placebo responses. Crossover designs have the advantage of requiring smaller numbers of patients than a parallel design but may not be truly blind if the drug in question has significant adverse effects that patients may be able to detect. One solution to unblinding of treatments by adverse effects is to include an additional study arm/treatment period with a positive control (such as codeine) or an active placebo. Because of the objective evidence that codeine is an effective anti-tussive is weak,[37] codeine may well be an ideal comparator (**Fig. 4**).[38]

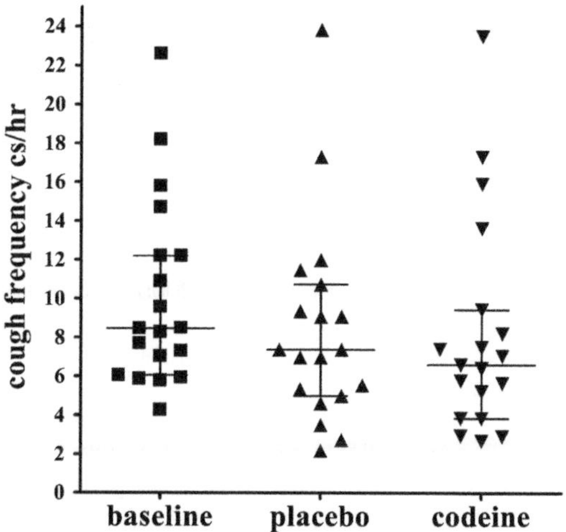

Fig. 4. Lack of effect of codeine over placebo on objective cough frequency in chronic obstructive pulmonary disease. (*Adapted from* Smith J, Owen E, Earis J, et al. Effect of codeine on objective measurement of cough in chronic obstructive pulmonary disease. J Allergy Clin Immunol 2006;117(4):833; with permission.)

In this author's opinion, the primary endpoint in a proof-of-concept study for a novel antitussive should be objective cough frequency. Secondary endpoints must include subjective scores of cough frequency and intensity and cough-specific quality of life, to explore whether any improvement in cough count observed is appreciated by subjects as significant, although the greater variability of these measures means larger follow-on studies are likely to be required to confirm an effect.

The study sample size required to test proof of concept for a novel antitussive will depend upon the variability of the endpoint used between subjects (for parallel designs) and within subjects (for crossover designs). Patients with chronic cough exhibit high objective cough frequencies,[35] facilitating the appreciation of changes, and are highly repeatable within subjects over a 1 month period.[39] The author's recent studies have suggested that similar cough frequencies and repeatability are seen in acute cough over a 2-day period (JA Smith, unpublished data, 2009).

The other parameter governing the number of patients required to test an antitussive treatment is the clinically important difference in objective cough frequency. This has been difficult to establish, as the drugs tested to date generally have failed to improve cough frequency. In a recent study, however, the author found that the presence of an esophageal catheter reduced cough frequency by 33%. This change was appreciated by the patients, as their cough VAS significantly improved. In contrast, a very large study (n = 710) testing the effects of dextromethorphan in patients with acute cough only reduced cough counts by 12% to 13%.[40] Unfortunately, the subjects' perception of cough severity was not assessed in this study. In this author's opinion, however, such small changes may be difficult to appreciate, and studies of novel antitussives should be powered to detect changes of at least 33% in cough frequency, based on current knowledge.

SUMMARY

In conclusion, the development of objective cough monitoring systems and cough-specific quality-of-life measures will revolutionize the testing of novel antitussive agents. A combination of both objective and subjective measures is required to fully assess responses to therapy, and hopefully these will facilitate the development of efficacious treatments.

REFERENCES

1. French CL, Irwin RS, Curley FJ, et al. Impact of chronic cough on quality of life. Arch Intern Med 1998;158(15):1657–61.
2. Proprietary Association of Great Britain. IRI 2005 OTC market size statistics. 2005. Available at: www.pagb.co.uk.
3. Morice AH, McGarvey L, Pavord I. Recommendations for the management of cough in adults. Thorax 2006;61(Suppl 1):i1–24.
4. Vernon M, Leidy NK, Nacson A, et al. Measuring cough severity: perspectives from the literature and from patients with chronic cough. Cough 2009;5:5.
5. Irwin RS, Zawacki JK, Wilson MM, et al. Chronic cough due to gastroesophageal reflux disease: failure to resolve despite total/near-total elimination of esophageal acid. Chest 2002;121(4):1132–40.
6. Decalmer SC, Webster D, Kelsall AA, et al. Chronic cough: how do cough reflex sensitivity and subjective assessments correlate with objective cough counts during ambulatory monitoring? Thorax 2007;62(4):329–34.

7. Birring SS, Prudon B, Carr AJ, et al. Development of a symptom specific health status measure for patients with chronic cough: Leicester Cough Questionnaire (LCQ). Thorax 2003;58(4):339–43.
8. Fletcher KE, French CL, Irwin RS, et al. A prospective global measure, the Punum Ladder, provides more valid assessments of quality of life than retrospective transition measures. J Clin Epidemiol, in press.
9. Hsu JY, Stone RA, Logan-Sinclair RB, et al. Coughing frequency in patients with persistent cough: assessment using a 24 hour ambulatory recorder. Eur Respir J 1994;7(7):1246–53.
10. Morice AH, Fontana GA, Belvisi MG, et al. ERS guidelines on the assessment of cough. Eur Respir J 2007;29(6):1256–76.
11. Dicpinigaitis PV, Alva RV. Safety of capsaicin cough challenge testing. Chest 2005;128(1):196–202.
12. Dicpinigaitis PV. Short- and long-term reproducibility of capsaicin cough challenge testing. Pulm Pharmacol Ther 2003;16(1):61–5.
13. Smith J, Woodcock A. New developments in the objective assessment of cough. Lung 2008;186(Suppl 1):S48–54.
14. Coyle MA, Keenan DB, Henderson LS, et al. Evaluation of an ambulatory system for the quantification of cough frequency in patients with chronic obstructive pulmonary disease. Cough 2005;1:3.
15. Gavriely N, Guryachev Y, Dekel D, et al. Simulated cough-based database for cough-counting algorithm validation [abstract]. Am J Respir Crit Care Med 2009;179:A4429.
16. Birring SS, Fleming T, Matos S, et al. The leicester cough monitor: preliminary validation of an automated cough detection system in chronic cough. Eur Respir J 2008;31(5):1013–8.
17. Morice AH, Kastelik JA, Thompson R. Cough challenge in the assessment of cough reflex. Br J Clin Pharmacol 2001;52(4):365–75.
18. Birring SS, Mann VM, Matos S, et al. The Leicester cough monitor: a semi-automated, semivalidated cough detection system? [erratum]. Eur Respir J 2009; 33(1):224.
19. Barry SJ, Dane AD, Morice AH, et al. The automatic recognition and counting of cough. Cough 2006;2:8.
20. McGuinness K, Morris J, Kelsall A, et al. The relationship between cough acoustics and the volume inspired prior to coughing. Am J Respir Crit Care Med 2007; 175:A381.
21. Smith J, Owen E, Earis J, et al. Cough in COPD: correlation of objective monitoring with cough challenge and subjective assessments. Chest 2006;130(2):379–85.
22. Eccles R. The powerful placebo in cough studies? Pulm Pharmacol Ther 2002; 15(3):303–8.
23. Smith JA, Earis JE, Woodcock AA. Establishing a gold standard for manual cough counting: video versus digital audio recordings. Cough 2006;2:6.
24. McGuinness K, Kelsall A, Lowe J, et al. Automated cough detection: a novel approach. Am J Respir Crit Care Med 2007;175:A381.
25. Smith JA, Owen EC, Jones AM, et al. Objective measurement of cough during pulmonary exacerbations in adults with cystic fibrosis. Thorax 2006;61(5):425–9.
26. French CT, Irwin RS, Fletcher KE, et al. Evaluation of a cough-specific quality-of-life questionnaire. Chest 2002;121(4):1123–31.
27. Baiardini I, Braido F, Fassio O, et al. A new tool to assess and monitor the burden of chronic cough on quality of life: chronic cough impact questionnaire. Allergy 2005;60(4):482–8.

28. Polley L, Yaman N, Heaney L, et al. Impact of cough across different chronic respiratory diseases: comparison of two cough-specific health-related quality of life questionnaires. Chest 2008;134(2):295–302.
29. McGuinness K, Morice A, Woodcock A, et al. The leicester cough monitor: a semi-automated, semivalidated cough detection system? Eur Respir J 2008;32(2): 529–30 [author reply: 530–1].
30. Ward K, Reilly C, McGuinness K, et al. Respiratory muscle activation during voluntary coughing in healthy volunteers [abstract]. Eur Respir J 2009;34(Suppl 53):229s.
31. Marsden PA, Smith JA, Kelsall AA, et al. A comparison of objective and subjective measures of cough in asthma. J Allergy Clin Immunol 2008;122(5):903–7.
32. French CT, Fletcher KE, Irwin RS. A comparison of gender differences in health-related quality of life in acute and chronic coughers. Chest 2005;127(6):1991–8.
33. Raj AA, Pavord DI, Birring SS. Clinical cough IV:what is the minimal important difference for the leicester cough questionnaire? Handb Exp Pharmacol 2009; 187:311–20.
34. Morice AH, Menon MS, Mulrennan SA, et al. Opiate therapy in chronic cough. Am J Respir Crit Care Med 2007;175(4):312–5.
35. Kelsall A, Decalmer S, McGuinness K, et al. Sex differences and predictors of objective cough frequency in chronic cough. Thorax 2009;64(5):393–8.
36. Woodcock A, McLeod RL, Sadeh J, et al. The efficacy Of A NOP1 agonist (Sch486757) in subacute cough. Lung, 2009. [Epub ahead of print].
37. Bolser DC, Davenport PW. Codeine and cough: an ineffective gold standard. Curr Opin Allergy Clin Immunol 2007;7(1):32–6.
38. Smith J, Owen E, Earis J, et al. Effect of codeine on objective measurement of cough in chronic obstructive pulmonary disease. J Allergy Clin Immunol 2006; 117(4):831–5.
39. Kelsall A, Jones H, Decalmer S, et al. The effect of oesophageal monitoring on objective and subjective measures of cough. Am J Respir Crit Care Med 2008; 177:A897.
40. Pavesi L, Subburaj S, Porter-Shaw K. Application and validation of a computerized cough acquisition system for objective monitoring of acute cough: a meta-analysis. Chest 2001;120(4):1121–8.

Unexplained Cough in the Adult

Richard S. Irwin, MD[a,b,*]

KEYWORDS

- Cough • Unexplained cough
- Management of unexplained cough • Idiopathic cough

As stated in the 2006 American College of Chest Physicians (ACCP) Evidenced-Based Clinical Practice Guidelines on diagnosis and management of cough[1]

> *"the diagnosis of unexplained (idiopathic) cough is a diagnosis of exclusion. It should not be made until a thorough diagnostic evaluation is performed, specific and appropriate treatment (according to the management protocols that have performed the best in the literature) has been tried and has failed, and uncommon causes have been ruled out"*

In essence, the unexplained cough is a variant of chronic cough (ie, a cough of more than 2 months duration) that has remained persistently troublesome to the patient. This article, expands upon this definition by discussing why unexplained cough is a better term than idiopathic cough to characterize treatment failures and then poses and answers a series of questions:

How often is chronic cough unexplained, and what are the potential explanations?
How should clinicians and researchers approach the problem?
What are the pitfalls in management, and have they been avoided?
How often will chronic cough remain truly unexplained after the recommended management protocol has been followed?

The article also discusses the potential pathogenetic mechanisms to explain the truly refractory unexplained cough and the available options to manage it.

UNEXPLAINED VERSUS IDIOPATHIC COUGH

I agree with the ACCP cough guidelines[1] that unexplained is a better descriptor than idiopathic when referring to the persistently troublesome cough and that the

[a] Division of Pulmonary, Allergy, and Critical Care Medicine, University of Massachusetts Medical School, 55 Lake Avenue North, Worcester, MA 01655, USA
[b] Critical Care Operations, UMass Memorial Medical Center, 55 Lake Avenue North, Worcester, MA 01655, USA
* Division of Pulmonary, Allergy, and Critical Care Medicine, University of Massachusetts Medical School, 55 Lake Avenue North, Worcester, MA 01655.
E-mail address: irwinr@ummhc.org

Otolaryngol Clin N Am 43 (2010) 167–180
doi:10.1016/j.otc.2009.11.009 oto.theclinics.com
0030-6665/10/$ – see front matter

distinction is important, because the difference in terms might affect how the problem is approached. For instance, the term unexplained implies that the cause is yet to be determined and that there might be multiple reasons to consider and reconsider; on the other hand, the term idiopathic implies that while the cause is unknown, it is likely due to a single condition that has yet to be described. This has the potential to truncate any further work-up. The literature supports the preferential use of the term unexplained, because it has suggested that some of the variation in successful treatment of chronic cough could be explained by investigators using inadequate management protocols.[1] For example, in some countries in Europe, the putatively most effective treatment for upper airway cough syndrome, the older first-generation H_1-antagonists, are generally unavailable, leading to the preferential prescribing of the newer-generation H_1-antagonists that are considered to be less effective,[2] or, in the case of cough caused by the common cold, ineffective.[2]

HOW OFTEN IS CHRONIC COUGH UNEXPLAINED, AND WHAT ARE THE POTENTIAL EXPLANATIONS?

Based upon the published results of prospective and retrospective before and after intervention trials, treatment failures for chronic cough have ranged from 0% to 46% of patients referred for specialist management.[1,3] Although there has been a wide range of unexplained cough reported in the literature, most of the time (approximately 90%) chronic cough has been explained and successfully treated. Possible explanations to account for coughs that remain persistently troublesome are multiple and include

- The previously mentioned failure to follow a successful, validated protocol (eg, failing to use the most effective medication)
- Failure of patients to follow treatment recommendations
- Patients not being willing to be contacted or refusing to complete evaluations
- Investigators reporting results in a group of patients with a different spectrum of pretreatment, presumptive causes
- Investigators reporting results in a group of patients with different phenotypic or airway histopathologic profiles or referral sources
- Development of serious, comorbid illnesses that force patients to drop out of studies or not follow prescribed treatment plans
- The diagnosis is correct, but the cough is refractory to the prescribed treatment regimen(s)
- Combinations of the above
- The cough is truly unexplained.

HOW SHOULD CLINICIANS AND RESEARCHERS APPROACH THE PROBLEM?

The first step in approaching the adult patient with an unexplained cough is to review the patient's work-up to be certain that an appropriate and comprehensive management protocol has been followed such as that shown in **Fig. 1**. This protocol was developed by the ACCP Cough Guideline Committee based upon

- The known relative frequency of the disorders (singly and in combination) that have been reported to cause chronic cough
- The known sensitivity and specificity of most diagnostic tests in predicting the cause(s) of chronic cough
- The known timeframe of response to appropriate therapy[4]

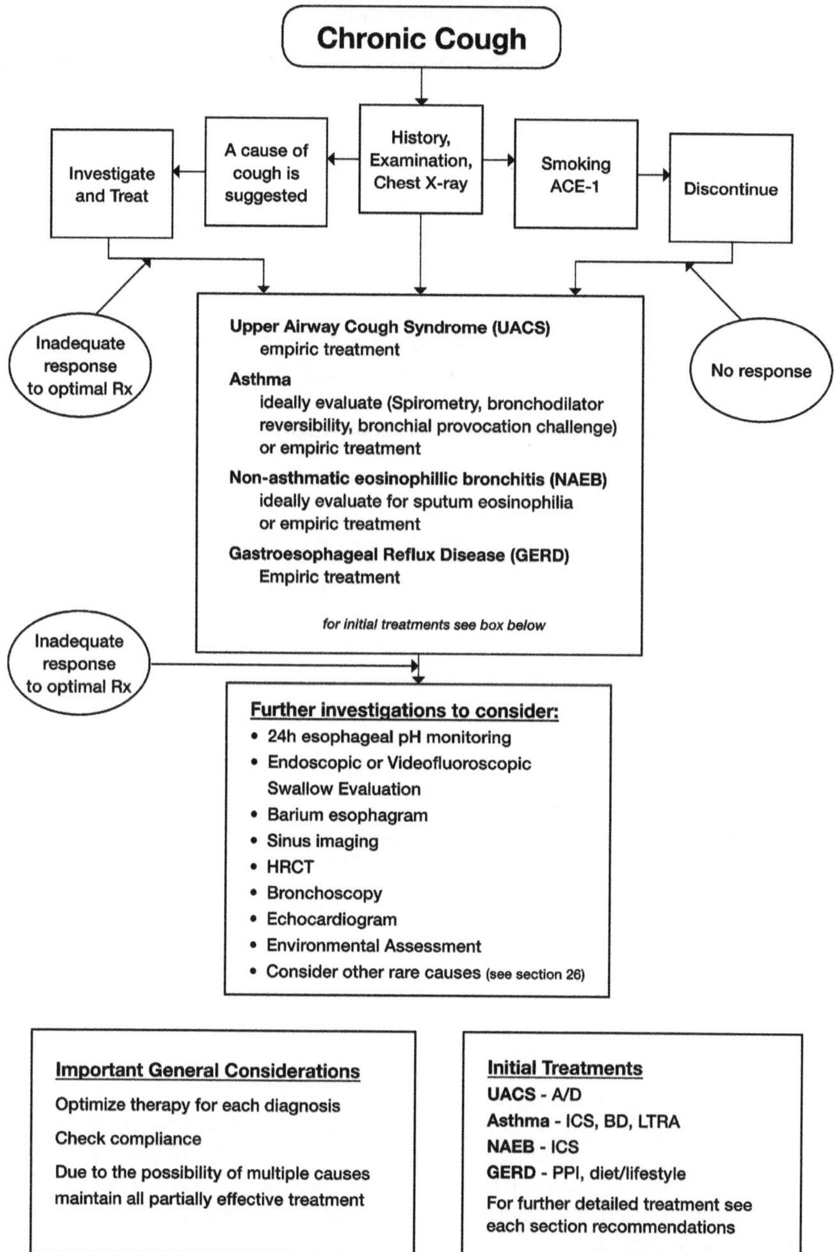

Fig. 1. Management algorithm for chronic cough in adult patients. *Abbreviations:* ACE-I, angiotensin inhibitor; A/D, antihistamine/decongestant; BD, bronchodilator; HRCT, high-resolution chest computed tomography (CT) scan; ICS, inhaled corticosteroid; LTRA, leukotriene receptor antagonist; PPI, proton pump inhibitor. Section 26 referred to in the figure begins on page 206S of the ACCP Cough Guidelines. (*From* Pratter MR, Brightling CE, Boulet L-P, et al. An empiric integrative approach to the management of cough: ACCP evidence-based clinical practice guidelines. Chest 2006;129:225S; with permission.)

This protocol summarizes guidance on how to effectively manage chronic cough by:

- Initially recommending that the commonest causes of chronic cough be sequentially evaluated and treated using a combination of selected diagnostic tests and empiric therapy
- Reminding that sequential and additive therapy is important, because more than one cause of cough is frequently present
- Considering evaluating for uncommon causes when the commonest causes have been adequately addressed
- Referral to a cough specialist or cough clinic when cough remains undiagnosed after all of the recommendations have been followed.

After determining that a protocol has been used that has been shown to lead to successful results, the next step to take when cough continues to remain troublesome, even when one thinks that the management has been appropriate and adequate, is to consider whether pitfalls in management have been avoided.

WHAT ARE THE PITFALLS IN MANAGEMENT, AND HAVE THEY BEEN AVOIDED?

Although a comprehensive discussion on how to use the protocol outlined in algorithmic form in **Fig. 1** can be found elsewhere,[4] the answers to this question reassure in specific terms whether specific and appropriate treatment has been prescribed or a thorough diagnostic evaluation work-up has been performed. While the author initially introduced this pitfall avoidance strategy in 1998[5] and revisited it in 2000[6] and 2002,[7] it is much more robustly expressed here.

Upper Airway Cough Syndrome (Previously Referred to as Postnasal Drip Syndrome) Caused by Various Rhinosinus Conditions

This condition may not be considered or correctly treated due to the following potential failures:

- Recognizing that it can present as a cough–phlegm syndrome[8] that can lead to the incorrect diagnose of chronic bronchitis
- Appreciating that all H_1-antagonists are not the same when treating cough. For example, the newer, relatively nonsedating agents are primarily useful when the upper airway cough syndrome (UACS) is caused by a histamine-mediated condition such as allergic rhinitis[2] and the older agents have been shown to be efficacious in conditions like the common cold when the newer agents failed[2]
- Considering sinusitis because it is silent (eg, no discolored nasal discharge, pain, or fever) from a clinical standpoint or the usefulness of endoscopy that might reveal its presence (**Fig. 2**)
- Considering allergic rhinitis or recommending the avoidance of allergens because symptoms are perennial
- Considering that this diagnosis can be silent (eg, no complaint of postnasal drip or throat clearing) up to 20% of the time[2]
- Considering aspirin-exacerbated disease or the usefulness of endoscopy that might uncover nasal polyposis (**Fig. 3**). In aspirin-sensitive patients, aspirin therapy following desensitization has been shown to be effective in preventing the reoccurrence of nasal polyposis.[9]

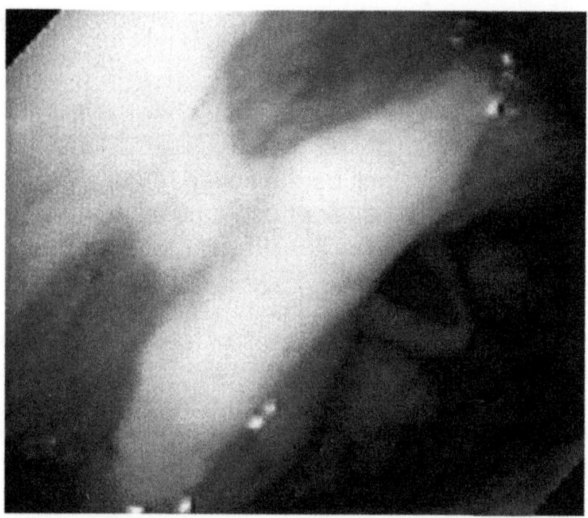

Fig. 2. Endoscopic view revealing evidence of suppuration due to sinusitis that was clinically silent and about to drip onto vocal cords.

Asthma

This disease may not be considered or correctly treated because of the following potential failures:

Recognizing that it can just present as a cough (cough variant asthma)[10] or as a cough–phlegm syndrome[8] that can lead to the incorrect diagnose of chronic bronchitis

Recognizing that inhaled medications may exacerbate cough[11]

Assuming that a positive methacholine challenge that is only consistent with asthma is actually diagnostic of asthma as the cause of cough. Cough can

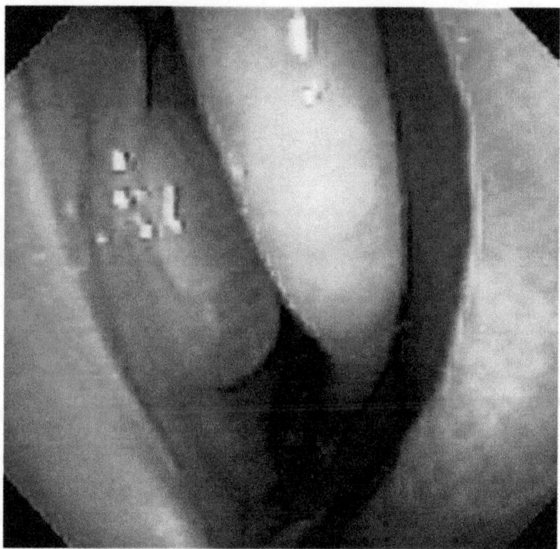

Fig. 3. Endoscopic view of a nasal polyp in a patient with chronic cough who was subsequently determined to have aspirin sensitivity during a monitored aspirin challenge.

only be diagnosed as being caused by asthma when the cough goes away with asthma treatment.[12]

Nonasthmatic Eosinophilic Bronchitis

Pitfalls in managing this condition include the failure to consider the diagnosis, order the correct tests to diagnose it, or consider occupational/environmental causes.[13]

Gastroesophageal Reflux Disease

Risks of misdiagnosis or improper treatment of gastroesophageal reflux disease (GERD) include the following potential failures:

- Recognizing that it can present as a cough–phlegm syndrome[8] that can lead to the incorrect diagnose of chronic bronchitis
- Appreciating that silent reflux disease can be the cause of cough,[14] that it may take 2 to 3 months of intensive medical treatment before cough starts to improve, and, on average, 5 to 6 months before cough resolves[14]
- Assuming that cough cannot be caused by GERD, because cough remains unchanged when gastrointestinal symptoms improve[15]
- Assuming that one can reliably make the diagnosis of GERD based upon the appearance of the vocal cords (**Fig. 4**)[16]
- Recognizing that coexisting diseases such as obstructive sleep apnea[17] or their treatment such as calcium channel blockers or nitrates for coronary artery

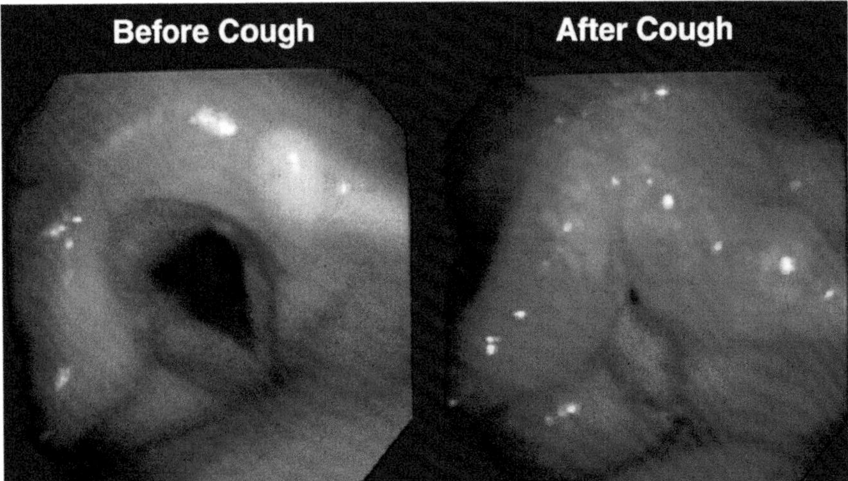

Fig. 4. Endoscopic views of supraglottic and glottic structures just before and immediately after an approximate 5-second paroxysm of spontaneous coughing in a patient being evaluated for chronic cough of 5 years duration. Before the coughing episode, mucosal surfaces were normal. Immediately after coughing, mucosal surfaces appear red and swollen. Because the coughing paroxysm occurred spontaneously and was not provoked by the instillation of fluid or trauma from the endoscope or regurgitation or vomiting, the changes noted were thought to be caused by the act of coughing itself and most likely represent venous congestion. (*From* Irwin RS, French CT. Cough and gastroesophageal reflux: identifying cough and assessing the efficacy of cough-modifying agents. Am J Med 2001;111(8A):45S–50S; with permission.)

disease or progesterone as hormone replacement therapy may be making GERD worse, because these drugs can relax the lower esophageal sphincter[17]

Considering nonacid reflux disease and assuming that cough always will respond to acid suppression[15,17]

Considering the importance of diet, avoiding intense exercising, and prokinetic therapy[17]

Treating adequately other coexisting causes of cough that perpetuate the cycle of cough and reflux, because coughing itself can provoke reflux events[17]

Recognizing that surgery may help when intensive medical therapy has failed.[17]

Triad of UACS, Asthma, and GERD

Because these three conditions commonly cause chronic cough singly or in combination,[18] it is also a pitfall in management to fail to

Consider that more than one of these conditions may be contributing simultaneously to the cough.

Consider these common conditions because the patient has a seemingly obvious pre-existing disease such as a chronic interstitial pneumonia (eg, idiopathic pulmonary fibrosis) that can cause cough. Approximately 50% of the time, in patients with a chronic interstitial pneumonia, the cause will be due to one of these common diseases.[19]

Appreciate that because these are chronic conditions, they will not be cured and will periodically flare especially with upper respiratory tract infections such as the common cold.

Re-evaluate the cough as a new problem when cough flares after a period of remission. For example, asthma may become a problem when it was not before, especially following a severe viral infection.

Angiotensin-Converting Enzyme Inhibitor

In patients taking angiotensin-converting enzyme inhibitors (ACEIs), it is a pitfall in management to fail to consider that these drugs may be causing cough, because the cough had already been present before the drug was initially prescribed or that stopping the drug for 1 to 3 weeks is enough time to see if cough is caused by the drug. The author advises always stopping the ACEIs in patients with chronic cough, because the original cause of the cough may have disappeared on its own or responded to treatment just when the ACEI was prescribed. Also, 4 weeks of abstinence from taking the ACEI may be required to start to see improvement or disappearance in ACEI-induced cough (**Fig. 5**).[20,21]

Unsuspected Airway Disease

In addition to missing the opportunity to diagnose unsuspected upper respiratory tract diseases such as silent sinusitis and nasal polyposis if nasopharyngoscopy or transnasal laryngoscopy is not performed in patients with unexplained cough, failure of diagnosing unsuspected lower airway diseases also may be a pitfall unless it is appreciated that the work-up of unexplained chronic cough is never completed unless and until bronchoscopy has been performed. If it is necessary to visualize the entire upper and lower airways during one procedure, bronchoscopy by the transnasal route will serve this purpose.

Because flexible bronchoscopy when routinely performed at the beginning of the work-up will have a low diagnostic yield of approximately 4% and almost always when the chest radiograph suggests the presence of neoplastic or active inflammatory

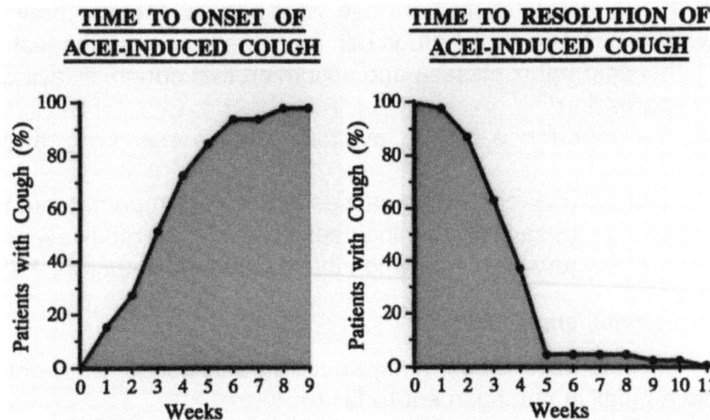

Fig. 5. Time course in development and resolution of ACEI-induced cough. By 4 weeks of discontinuing the ACEI, cough had disappeared in 62% of patients; it remarkably had improved in the remaining patients.

disease,[22] the procedure should not be performed initially in the context of a normal chest radiograph. The diagnostic yield, however, may be much greater, up to 28%,[23] when the procedure is performed at the end of the work-up, even when the chest radiograph is normal. For example, various partial or nonobstructing malignant (eg, squamous cell carcinoma) and benign airway lesions (eg, carcinoid tumors, endobronchial cysts **Fig. 6**) have been diagnosed as the cause of what had been considered a chronic, persistently troublesome cough until the procedure had been done.

Unsuspected suppurative lower airway disease is another benign disease that may be diagnosed only at the time of endoscopy (**Fig. 7**).[24] Although a clue to the diagnosis is hearing rhonchi or crackles on auscultation of the lungs, these physical findings may be absent, and chest imaging studies including high-resolution chest computed

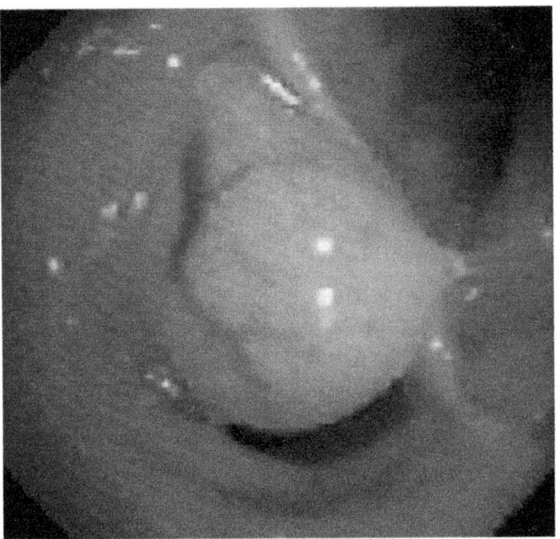

Fig. 6. Endoscopic view of a benign, endobronchial cyst that is partially obstructing the opening of the airway to the anterior segment of the right upper lobe. Following resection, the patient's persistently troublesome cough disappeared.

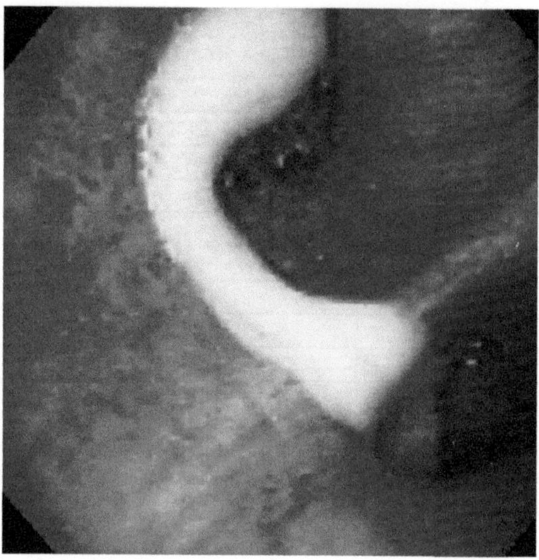

Fig. 7. Endoscopic view of unsuspected suppurative lower airway disease.

tomography (CT) scanning may be entirely normal. A pitfall in managing this condition is failing to appreciate that intravenous therapy for a prolonged period of time may be successful when the same drug given orally failed to improve cough.

Psychogenic Cough

There is a temptation to diagnose patients with unexplained coughs as having psychogenic cough, because they appear depressed, anxious, and agitated.[25,26] Because there are no reliable clinical characteristics of psychogenic cough,[25] and chronic coughing leads to psychological and physical complaints that adversely affect health-related quality of life,[25] it is a pitfall in management to ascribe unexplained cough to psychogenic cough unless an extensive evaluation has been performed that includes ruling out tic disorders and uncommon causes of chronic cough and, very importantly, cough improves with behavior modification or psychiatric therapy.[25]

HOW OFTEN WILL CHRONIC COUGH REMAIN TRULY UNEXPLAINED AFTER THE RECOMMENDED MANAGEMENT PROTOCOL HAS BEEN FOLLOWED?

The author essentially has been following the core of the ACCP cough guidelines for the past 40 years and has prospectively studied the putative reasons for success and failure in the eight series of patients with chronic cough that he has published (**Table 1**).[3,8,27–32] Because of this, it can be reported that chronic cough in the author's experience that failed to respond to treatment after following the ACCP Cough Guideline has averaged 5.7% (27/472). If one excludes the 2006 study, because there were suspicions that failure to improve was due in many instances to patients failing to follow treatment recommendations (eg, many of those who failed to get better refused to complete evaluations or were not willing to be contacted), the frequency of truly unexplained cough in the author's experience has ranged between 0 and 10%. These numbers have remained stable despite a referral source from around the globe, an increase over the years in the multiplicity of causes, and some variation in the spectrum and frequency of causes. In the author's experience, one now diagnoses unsuspected

Table 1
Outcomes of managing chronic cough: the UMass Memorial experience

Year	Treatment Failure n	%	References
1981	1/49	2%	27
1990	1/102	2%	28
1995	2/71	3%	8
1996	2/88	2%	29
1998	0/11	0%	30
2002	0/24	0%	31
2006	11/24	46%	3
2010	10/103	10%[a]	32

[a] Based upon total cough quality of life questionnaire (CQLQ) scores for subjects who had scores for both time periods, 93 of 103 or 90.3% of subjects showed improvement from baseline to 6 months follow-up.

suppurative airway disease as the cause of chronic cough, and this condition was only described in 2003.[24] Moreover, the disease the author most commonly diagnoses as the cause of chronic cough since the beginning of the new millennium has been GERD, and it is almost always predominantly or solely nonacidic in nature.

WHAT ARE THE POTENTIAL PATHOGENIC MECHANISMS TO EXPLAIN THE TRULY REFRACTORY, UNEXPLAINED COUGH?

The potential mechanisms are multiple and include an overly sensitive cough reflex, coexistence of autoimmune diseases, existing diseases that require discovery of better treatments, and a different airway histopathologic profile.

Because an overly sensitive cough reflex has been demonstrated in many subjects with chronic cough whether or not their coughs respond to treatment or remain unexplained, the mere presence of an overly sensitive cough reflex does not by itself explain the difference in outcomes. Although it is possible that the heightened cough reflex in the unexplained cough is caused by a different mechanism, none, to date, has been implicated. For example, while the role of neurogenic inflammation has been shown to be important in experimental animals, such has not been the case in people[33] as of yet. Although some have postulated that female sex hormones may be playing a role based upon the knowledge that women have a heightened cough reflex compared with males[34] and women have outnumbered men in series of subjects with unexplained cough, I think this an unlikely explanation for several reasons. Women have almost always outnumbered men in series of coughers whether or not coughs responded to therapy or remained unexplained. Furthermore, in the author's series of reports, men outnumbered the women in the one study in which there was the largest number of subjects with persistently troublesome coughs.[3]

Although the role of the transient receptor potential (TRP) family of ion channels and especially overexpression of TRPV1 (the capsaicin receptor) may explain the overly sensitive cough reflex in unexplained cough, experimental work in this area is just beginning.[35,36] Lastly, it is possible that a vagal sensory neuropathy may have been provoked by a stimulus such as a preceding viral infection. Speculation regarding this has been suggested most commonly in the otolaryngology literature in the context of a diagnosis of laryngeal sensory neuropathy or irritable larynx syndrome.[37,38]

However, because a preceding upper respiratory tract infection often predates the beginning of all chronic coughs, and most subjects improve, it is not known if a vagal sensory neuropathy explains the overly sensitive cough reflex in the persistently troublesome cough.

Although a case–control study showed that patients with unexplained cough were eight times more likely to have the coexistence of an organ-specific autoimmune disease, particularly hypothyroidism,[39] it is not clear how this relates to pathogenesis, and it has not been helpful, for the most part, in management.

Patients with unexplained cough can present with clinical manifestations that suggest a condition known to cause chronic cough such as UACS or with laboratory studies that suggest GERD but do not respond to conventional treatment for these conditions. An explanation to explain failure to respond to therapy in these conditions is that they have these existing diseases but require discovery of better treatments such as more effective and safe prokinetic agents for GERD of a nonacid nature.

Lastly, although it had been suggested that patients with unexplained cough had a different airway histopathologic profile composed primarily of lymphocytic inflammation and that autoimmunity might be responsible,[34] it is now thought that the trauma from the chronic cough itself is the most likely cause of the lymphocytic inflammation, and this lymphocytic inflammation is present in the airways of all patients with chronic cough, whether or not it responds to treatment.

WHAT MANAGEMENT OPTIONS ARE AVAILABLE FOR THE TRULY REFRACTORY UNEXPLAINED COUGH?

The options include:

- Referral to a cough clinic with interdisciplinary expertise (eg, pulmonary, allergy, gastrointestinal, otolaryngologic, speech, and swallowing) in managing cough
- Referral for a specific trial of speech therapy that has been shown to be helpful in this group of patients[40]
- A self-limited trial of drugs such as certain opiates[41] that have been shown to be effective in double-blind randomized placebo-controlled studies and consideration of a trial of drugs that have been suggested but not proven to be of benefit such as nebulized local anesthetics,[42,43] gabapentin,[37] or amitriptyline.[44]

Because opiates have a high potential to lead to an addiction problem, the author uses them in short-term trials for a few months to help determine if they can block a potential cough perpetuating cough cycle. The author's practice is based upon the knowledge that the act of coughing itself can lead to airway inflammatory changes that might provoke cough[3] and, in the case of GERD, potentially can maintain a reflux problem by provoking reflux events.[45]

Although the data supporting the use of nebulized local anesthetics with agents such as lidocaine and mepivacaine, and enteral gabapentine and amitriptyline are much less convincing than for morphine, it is reasonable to try them to see if they might block a cough begetting cough cycle. Gabapentin, a drug that has been used to treat seizures and neuropathic pain, has been tried in patients with unexplained cough due to presumed laryngeal sensory neuropathy, because this condition had some similarities to patients with seizures and neuropathic pain.[37] Amitriptyline was tried in another group of similar patients with presumed postviral vagal neuropathy because of its potential benefit in treating neuropathic pain.[44] This latter study was designed as a prospective, randomized, controlled trial comparing the effects of 10 mg amitriptyline at bedtime versus 10 to 100 mg/5 mL of codeine/guaifenesin every

6 hours while awake for 10 days on cough-specific quality of life. Although the authors state that they showed that amitriptyline was effective, we are not able to determine this from the data that were published; and, my colleagues and I are the developers of the cough-specific quality of life instrument that was used by these authors as their sole outcome measure. Moreover, if the amitriptyline was effective, there is a more plausible alternative explanation on how it might have worked so quickly. Because the description of their subjects suggested that they might have had an UACS, amitriptyline might have been effective by virtue of its ability to block muscarinic cholinergic or H_1 histaminergic receptors rather than by blocking neuropathic pain fiber transmission. Consequently, I would caution others not to try amitriptyline before an older antihistamine plus decongestant agent in patients with presumed upper airway postviral vagal neuropathy. If gabapentin or amitriptyline truly appears to help, the decision to continue them must be based upon a risk–benefit discussion with the patient.

While unilateral superselective vagotomy appears to have been of benefit in selected patients with refractory cough caused by unresectable, unilateral bronchogenic carcinoma,[46] the author is not aware that this radical treatment option has been tried in patients with unexplained chronic cough. Before considering this as a possible, viable option in patients with unexplained chronic cough, however, future studies will need to be done that show that bilateral superselective vagotomy will not lead to disastrous complications. Although the double lung transplant experience suggests that the lack of a cough reflex might contribute to more infections, the author is not aware that this has been prospectively assessed in a controlled fashion. Perhaps, it is also possible that superselective vagotomies may become pharmacologically feasible and become part of the indications (eg, superselective vagal nerve block) for interventional pulmonology.

Lastly, the author encourages in the strongest possible terms research devoted to the development of better treatment agents such as effective and safe prokinetic agents for treating GERD and for attenuating an overly sensitive cough reflex.

SUMMARY

The author recommends the following strategy for managing unexplained chronic cough:

Faithfully follow a validated systematic management protocol that has been reported to be successful.

Systematically consider and evaluate the multiple potential pitfalls in management.

Before choosing a management option such as opiates, amitriptyline, or bilateral superselective vagotomy for the truly refractory cough, remember the Latin phrase: "primum non nocere" or "above all, do no harm."

While advocating for continued cough research, remember the progress that has been made over the past 30 years and that it is the minority of patients whose chronic coughs remain persistently troublesome.

REFERENCES

1. Pratter MR. Unexplained (idiopathic) cough: ACCP evidence-based clinical practice guidelines. Chest 2006;129(1):220S–1S.
2. Pratter MR. Chronic upper airway cough syndrome secondary to rhinosinus diseases (previously referred to as postnasal drip syndrome): ACCP evidence-based clinical practice guidelines. Chest 2006;129:63S–71S.

3. Irwin RS, Ownbey R, Cagle PT, et al. Interpreting the histopathology of chronic cough: a prospective, controlled, comparative study. Chest 2006;130:362–70.
4. Pratter MR, Brightling CE, Boulet L-P, et al. An empiric integrative approach to the management of cough: ACCP evidence-based clinical practice guidelines. Chest 2006;129:222S–31S.
5. Irwin RS, Boulet L-P, Cloutier MM, et al. Managing cough as a defense mechanism and as a symptom. A consensus panel report of the American College of Chest Physicians. Chest 1998;114:133S–81S.
6. Irwin RS, Madison JM. The diagnosis and management of cough. N Engl J Med 2000;343:1715–21.
7. Irwin RS, Madison JM. The persistently troublesome cough. Am J Respir Crit Care Med 2002;165:1469–74.
8. Smyrnios NA, Irwin RS, Curley FJ. Chronic cough with a history of excessive mucus mucus production: the spectrum and frequency of causes, key components of the diagnostic evaluation, and outcome of specific therapy. Chest 1995;108:991–7.
9. Berges-Gimeno MP, Stevenson DD. Nonsteroidal anti-inflammatory drug-induced reactions and desensitization. J Asthma 2004;41:375–84.
10. Corrao WM, Braman SS, Irwin RS. Chronic cough as the sole presenting manifestation of bronchial asthma. N Engl J Med 1979;300:633–7.
11. Shim CS, Williams MH Jr. Cough and wheezing from beclomethasone aerosol. Chest 1987;91:207–9.
12. Dicpinigaitis PV. Chronic cough due to asthma: ACCP evidence-based clinical practice guidelines. Chest 2006;129:75S–9S.
13. Brightling CE. Chronic cough due to nonasthmatic eosinophilic bronchitis: ACCP evidence-based clinical practice guidelines. Chest 2006;129:116S–21S.
14. Irwin RS, Zawacki JK, Curley FJ, et al. Chronic cough as the sole presenting manifestation of gastroesophageal reflux. Am Rev Respir Dis 1989;140:1294–300.
15. Irwin RS, Zawacki JK, Wilson MM, et al. Chronic cough due to gastroesophageal reflux disease: failure to resolve despite total/near total elimination of esophageal acid. Chest 2002;121:1132–40.
16. Irwin RS, French CT. Cough and gastroesophageal reflux: identifying cough and assessing the efficacy of cough-modifying agents. Am J Med 2001;111(8A): 45S–50S.
17. Irwin RS. Chronic cough due to gastroesophageal reflux disease: ACCP evidence-based clinical practice guidelines. Chest 2006;129:80S–94S.
18. Palombini BC, Villanova CAC, Araujo E, et al. A pathogenic triad in chronic cough: asthma, postnasal drip syndrome, and gastroesophageal reflux disease. Chest 1999;116:279–84.
19. Madison JM, Irwin RS. Chronic cough in adults with interstitial lung disease. Curr Opin Pulm Med 2005;11:412–6.
20. Dicpinigaitis PV. Angiotensin-converting enzyme inhibitor-induced cough: ACCP evidence-based clinical practice guidelines. Chest 2006;129:169S–73S.
21. Lacourciere Y, Brunner H, Irwin RS, et al. Effects of modulators of the renin-angiotensin-aldosterone system on cough. J Hypertens 1994;12:1387–93.
22. Markowitz DH, Irwin RS. Is bronchoscopy overused in the evaluation of chronic cough? J Bronchol 1997;4:332–6.
23. Sen RP, Walsh TE. Fiberoptic bronchoscopy for refractory cough. Chest 1991;99: 33–5.
24. Schaefer OP, Irwin RS. Unsuspected bacterial suppurative disease of the airways presenting as chronic cough. Am J Med 2003;114:602–6.

25. Irwin RS, Glomb WB, Chang AB. Habit cough, tic cough, and psychogenic cough in adult and pediatric populations: ACCP evidence-based clinical practice guidelines. Chest 2006;129:174S–9S.
26. Dicpinigaitis PV, Tso R, Banauch G. Prevalence of depressive symptoms among patients with chronic cough. Chest 2006;130:1839–43.
27. Irwin RS, Corrao WM, Pratter MR. Chronic persistent cough in the adult: the spectrum and frequency of causes and successful outcome of specific therapy. Am Rev Respir Dis 1981;123:413–7.
28. Irwin RS, Curley FJ, French CL. Chronic cough: the spectrum and frequency of causes, key components of the diagnostic evaluation, and outcome of specific therapy. Am Rev Respir Dis 1990;141:640–7.
29. Mello CJ, Irwin RS, Curley FJ. Predictive values of the character, timing, and complications of chronic cough in diagnosing its cause. Arch Intern Med 1996; 156:997–1003.
30. French CL, Irwin RS, Curley FJ, et al. Impact of chronic cough on quality of life. Arch Intern Med 1998;158:1657–61.
31. French CT, Irwin RS, Fletcher KE, et al. Evaluation of a cough-specific quality-of-life questionnaire. Chest 2002;121:1123–31.
32. Fletcher KE, French CT, Irwin RS, et al. A prospective global measure, the Punum Ladder, provides more valid assessments of quality of life than retrospective transition measures. J Clin Epidemiol, in press.
33. Barnes PJ. Neurogenic inflammation in the airways. Respir Physiol 2001;125: 145–54.
34. McGarvey LPA. Does idiopathic cough exist? Lung 2008;186(Suppl 1):S78–81.
35. Undem BJ, Lee M-G. Basic mechanisms of cough: current understanding and remaining questions. Lung 2008;186(Suppl 1):S10–6.
36. McLeod RL, Correll CC, Jia Y, et al. TRPV1 antagonists as potential antitussive agents. Lung 2008;186(Suppl 1):S59–65.
37. Lee H, Woo P. Chronic cough as a sign of laryngeal sensory neuropathy: diagnosis and treatment. Ann Otol Rhinol Laryngol 2005;114:253–7.
38. Morrison M, Rammage L, Emami AJ. The irritable larynx syndrome. J Voice 1999; 13:447–55.
39. Birring SS, Murphy AC, Scullion JE, et al. Idiopathic chronic cough and organ-specific autoimmune diseases: a case–control study. Respir Med 2004;98: 242–6.
40. Vertigan AE, Theodoros DG, Gibson PG, et al. Efficacy of speech pathology management for chronic cough: a randomized placebo controlled trial of treatment efficacy. Thorax 2006;61:1065–9.
41. Morice AH, Menon MS, Mulrennan SA, et al. Opiate therapy in chronic cough. Am J Respir Crit Care Med 2007;175:312–5.
42. Hunt LW, Swedlung HA, Gleich GJ. Effect of nebulized lidocaine on severe glucocorticoid-dependent asthma. Mayo Clin Proc 1996;71:361–8.
43. Almansa-Pastor A. Treating refractory cough with aerosols of mepivacine. Chest 1966;110:1374–5.
44. Jeyakumar A, Brickman T, Haben M. Effectiveness of amitriptyline versus cough suppressants in the treatment of chronic cough resulting from postviral vagal neuropathy. Laryngoscope 2006;116:2108–12.
45. Laukka MA, Cameron AJ, Schei AJ. Gastroesophageal reflux and chronic cough: which comes first? J Clin Gastroenterol 1994;19:100–4.
46. Andrews NC, Curtis GM, Klassen KP, et al. Palliative vagotomy for nonresectable bronchogenic carcinoma. Ill Med J 1956;110:167–71.

Cough in the Pediatric Population

Anne B. Chang, MBBS, FRACP, PhD[a,b,*],
Robert G. Berkowitz, MBBS, MD, FRACS[c]

KEYWORDS

- Pediatric cough • Chronic cough • Otolaryngology
- Nonspecific cough

Otolaryngologists are sometimes referred children with cough as cough is the most common symptom that results in medical consultations.[1–3] In the United States, 29.5 million visits to doctors are for cough.[4] Although most of these consultations are likely for acute cough (cough lasting less than 2 weeks[5]), a significant number of consults are for chronic cough. Otolaryngologists are unlikely to encounter children with acute cough, however, other than in the context of an aspiration of a foreign body. Hence, this article concentrates on chronic cough defined as cough present for more than 4 weeks.[5] The time-length definition of chronic cough in children differs from that used in adults (more than 8 weeks), primarily based on the natural history of acute respiratory infection–associated cough in children.[6] It also takes into consideration child-specific safety issues, such as aspiration of foreign body, where delayed diagnosis can lead to long-term significant consequences.

In general, although children and adults share some commonalities, there are significant differences.[5,7,8] An example pertinent to cough is the marked difference between adults and children in the likelihood of chronic cough being a symptom of bronchial carcinoma. Cough-related issues related to adults are discussed elsewhere in articles in this issue. This article highlights and focuses the discussion on the cough issues relevant to otolaryngologists.

Work was supported by Australian National Health and Medical Research Council grants 490321 and 545216; Royal Children's Hospital Foundation, Brisbane; and Queensland Smart State Fellowship.

[a] Queensland Children's Respiratory Centre, Children's Medical Research Institute, Royal Children's Hospital, Herston, Brisbane, Queensland 4029, Australia

[b] Child Health Division, Menzies School of Health Research, Charles Darwin University, NT, Australia

[c] Department of Otolaryngology, Royal Children's Hospital, Parkville, Melbourne, Vic 3052, Australia

* Corresponding author. Queensland Children's Respiratory Centre, Queensland's Children's Medical Research Institute, Royal Children's Hospital, Herston, Brisbane, Queensland 4029, Australia.

E-mail address: annechang@ausdoctors.net (A.B. Chang).

Otolaryngol Clin N Am 43 (2010) 181–198
doi:10.1016/j.otc.2009.11.010 **oto.theclinics.com**
0030-6665/10/$ – see front matter

EPIDEMIOLOGY DATA

Prevalence

There are few accurate data on the prevalence of chronic cough in children as questionnaires for chronic cough assessment have limited validity. Published data describe community prevalence of chronic cough in primary school–aged children (6–12 years) as 5% to 10%.[9] The prevalence is likely higher in preschool-aged children as retrospective[10] and prospective[11] studies have shown that the majority of children with chronic cough seen in clinics were young (median age 2 to 3 years).

Burden of Illness

Chronic cough is considered trivial to some medical practitioners; however, the symptom is associated with significant morbidity in children and their parents.[9,12] The burden of cough is also reflected in the use of over-the-counter (OTC) cough medications consumed worldwide. Approximately 10% of US children use a cough and cold medication in a given week.[13] The cost of prescribed medicines (eg, those for asthma, gastroesophageal reflux, and so forth) used for cough is unknown. Furthermore, people report a high number of medical visits for cough before they visit a specialist. In one study that assessed the number of prior medical consultations for coughing illness in the 12 months before children first presented to a respiratory pediatrician, more than 80% of children had five or more doctor visits and 53% had more than 10.[12]

Understanding why parents consult is helpful in evaluating children with chronic cough. There are only three studies of children that have examined parental evaluations or concerns of their children's coughing illness. In the two older studies, parents' main concerns were related to disturbed sleep, discomfort, and fear that cough would cause permanent chest damage.[14,15] A recent Australian study involving 190 families described that the most significant concerns and worries expressed by parents were feelings of frustration, being upset, sleepless nights, awakenings at night, helplessness, stress, and feeling sorry for the child. Specific issues that bothered parents most were the cause of cough, cough relating to a serious illness, their child not sleeping well, and cough causing damage.[12] These concerns and worries of parents were significantly reduced when the child's cough resolved.[12]

Unlike adults with chronic cough, children with chronic cough did not have symptoms of anxiety.[12] Also parents of children with chronic cough did not have symptoms of anxiety or depression but were under stress.[12] This is in contrast to the data in adults with chronic cough, which showed associated anxiety or depression symptoms.[16–19]

PATHOPHYSIOLOGY

There is direct and indirect evidence that age influences the physiologic domains that influence the clinical manifestation of conditions where cough is a dominant feature. These physiologic domains can be simplified:

1. Cough-specific physiology
2. General respiratory physiology
3. Other direct systems, such as the immune system, that influence the respiratory system
4. Other general physiology.

Much of these data are available elsewhere.[20] Examples of cough-specific physiologic differences include age- and gender-related variations in cough sensitivity.[21–23] In children, gender does not influence cough sensitivity,[23] whereas in postpubertal adolescents and adults, girls and women have significantly increased sensitivity.[21,22] Also, the cough reflex is weak in premature infants and develops with maturity.[24] Exactly when the cough reflex is fully matured is unknown but it is likely at approximately age 5, which is the cutoff age for risk of accidental nut inhalation; thus, parents are advised not to give nuts to their children prior to age 5. Also, adults easily expectorate when airway secretions are present whereas children do not, even when secretions are abundant.[25] Thus classical adult terms, such as productive cough, cannot be applied to young children.[26]

Examples of general respiratory physiology include differences in caliber of large and small airways and percentage of time spent in rapid eye movement sleep, which influences cough frequency.[27] Smaller airway caliber (which influences air flow exponentially as opposed to linearly) and lack of collateral ventilation in immature lungs influence the likelihood of presence of wheeze and atelectasis in respiratory conditions in which chronic cough is common, such as chronic suppurative lung disease and right middle lobe syndrome.[26,28]

The immune system, which has its own developmental physiology,[29] affects the degree and frequency of respiratory infections, hence, presentations to doctors for cough. Other general physiology that influences the pathophysiology and management in children compared to adults includes differences in cognitive function, ability to self-express, and so forth.

Thus, there are observed differences in cause, management, and measurement of response between children and adults. Cough quality (eg, brassy cough and wet cough) used in children as a marker of some conditions[25,30] is less useful in adults.[31] Also, although empirical therapy (for asthma, gastroesophageal reflux disease [GERD], and upper airway disease) for chronic cough is widely advocated in adults,[7] such an approach is not advocated in children.[5,32,33] There is some evidence that an empirical approach is potentially harmful, related to the use of medications[10,34,35] and the delay in obtaining a correct diagnosis, such as missed foreign body aspiration, that lead to bronchiectasis. The differences between adults and children are also exemplified in child-specific diagnoses, such as protracted bacterial bronchitis and evidence-based cough guidelines.[5,7,36]

ETIOLOGIC FACTORS

Common etiologic causes are dependent on the setting or practice and consideration of whether or not coexistent symptoms are taken into account. For example, in Iran, pediatric chronic cough is not uncommonly associated with eosinophilia related to parasitic infestation.[37] In Indigenous settings in rural Australia, the most common cause of chronic cough is bronchiectasis.[38] In affluent urban settings, these diagnoses for chronic cough are rare.[39] Also, common etiology depends on whether or not isolated cough is considered (ie, cough without other symptoms or nonspecific cough) or cough in association with other symptoms (specific cough). In a Turkish study, 25% of the children with chronic cough managed in accordance with American College of Chest Physicians guidelines had asthma. This was not surprising, as the cohort included children without isolated cough; 18.5% of children had airway reversibility at the first assessment.[40] In contrast, most children with isolated cough do not have asthma.[5,41,42] Thus, although an otolaryngologist may encounter any underlying cause of a child's chronic cough, the frequency of the etiologic factors is likely different from that seen by pulmonologists. **Table 1** highlights common etiologic factors in children, including differences from adults and level of evidence defining cause and effect.

Table 1
Etiologic factors[a] of chronic cough in children, including differences from adults and level of evidence defining cause and effect

	Type of Cough[b]	Key Difference Between Children and Adults	Best Method for Confirmation of Diagnosis	Alternative Method for Confirmation of Diagnosis	Highest Level of Evidence[c]	Limitation
Asthma	Dry[80]	Nonspecific cough in children is unlikely asthma.[80] In adults, isolated cough is commonly asthma.[81]	Reversibility of FEV_1 demonstrated on spirometry	Indirect challenge for airway hyper-responsiveness^	RCT for cough associated with other symptoms.[80]	Asthma medications for nonspecific cough not effective.[58,59]
Protracted bronchitis	Wet[30]	Not described in adults	Bronchoscopy and response to antibiotics[11]	Response to antibiotics	Meta-analysis[47] cohort[11,30]	
Tracheobron-chomalacia	Brassy for tracheomalacia[25]	Not known if useful in adults (no studies)	Bronchoscopy	Airway screen (no data on specificity or sensitivity)	Cohort[82]	
Tonsillar hypertrophy	Dry[43]	In adults, snoring is associated with bronchitis.[83] In otherwise normal children with OSA, most do not have a cough.	Direct visualization		Case series[43]	
Rhinitis	Dry	Consideration of immune testing, CF screen, etc recommended in children with persistent rhinitis[84]	Defined by AAAAI and ACAAI as "characterised by one or more of following symptoms: nasal congestion, rhinnorhea, sneezing, itching[84]"	No diagnostic tests but in some skin testing (preferred method), IgE immunoassays or nasal endoscopy are required[84]	RCT[56] but meta-analysis of studies of antihistamines for seasonal allergic rhinitis shows different results to single positive RCT.[55]	Change in cough marginal compared to other symptoms and no difference seen in night-time cough[56]

Chronic rhinosinusitis	Wet or dry	Consideration of immune testing, CF screen, etc recommended in children with persistent rhinitis.[84] Different sinus develops at different ages with adult sizes attained usually by 14 years to late adolescents.[85]	Major symptoms (nasal congestion or obstruction, nasal discharge with or without facial pain/ pressure, olfactory disturbance) and either endoscopic signs (polyps, mucopurulent discharge, edema, obstruction at meatus) or CT changes[86]	Clinical diagnosis primarily with limited role for radiology as CT scans are abnormal in a third of population[86]	Descriptive studies.[85] Cough inconsistently mentioned in guidelines as a symptom.[85,86]	Other studies have shown that while there was a significant difference in rhinitis-specific symptoms, there was no significant difference in cough.[87]
Aspiration	Wet[88]	In children, aspiration is associated with those with multisystem dysfunction (ie, not only neurology problems[89]). In adults, aspiration most common in those with stroke	Videofluoroscopy[88]	Speech pathology clinical evaluation	Case series[88]	
GERD and laryngophargngeal reflux	Dry unless associated with aspiration	GERD as cause of nonspecific cough is uncommon in children[11,90] but common in adults[91]	pH monitoring with limitations[92]	Role of barium meal and esophageal impedence monitoring uncertain	Case series[93] Gastroenterology-based guidelines are less definitive about the association between cough and GERD.[66,94,95]	Increased respiratory problems in infants with GERD treated with proton pump inhibitors[34]

(*continued on next page*)

Table 1
(continued)

	Type of Cough[b]	Key Difference Between Children and Adults	Best Method for Confirmation of Diagnosis	Alternative Method for Confirmation of Diagnosis	Highest Level of Evidence[c]	Limitation
Underlying lung disease, such as bronchiectasis, interstitial lung disease	Depends on cause		High-resolution CT scan[96]	Depends on cause	Depends on cause, meta-analysis for bronchiectasis[97]	
Pulmonary infections (eg mycoplasma, pertussis, chlamydia, tuberculosis)	Depends on cause. In pertussis with or without whoop and vomiting. Generally dry post acute phase.	Adults with pertussis rarely whoop or have post-tussive vomiting[98]	Bronchoalveolar lavage, nasopharyngeal specimen (PCR or culture)	Sputum or bloods when specific tests available		
Habit and psychogenic cough	Dry	Characteristic cough recognized in children but not in adults[99]	No diagnostic test	Response to psychologic based Rx	Cohort studies[99]	

Abbreviations: AAAAI, American Academy of Allergy Asthma & Immunology; ACAAI, American College of Allergy, Asthma & Immunology; CF, cystic fibrosis; FEV_1, forced expiratory volume in the first second of expiration; OSA, obstructive sleep apnea; PCR, polymerase chain reaction; Rx, therapy or therapies.

[a] More rare causes associated with cough are not included (ie, almost all pulmonary and some cardiac disorders can present with chronic cough).

[b] Type of cough refers to quality of spontaneous cough. When a child has not coughed spontaneously during the consultation, the child's cough character may be elicited by requesting the child to cough several times.[25] There is sometimes a difference, however, between spontaneous cough and volunteered cough.

[c] Highest level of evidence is evidence that refers to whether not cough resolves with treatment specific for cause in pediatric studies.

Conditions that otolaryngologists may encounter in the evaluation of children with chronic cough include the conditions listed in **Table 1**.[43,44]

EVALUATION OF CHILDREN WITH CHRONIC COUGH

Etiologically based diagnosis is the main strategy for treating cough in adults and children; however, although an integrative empirical treatment strategy works well in adults, an etiologically based treatment is best for children.[5,8,33] Thus, defining the cause is an important component of the evaluation. In defining the cause, it is helpful to define cough types in accordance with different constructs. Pediatric chronic cough can be classified in several constructs based on (1) likelihood of an identifiable underlying primary cause (specific and nonspecific cough) or (2) characteristic (moist versus dry). Specific cough refers to cough associated with other symptoms and signs that are suggestive of an associated or underlying problem, and nonspecific cough is dry cough in the absence of any identifiable respiratory disease or known cause. These classifications are, however, not mutually exclusive.

Wet/Moist/Productive Cough Versus Dry Cough

Even when airway secretions are present, young children rarely expectorate sputum. Hence, wet/moist cough is a preferable to productive cough.[45,46] The distinction of dry and wet/moist cough has been shown to be valid and reliable. In a study of 106 children, cough quality (wet/dry) assessed by clinicians had good agreement with parents assessment ($\kappa = 0.75$; 95% CI, 0.58–0.93) and had good sensitivity (0.75) and specificity (0.79) when compared to bronchoscopy findings.[25] The use of wet versus dry cough for predicting cause of cough or response to treatment has not been shown in children, except in protracted bronchitis.[47]

Specific and Nonspecific Chronic Cough

Clinical signs and symptoms that are suggestive of an underlying pulmonary or systemic disorder are termed specific cough pointers (**Box 1**). When any of these pointers are present, the cough is referred to as specific cough.[48] If specific cough pointers are present, further investigations and management of the primary pulmonary pathology are usually warranted. If not, a counsel, watch, wait, and review approach is suggested. This approach is suggested for nonspecific cough (dry cough in the absence of specific cough pointers). Such a cough is more likely to undergo natural resolution[30]; however, a dry cough may be the early phase of a wet cough,[49] so children should be reviewed and attention to exacerbation factors and parental concerns is warranted (discussed later).

In selected children with nonspecific cough, diagnoses with simple treatment options (eg, asthma and complications of upper respiratory tract infections, such as sinusitis and bronchitis, may be considered). The evidence for the association between asthma[26,48] and upper airway disorders and cough, however, is not as straightforward in children as it is in adults.[8,50] The use of isolated cough as a marker of asthma is controversial, with more recent evidence (clinical and community epidemiologic studies) showing that in most children, isolated cough or nonspecific cough does not represent asthma.[41,48,51]

Investigations

At minimum, all children with chronic cough should have a spirometry (if age appropriate) and chest radiograph performed.[5,6] The validity of these has been shown.[30] When a chest radiograph taken for chronic cough is abnormal, the odds ratio of

Box 1
Pointers for presence of specific cough

Auscultatory findings (wheeze, crepitations/crackles, differential breath sounds, stridor)

Cough characteristics (eg, cough with choking, cough quality cough starting from birth)

Cardiac abnormalities (including murmurs)

Chest pain

Chest wall deformity

Daily moist or productive cough

Digital clubbing

Dyspnea (exertional or at rest)

Exposure to pertussis, tuberculosis, etc

Failure to thrive

Feeding difficulties or dysphagia (including choking/vomiting)

Hemoptysis

Immune deficiency

Medications or drugs (angiotensin-converting enzyme inhibitor)

Neurodevelopmental abnormality

Recurrent pneumonia

Data from Chang AB, Landau LI, van Asperen PP, et al. The Thoracic Society of Australia and New Zealand. Position statement. Cough in children: definitions and clinical evaluation. Med J Aust 2006;184:398–403.

a specific cause was 3.16 (95% CI, 1.32–7.62).[30] Other tests to identify the cause of nonspecific cough have limited applicability in pediatrics (but are included in **Table 1**). Identification of airway hyper-responsiveness, diagnostic for asthma in adults, is of limited use in children because of interpretation difficulties, and reliable tests can only be performed in older children in whom cough is less common. The three most common causes of chronic cough in adults (GERD, asthma, and upper airways syndrome)[7] are not as common in children.[11,33] Increased cough sensitivity is found in most conditions causing chronic cough but its utility is limited to research.[5]

Except when classical asthma is the cause, children with specific cough usually require additional tests (chest high-resolution CT scan, bronchoscopy, videofluoroscopy, echocardiograph, sleep polysomnography, nuclear medicine scans, immunologic assessment, and so forth). Brief points on the role of selected investigations for the more common causes of chronic cough are summarized in **Table 1**. A comprehensive role of all available tests for evaluation of lung disease is beyond the scope of this article, as it would encompass the entire spectrum of pediatric respiratory illness.

Medications

Treatment of chronic cough should be etiologically based, which for specific cough (which includes almost all respiratory diseases) is beyond the scope of this article. Clinicians should be cognizant that cough is subjected to the period effect (ie, spontaneous resolution of cough); the benefit of placebo treatment of cough has been reported to be as high as 85% and, therefore, nonplacebo-controlled intervention studies have to be interpreted with caution.[48] Evidence (or lack of) for efficacy of treatment trials for nonspecific cough is summarized in **Table 2**. Systematic reviews have concluded that cough OTCs have little benefit in the symptomatic control of childhood cough. Significant morbidity and mortality[52] from cough OTCs can occur and OTCs are common unintentional ingestions in children aged under age 5.[53] Cochrane reviews of symptomatic treatment of cough have shown that diphenhyramine is not beneficial for pertussis-related cough; cromones and anticholinergics have little, if any, role in nonspecific chronic childhood cough; and, 10 days of antimicrobials reduces persistent cough in children with chronic nasal discharge but benefits are modest (number needed to treat was eight). Antimicrobials may be indicated for subacute/chronic moist cough; two randomized controlled trials (RCTs) showed predominance of *Moraxella catarrhalis*. Meta-analysis of antimicrobials for acute bronchitis in older children (age older than 8 years) and adults showed a small benefit of 0.58 days but with significantly more adverse events. Systematic review of uncomplicated sinusitis in children showed that the clinical improvement rate was 88% with antimicrobial and 60% with no antimicrobial. Observational studies show an improvement in cough associated with rhinitis.[54] A single small (n = 20) RCT in children with allergic rhinitis treated with antihistamines showed benefit but larger safety studies (combined n = 793) did not.[55] In comparison, a large difference between groups was found for nasal symptoms and there was no difference in nighttime cough.[56] An earlier study in children with asthma and nasal obstruction showed decreased cough in addition to asthma severity in those randomized to intranasal budesonide.[57] There are only two published RCTs on inhaled corticosteroids for nonspecific cough in children and both groups cautioned against its prolonged use.[58,59]

Laryngopharyngeal reflux is widely regarded by some people as a cause of chronic cough related to GERD. To date, however, all but one RCT with subjects enrolled from ear, nose, and throat clinics where cough was an outcome measure have shown that proton pump inhibitors (the main stay of GERD treatment) are not efficacious when compared to placebo.[60,61] This includes the largest (n = 145) of these studies involving GERD therapy with cough as an outcome measure.[62] Two independent systematic reviews found that high-dose proton pump inhibitor was no more effective than placebo in producing symptomatic improvement or resolution of cough presumed related to laryngopharyngeal reflux.[60,63] Furthermore, a controlled non-randomized study showed that fundoplication was not efficacious for cough either.[64] In contrast, "uncontrolled studies suggest that 40%–100% of patients who have suspected acid-related ear, nose, and throat symptoms improve on aggressive anti-reflux therapy."[65] In the North American Society for Pediatric Gastroenterology and Nutrition guidelines for pediatric gastroesophageal reflux, the conclusion on cough and GERD section was "there is insufficient evidence and experience in children for a uniform approach to diagnosis and treatment."[66]

If medications are trialed for nonspecific cough, children should be reviewed and time to response considered. For example, in asthma-related cough, earlier non-RCT studies in adults and children that utilized medications for asthma for the era (ie, nonsteroids, theophylline, terbutaline, and major tranquillizers) reported that cough completely resolved by 2 to 7 days.[48] Time to response is defined as the expected length of time cough resolution occurred in studies where the cough treated was related to the defined cause.

Defining Exacerbation Factors

When reviewing any child with cough irrespective of the cause, exacerbation factors should be explored, although no RCTs have examined the effect of cessation of environmental pollutants on cough. There is little doubt that children with environmental

Table 2
Recommendations for possible interventions for nonspecific cough in children

Therapy	Recommendation	Type and Strength of Evidence	Time to Response*
Antihistamines Nonsedating Sedating	Not generally recommended unless symptoms of rhinitis coexist Sedating antihistamines should not be used	SR with RCTs[55,100]	1 week Not relevant
Antimicrobials	For wet cough only	SR with RCTs[47]	1–2 wk
Asthma-type therapy			
Cromones	Not recommended	SR with single open trial[101]	2 wk
Anticholinergics	Not recommended	SR, no studies in children RCTs[102]	No data
Inhaled CS	Not generally recommended unless symptoms of asthma present	SR with RCTs[58,59]	2–4 wk
Oral CS	Not recommended	No data	
β_2-Agonist (oral or inhaled)	Not generally recommended unless symptoms of asthma present	SR with RCTs[103] RCT[58]	Not relevant
Theophylline	Not recommended	SR, no studies[104]	1–2 wk
Leukotriene receptor antagonist	Not recommended unless symptoms of asthma present	SR, observational study[105]	2–3 wk
GORD therapy			
Motility agents	Not recommended as empirical therapy	SR with single trial[60]	Not relevant

Acid suppression	Not recommended as empirical therapy	SR with no RCTs in children[60]	
Food thickening or antireflux formula	Consider if other symptoms of reflux present (infants only)	SR with RCTs[60]	1 wk
Fundoplication		SR[60]	
Herbal antitussive therapy	Not recommended	No data	
Nasal therapy			
Nasal steroids	Not generally recommended unless symptoms of rhinitis coexist.	RCT[56] beneficial when combined with antibiotics for sinusitis[106]	1–2 wk
Other nasal sprays	Not recommended	No data	
OTC cough medications	Not recommended	SR with RCTs[100,107,108]	Not relevant
Other therapies			
Steam, vapor, rubs	Consider rubs but not vapor or steam	No data	
Honey	Recommended if no contraindications for using of honey	Single RCT on acute cough[109]	One day
Physiotherapy	Not recommended unless cough related to suppurative lung disease	No data in cough that is unrelated to suppurative-like lung diseases	

Abbreviations: CS, corticosteroids; SR, systematic review.
* Time taken for cough to resolve as reported by triallist.

tobacco smoke (ETS) exposure have increased risk of having chronic[67,68] and recurrent cough.[69] Cough resolution was achieved in children exposed to ETS, however, in several studies,[11,40] which suggests that ETS alone is not the sole cause. The American Academy of Pediatrics policy on tobacco includes recommendations for tobacco cessation.[70] Other exacerbation factors include exposure to pollutants and secondary gains from having a cough.

Defining Effect on Child and Parent

As discussed previously, parents presenting to doctors for their children's cough have significant concerns, which causes parental stress.[12] Exploration of parental expectations and fears is valuable when managing children with a chronic cough. Providing parents with information on the expected time length of resolution of respiratory tract infections respiratory tract infections may reduce anxiety in parents and the need for medication use.[71] Parental and professional expectations and doctors' perceptions of patients' expectations influence consulting rates and prescription of medications in respiratory tract infections.[72,73] It is also known that information available from the Internet provides incorrect advice on the home management of cough in children.[74]

Assessing Response to Therapy

Several methods are available to objectively assess cough frequency, cough severity, and a cough's response to therapy. Child-specific assessment tools are required in children as the adult assessment tools have limited applicability in children.[8] For example, in the assessment of cough sensitivity, inspiratory flow significantly influences results,[75] and inclusion of questions about urinary incontinence and other adult-specific issues render adult cough-specific quality-of-life questionnaires inapplicable to children.[76] Adult-based cough counters cannot be assumed to be reliable in children without validation studies as young children generate lower-amplitude electromyographic and cough audio signals. The choice of the quantitative and objective cough indices performed is dependent on the setting and reason for performing the measurement.[77] In a research setting, outcome of response to therapy ideally includes objective measures (eg, cough counters) in addition to patient-orientated outcomes (quality-of-life and subjective scores). Pediatric studies have documented that objectively measured cough frequency relates to subjective cough scores and cough sensitivity.[77,78] Also, the change in cough frequency relates to the changes between cough scores and cough sensitivity.[77,78] Similar data have also recently been found in adults.[79]

In summary, when children with chronic cough present, undertake:

1. A complete medical examination, with particular attention to the cardiorespiratory systems and a focus on
   a. The clinical pattern
      - Characteristic cough (eg, pertussis, brassy/tracheomalacic cough)
      - Wet or dry cough? Protracted bronchitis?
      - Presence of specific cough pointers to differentiate specific from nonspecific cough, (see **Box 1**)
   b. Presence of exacerbation factors (such as ETS, curtailment of physical activity)
   c. Defining effect of the cough on children and parents and exploring their concerns (discussed previously)
2. All children should undergo
   a. Chest radiograph

   b. Spirometry (if older than age 3 years in a respiratory center or older than age 6 in other centers)
3. Children should be further investigated and likely require referral to a pulmonologist if
   a. Specific cough pointers are present, other than asthma (see **Box 1**)
   b. Cough has not resolved with treatment trials
4. Assessment by an otolaryngologist should be considered when there are coexistent symptoms or signs that suggest an upper airway cause for a child's cough or if a foreign body is suspected. These include presence of stridor, snoring, obstructive sleep symptoms, laryngeal disorders causing aspiration (eg, laryngeal cleft), and persistent rhinitis/rhinosinusitis symptoms.
5. A wait, reassess, and review approach is recommended for children with nonspecific cough as medications are generally not efficacious for nonspecific cough (see **Table 2**). If medications are trialed, a reassessment is recommended in 2 to 3 weeks, which is the time to response for most medications.[5,6]

REFERENCES

1. Britt H, Miller GC, Knox S, et al. General practice activity in Australia 2003–2004. Australian Institute of Health and Welfare; 2004. Canberra: AIHW Cat. No. GEP 16.
2. Morice AH. Epidemiology of cough. Pulm Pharmacol Ther 2002;15:253–9.
3. Britt H, Miller GC, Knox S, et al. Bettering the evaluation and care of health - a study of general practice activity. Australian Institute of Health and Welfare; 2002. Canberra: AIHW Cat. No. GEP-10.
4. Irwin RS. Introduction to the diagnosis and management of cough: ACCP evidence-based clinical practice guidelines. Chest 2006;129:25S–27.
5. Chang AB, Glomb WB. Guidelines for evaluating chronic cough in pediatrics: ACCP evidence-based clinical practice guidelines. Chest 2006;129:260S–283.
6. Chang AB, Landau LI, van Asperen PP, et al. The Thoracic Society of Australia and New Zealand. Position statement. Cough in children: definitions and clinical evaluation. Med J Aust 2006;184:398–403.
7. Irwin RS, Baumann MH, Bolser DC, et al. Diagnosis and management of cough executive summary: ACCP evidence-based clinical practice guidelines. Chest 2006;129:1S–23.
8. Chang AB. Cough: are children really different to adults? Cough 2005;1:7.
9. Faniran AO, Peat JK, Woolcock AJ. Persistent cough: is it asthma? Arch Dis Child 1998;79:411–4.
10. Thomson F, Masters IB, Chang AB. Persistent cough in children—overuse of medications. J Paediatr Child Health 2002;38:578–81.
11. Marchant JM, Masters IB, Taylor SM, et al. Evaluation and outcome of young children with chronic cough. Chest 2006;129:1132–41.
12. Marchant JM, Newcombe PA, Juniper EF, et al. What is the burden of chronic cough for families? Chest 2008;134:303–9.
13. Vernacchio L, Kelly JP, Kaufman DW, et al. Cough and cold medication use by US children, 1999–2006: results from the slone survey. Pediatrics 2008;122: e323–9.
14. Cornford CS, Morgan M, Ridsdale L. Why do mothers consult when their children cough? Fam Pract 1993;10:193–6.
15. Davies MJ, Cane RS, Ranganathan SC, et al. Cough, wheeze and sleep. Arch Dis Child 1998;79:465.
16. Dicpinigaitis PV, Tso R, Banauch G. Prevalence of depressive symptoms among patients with chronic cough. Chest 2006;130:1839–43.

17. Ludviksdottir D, Bjornsson E, Janson C, et al. Habitual coughing and its associations with asthma, anxiety, and gastroesophageal reflux. Chest 1996;109:1262–8.
18. McGarvey LP, Carton C, Gamble LA, et al. Prevalence of psychomorbidity among patients with chronic cough. Cough 2006;2:4.
19. French CT, Irwin RS, Fletcher KE, et al. Evaluation of a cough-specific quality-of-life questionnaire. Chest 2002;121:1123–31.
20. Chang AB, Widdicombe JG. Cough throughout life: children, adults and the senile. Pulm Pharmacol Ther 2006;20:371–82.
21. Kelsall A, Decalmer S, McGuinness K, et al. Sex differences and predictors of objective cough frequency in chronic cough. Thorax 2009;64:393–8.
22. Varechova S, Plevkova J, Hanacek J, et al. Role of gender and pubertal stage on cough sensitivity in childhood and adolescence. J Physiol Pharmacol 2008;59(Suppl 6):719–26.
23. Chang AB, Phelan PD, Sawyer SM, et al. Cough sensitivity in children with asthma, recurrent cough, and cystic fibrosis. Arch Dis Child 1997;77:331–4.
24. Burns Y, Rogers Y, Neil M, et al. Development of oral function in pre-term infants. Physiotherapy Pract 1987;3:168–78.
25. Chang AB, Eastburn MM, Gaffney J, et al. Cough quality in children: a comparison of subjective vs. bronchoscopic findings. Respir Res 2005;6:3.
26. Chang AB, Redding GJ, Everard ML. Chronic wet cough: protracted bronchitis, chronic suppurative lung disease and bronchiectasis. Pediatr Pulmonol 2008; 43:519–31.
27. Widdicombe J, Eccles R, Fontana G. Supramedullary influences on cough. Respir Physiol Neurobiol 2006;152:320–8.
28. Everard M. New respect for old conditions. Pediatr Pulmonol 2007;42:400–2.
29. Tulic MK, Fiset PO, Manuokion JJ, et al. Roll of toll like receptor 4 in protection by bacterial lipopolysaccharide in the nasal mucosa of children but not adults. Lancet 2004;363:1689–98.
30. Marchant JM, Masters IB, Taylor SM, et al. Utility of signs and symptoms of chronic cough in predicting specific cause in children. Thorax 2006;61:694–8.
31. Mello CJ, Irwin RS, Curley FJ. Predictive values of the character, timing, and complications of chronic cough in diagnosing its cause. Arch Intern Med 1996;156:997–1003.
32. Chang AB. Cough. Pediatr Clin North Am 2009;56:19–31.
33. Shields MD, Bush A, Everard ML, et al. British Thoracic Society Guidelines Recommendations for the assessment and management of cough in children. Thorax 2008;63:iii1–15.
34. Orenstein SR, Hassall E, Furmaga-Jablonska W, et al. Multicenter, double-blind, randomized, placebo-controlled trial assessing the efficacy and safety of proton pump inhibitor lansoprazole in infants with symptoms of gastroesophageal reflux disease. J Pediatr 2009;154:514–20.
35. Russell G. Very high dose inhaled corticosteroids: panacea or poison? Arch Dis Child 2006;91:802–4.
36. Chang AB. ACCP cough guidelines for children: can its use improve outcomes? Chest 2008;134:1111–2.
37. Alavi SM, Sefidgaran G. Frequency of anti Toxocara antibodies in schoolchildren with chronic cough and eosinophilia in Ahwaz, Iran, 2006. Pak J Med Sci 2008; 24:360–3.
38. Anderson SD, Brannan JD. Methods for "indirect" challenge tests including exercise, eucapnic voluntary hyperpnea, and hypertonic aerosols. Clin Rev Allergy Immunol 2003;24:27–54.

39. Marchant JM, Chang AB. Re: evaluation and outcome of young children with chronic cough. Chest 2006;130:1279–80.
40. Asilsoy S, Bayram E, Agin H, et al. Evaluation of chronic cough in children. Chest 2008;134:1122–8.
41. McKenzie S. Cough—but is it asthma? Arch Dis Child 1994;70:1–2.
42. de Benedictis FM, Selvaggio D, de Benedictis D. Cough, wheezing and asthma in children: lesson from the past. Pediatr Allergy Immunol 2004;15:386–93.
43. Gurgel RK, Brookes JT, Weinberger MM, et al. Chronic cough and tonsillar hypertrophy: a case series. Pediatr Pulmonol 2008;43:1147–9.
44. Litman DA, Shah UK, Pawel BR. Isolated endobronchial atypical mycobacterium in a child: a case report and review of the literature. Int J Pediatr Otorhinolaryngol 2000;55:65–8.
45. Chang AB, Masel JP, Boyce NC, et al. Non-CF bronchiectasis-clinical and HRCT evaluation. Pediatr Pulmonol 2003;35:477–83.
46. De Jongste JC, Shields MD. Chronic cough in children. Thorax 2003;58: 998–1003.
47. Marchant JM, Morris P, Gaffney J, et al. Antibiotics for prolonged moist cough in children. Cochrane Database Syst Rev 2005;4:CD004822.
48. Chang AB. State of the art: cough, cough receptors, and asthma in children. Pediatr Pulmonol 1999;28:59–70.
49. Chang AB, Faoagali J, Cox NC, et al. A bronchoscopic scoring system for airway secretions-airway cellularity and microbiological validation. Pediatr Pulmonol 2006;41:887–92.
50. Kemp AS. Does post-nasal drip cause cough in childhood? Paediatr Respir Rev 2006;7:31–5.
51. Gibson PG, Simpson JL, Chalmers AC, et al. Airway eosinophilia is associated with wheeze but is uncommon in children with persistent cough and frequent chest colds. Am J Respir Crit Care Med 2001;164:977–81.
52. Gunn VL, Taha SH, Liebelt EL, et al. Toxicity of over-the-counter cough and cold medications. Pediatrics 2001;108:E52.
53. Chien C, Marriott JL, Ashby K, et al. Unintentional ingestion of over the counter medications in children less than 5 years old. J Paediatr Child Health 2003;39:264–9.
54. Cassano M, Maselli A, Mora F, et al. Rhinobronchial syndrome: pathogenesis and correlation with allergic rhinitis in children. Int J Pediatr Otorhinolaryngol 2008;72:1053–8.
55. Chang AB, Peake J, McElrea M. Anti-histamines for prolonged non-specific cough in children. Cochrane Database Syst Rev 2008;2:CD005604.
56. Gawchik S, Goldstein S, Prenner B, et al. Relief of cough and nasal symptoms associated with allergic rhinitis by mometasone furoate nasal spray. Ann Allergy Asthma Immunol 2003;90:416–21.
57. Henriksen JM, Wenzel A. Effect of an intranasally administered corticosteroid (budesonide) on nasal obstruction, mouth breathing, and asthma. Am Rev Respir Dis 1984;130:1014–8.
58. Chang AB, Phelan PD, Carlin J, et al. Randomised controlled trial of inhaled salbutamol and beclomethasone for recurrent cough. Arch Dis Child 1998;79:6–11.
59. Davies MJ, Fuller P, Picciotto A, et al. Persistent nocturnal cough: randomised controlled trial of high dose inhaled corticosteroid. Arch Dis Child 1999;81: 38–44.
60. Chang AB, Lasserson T, Gaffney J, et al. Gastro-oesophageal reflux treatment for prolonged non-specific cough in children and adults. Cochrane Database Syst Rev 2005;2:CD004823.

61. Chang AB, Lasserson TJ, Kiljander TO, et al. Systematic review and meta-analysis of randomised controlled trials of gastro-oesophageal reflux interventions for chronic cough associated with gastro-oesophageal reflux. BMJ 2006;332: 11–7.
62. Vaezi MF, Richter JE, Stasney CR, et al. Treatment of chronic posterior laryngitis with esomeprazole. Laryngoscope 2006;116:254–60.
63. Gatta L, Vaira D, Sorrenti G, et al. Meta-analysis: the efficacy of proton pump inhibitors for laryngeal symptoms attributed to gastro-oesophageal reflux disease. Aliment Pharmacol Ther 2008;25:385–92.
64. Swoger J, Ponsky J, Hicks DM, et al. Surgical fundoplication in laryngopharyngeal reflux unresponsive to aggressive acid suppression: a controlled study. Clin Gastroenterol Hepatol 2006;4:433–41.
65. Richter JE. Ear, nose and throat and respiratory manifestations of gastro-esophageal reflux disease: an increasing conundrum. Eur J Gastroenterol Hepatol 2004;16:837–45.
66. Rudolph CD, Mazur LJ, Liptak GS, et al. Guidelines for evaluation and treatment of gastroesophageal reflux in infants and children: recommendations of the North American Society for Pediatric Gastroenterology and Nutrition. J Pediatr Gastroenterol Nutr 2001;32(Suppl 2):S1–31.
67. Holscher B, Heinrich J, Jacob B, et al. Gas cooking, respiratory health and white blood cell counts in children. Int J Hyg Environ Health 2000;203:29–37.
68. Jaakkola JJ, Jaakkola MS. Effects of environmental tobacco smoke on the respiratory health of children. Scand J Work Environ Health 2002;28(Suppl 2):71–83.
69. Hermann C, Westergaard T, Pedersen BV, et al. A comparison of risk factors for wheeze and recurrent cough in preschool children. Am J Epidemiol 2005;162: 345–50.
70. American Academy of Pediatrics: Tobacco's toll: implications for the pediatrician. Pediatrics 2001;107:794–8.
71. Butler CC, Kinnersley P, Hood K, et al. Clinical course of acute infection of the upper respiratory tract in children: cohort study. BMJ 2003;327:1088–9.
72. Cockburn J, Pit S. Prescribing behaviour in clinical practice: patients' expectations and doctors' perceptions of patients' expectations questionnaire study. BMJ 1997;315:520–3.
73. Little P, Gould C, Williamson I, et al. Reattendance and complications in a randomised trial of prescribing strategies for sore throat: the medicalising effect of prescribing antibiotics. BMJ 1997;315:350–2.
74. Morris P, Leach A. Antibiotics for persistent nasal discharge (rhinosinusitis) in children. Cochrane Database Syst Rev 2002;2:CD001094.
75. Chang AB, Phelan PD, Roberts RGD, et al. Capsaicin cough receptor sensitivity test in children. Eur Respir J 1996;9:2220–3.
76. Newcombe PA, Sheffield JK, Juniper EF, et al. Development of a parent-proxy quality-of-life chronic cough-specific questionnaire: clinical impact vs psychometric evaluations. Chest 2008;133:386–95.
77. Chang AB, Phelan PD, Robertson CF, et al. Relationship between measurements of cough severity. Arch Dis Child 2003;88:57–60.
78. Chang AB, Phelan PD, Robertson CF, et al. Frequency and perception of cough severity. J Paediatr Child Health 2001;37:142–5.
79. Decalmer SC, Webster D, Kelsall AA, et al. Chronic cough: how do cough reflex sensitivity and subjective assessments correlate with objective cough counts during ambulatory monitoring? Thorax 2007;62:329–34.

80. British Thoracic Society. British Guideline on the Management of Asthma. Thorax 2008;63:iv1–121.
81. Irwin RS, Curley FJ, French CL. Chronic cough. The spectrum and frequency of causes, key components of the diagnostic evaluation, and outcome of specific therapy. Am Rev Respir Dis 1990;141:640–7.
82. Masters IB, Zimmerman PV, Pandeya N, et al. Quantified tracheobronchomalacia disorders and their clinical profiles in children. Chest 2007;133:461–7.
83. Baik I, Kim J, Abbott RD, et al. Association of snoring with chronic bronchitis. Arch Intern Med 2008;168:167–73.
84. Wallace DV, Dykewicz MS, Bernstein DI, et al. The diagnosis and management of rhinitis: an updated practice parameter. J Allergy Clin Immunol 2008;122:S1–84.
85. Slavin RG, Spector SL, Bernstein IL, et al. The diagnosis and management of sinusitis: a practice parameter update. J Allergy Clin Immunol 2005;116: S13–47.
86. Scadding GK, Durham SR, Mirakian R, et al. BSACI guidelines for the management of rhinosinusitis and nasal polyposis. Clin Exp Allergy 2008;38:260–75.
87. Lusk RP, Bothwell MR, Piccirillo J. Long-term follow-up for children treated with surgical intervention for chronic rhinosinusitis. Laryngoscope 2006;116: 2099–107.
88. Weir K, McMahon S, Barry L, et-al. Clinical signs and symptoms of oropharyngeal aspiration and dysphagia in children. Eur Respir J 2009;33:604–11.
89. Weir K, McMahon S, Barry L, et al. Oropharyngeal aspiration and pneumonia in children. Pediatr Pulmonol 2007;42:1024–31.
90. Chang AB, Cox NC, Faoagali J, et al. Cough and reflux esophagitis in children: their co-existence and airway cellularity. BMC Pediatr 2006;6:4.
91. Irwin RS. Chronic cough due to gastroesophageal reflux disease: ACCP evidence-based clinical practice guidelines. Chest 2006;129:80S–94S.
92. Eastburn MM, Katelaris PH, Chang AB. Defining the relationship between gastroesophageal reflux and cough: probabilities, possibilities and limitations. Cough 2007;3:4.
93. Chang AB, Lasserson TJ, Gaffney J, et al. Gastro-oesophageal reflux treatment for prolonged non-specific cough in children and adults. Cochrane Database Syst Rev 2006;4:CD004823.
94. Katelaris P, Holloway R, Talley N, et al. Gastro-oesophageal reflux disease in adults: guidelines for clinicians. J Gastroenterol Hepatol 2002;17:825–33.
95. Vakil N, van Zanten SV, Kahrilas P, et al. The Montreal definition and classification of gastroesophageal reflux disease: a global evidence-based consensus. Am J Gastroenterol 2006;101:1900–20.
96. Webb WR, Muller NL, Naidich DP. High-resolution computed tomography findings of lung disease. Philadelphia: Lippincott, Williams & Wilkins; 2001. p. 467–546.
97. Evans DJ, Bara AI, Greenstone M. Prolonged antibiotics for purulent bronchiectasis. Cochrane Database Syst Rev 2007;2:CD001392.
98. Marchant JM, Chang AB. Managing pertussis in adults. Aust Prescriber 2009; 32:36–8.
99. Irwin RS, Glomb WB, Chang AB, et al. Habit cough, Tic cough, and psychogenic cough in adult and pediatric populations: ACCP evidence-based clinical practice guidelines. Chest 2006;129:174S–179.
100. Schroeder K, Fahey T. Should we advise parents to administer over the counter cough medicines for acute cough? Systematic review of randomised controlled trials. Arch Dis Child 2002;86:170–5.

101. Chang AB, Marchant JM, Morris P. Cromones for prolonged non-specific cough in children. Cochrane Database Syst Rev 2004;1:CD004436.
102. Chang AB, McKean M, Morris P. Inhaled anti-cholinergics for prolonged non-specific cough in children. Cochrane Database Syst Rev 2003;4: CD004358.
103. Smucny JJ, Flynn CA, Becker LA, et al. Are beta2-agonists effective treatment for acute bronchitis or acute cough in patients without underlying pulmonary disease? A systematic review. J Fam Pract 2001;50:945–51.
104. Chang AB, Halstead RA, Petsky HL. Methylxanthines for prolonged non-specific cough in children. Cochrane Database Syst Rev 2005;3:CD005310.
105. Chang AB, Winter D, Acworth JP. Leukotriene receptor antagonist for prolonged non-specific cough in children. Cochrane Database Syst Rev 2006;2: CD005602.
106. Barlan IB, Erkan E, Bakir M, et al. Intranasal budesonide spray as an adjunct to oral antibiotic therapy for acute sinusitis in children. Ann Allergy Asthma Immunol 1997;78:598–601.
107. Schroeder K, Fahey T. Over-the-counter medications for acute cough in children and adults in ambulatory settings. Cochrane Database Syst Rev 2004;4: CD001831.
108. Paul IM, Yoder KE, Crowell KR, et al. Effect of dextromethorphan, diphenhydramine, and placebo on nocturnal cough and sleep quality for coughing children and their parents. Pediatrics 2004;114:e85–90.
109. Paul IM, Beiler J, McMonagle A, et al. Effect of honey, dextromethorphan, and no treatment on nocturnal cough and sleep quality for coughing children and their parents. Arch Pediatr Adolesc Med 2007;161:1140–6.

Future Directions in Treating Cough

Lorcan P.A. McGarvey, MD, MRCP[a,b,*], Jennifer Elder, MB, MRCP[b]

KEYWORDS

• Cough • Treatment • Novel therapy

Over the last four decades, considerable advances in basic and applied science have improved the understanding of the physiology and pathophysiology of cough. During this time, there also have been advances in the clinical management of cough with the development of systematic and protocol-based algorithms for diagnosing and treating cough.[1,2] This approach has formed the basis of current management guidelines for both adult and pediatric patients with cough.[3–6] In recent years, however, there has been a sense that progress has slowed with debate over the strength of the evidence base for current treatment recommendations,[7,8] the withdrawal of some established therapies following safety concerns,[9] and the recognition in both primary and secondary care of greater proportions of symptomatic patients with idiopathic or unexplained cough.[10–13] Such pessimism, however, seems misplaced given the number of developments over this time in diagnostic and experimental techniques relevant to cough. This article provides the authors' opinion on the future direction of the treatment of cough. The authors suggest that this requires a refinement of existing management protocols and fresh thinking on the clinical syndrome of cough with more emphasis on the common triggers and aggravating factors. Therefore, this article focuses on two main areas: the optimization of existing recommendations for the management of cough and the clinical features and consequences of cough reflex hypersensitivity associated with common acute and chronic cough syndromes. Throughout this article, to the authors highlight important gaps in knowledge and identify areas where advances may be made to improve the treatment of cough in the future.

ACUTE AND CHRONIC COUGH—THE EXTENT OF THE PROBLEM

The exact prevalence of cough in the general population is difficult to quantify with certainty, but depending on the population surveyed and the tools used, reported figures range from 3.3% to 33%. Cough remains the most common reason for which

[a] Respiratory Medicine Research Group, Centre for Infection and Immunity, The Queen's University of Belfast, Grosvenor Road, Belfast, BT12 6BN, Northern Ireland, UK
[b] The Royal Group Hospitals, Grosvenor Road, Belfast, Northern Ireland, UK
* Corresponding author. Respiratory Medicine Research Group, Centre for Infection and Immunity, The Queen's University of Belfast, Grosvenor Road, Belfast, BT12 6BN, Northern Ireland.
E-mail address: l.mcgarvey@qub.ac.uk (L.P.A. McGarvey).

Otolaryngol Clin N Am 43 (2010) 199–211
doi:10.1016/j.otc.2009.11.011 **oto.theclinics.com**

patients seek medical advice, with an estimated 84 million consultations in the United States during 1 year alone.[14] Cough associated with the common cold is usually self-limiting, but many individuals self-medicate, as reflected in the considerable expenditure on over-the-counter (OTC) preparations. In 2008, a total of £102.9 million was spent in the United Kingdom on cough syrups alone, and in the United States, the figure for OTC cold remedies has been estimated in the range of $3 billion.[15] The social and financial burden of cough may be even greater if school and work absenteeism associated with the common cold (estimated at between 40 and 100 million absences per year) are considered.[16] A more complete review of the worldwide problem of cough is covered elsewhere in this series.

OPTIMIZING THE EXISTING PROTOCOLS FOR THE MANAGEMENT OF COUGH

Several consensus statements have been produced to help physicians assess and treat patients with cough. In general, the recommended approach in both adult and pediatric settings is to undertake a systematic, integrated evaluation of the patient beginning with history and physical examination, baseline investigations followed by a combination of diagnostic tests, and therapeutic trials based on a suspected cause(s).[3–6,17,18] At present, there is no agreement as to the optimal sequence of tests or empiric trials and no strong evidence that such protocols are associated with superior outcomes to a nonprotocolized approach. A cost-effectiveness analysis of the contrasting management strategies suggested that the test all then treat approach, although the most expensive, had the shortest duration to treatment success compared with a protocol of sequential trials of empiric therapy.[19]

Concerns over health care costs may become the major driver for change in the management of patients with cough. The use of allied health care professionals to manage clinical problems has been suggested as a means of controlling health care expenditure.[20] Arguing that such an approach could reduce the physician workload, decrease patient wait times, and prove cost-effective, Field and colleagues undertook a study comparing the outcomes of patients with chronic cough (defined as greater than 4 weeks duration) managed by physicians with those managed by certified respiratory educators (CREs, ie, a group of allied health care professionals with specialist training and knowledge in respiratory diseases).[21] Patients initially were screened, and those with potentially serious underlying disease were excluded. The primary endpoint was the number of patients reporting cough resolution (subjective improvement) at the 8-week follow-up. The authors reported a greater number reporting improvement in cough (although similar improvements in quality of life), a shorter referral wait time, and lower costs per successfully treated patient in the CRE arm compared with physician-treated arm. Although limited in its design, this study demonstrates that randomized controlled clinical trials of cough management protocols can be undertaken. In the future, such studies will need to be conducted to establish the most practical and cost-effective approach to managing cough. Widespread access to the World Wide Web also has influenced the manner in which the general population access health care information. Dettmar and colleagues[22] reported their initial findings of a prospective cohort study of patients accessing an Internet-based cough clinic diagnostic site designed to suggest a probable diagnosis and offer treatment advice based along international recommendations. Over 8500 individuals completed the online 16-item diagnostic questionnaire and based on responses the causes for cough were identified as reflux (46%), asthma/asthma syndrome (39%), or rhinitis (15%). Unfortunately, the authors were only able to report follow data on a minority (approximately 12%) of participants, and while most of those found the site easy to use, less than two thirds took the recommended treatment. The online cough clinic represents a novel departure from current management of cough, but it may only prove useful for suitably motivated cough patients.

DEVELOPMENTS IN THE DIAGNOSIS AND TREATMENT OF THE COMMON TRIAD OF COUGH ETIOLOGIES

Asthma, gastroesophageal reflux disease (GERD), and upper airway cough syndrome (UACS) remain the most commonly recognized causes of cough presenting to primary and secondary care physicians. Over the last few decades, there have been few if any changes in the treatment options available for these patients. This is unlikely to change in the immediate future, but several technological developments (in particular noninvasive diagnostic tools) may improve the capacity to accurately identify patients most likely to respond to disease specific therapies. Success in this area would represent a significant advance and influence the approach to treatment of cough in the future. The new developments relevant to each condition in the common triad of cough etiologies will be discussed below.

Asthma/Eosinophilic Airway Cough Syndromes

A trial of inhaled corticosteroids or a short course of oral steroids remains an important strategy in the management of chronic cough. Current guidelines suggest assessing airway inflammation in all patients presenting with cough and giving trials of corticosteroids. This is based on strong evidence that asthma/eosinophilic airway syndromes commonly cause cough.[23–25] Cough variant asthma (CVA) is characterized by normal spirometry, evidence of bronchial hyper-responsiveness on bronchoprovocation challenge testing, and improvement in cough with bronchodilators or corticosteroids; CVA accounts for between 24 to 35% of those referred to specialist cough clinics.[26] Eosinophilic bronchitis (EB) is characterized by eosinophilic airway inflammation and a steroid responsive cough; unlike asthma, however, it is not associated with bronchial hyper-reactivity or variable airflow obstruction.[27] There is no consensus on the optimal method of assessing airway inflammation, the dose and duration of oral corticosteroid trials, and the required length of treatment with inhaled corticosteroids.

Although well described,[28] the routine use of induced sputum for the assessment of airway inflammation in cough clinics has not been adopted widely. Some of the reluctance to do so relates to the costs and technical expertise required to provide a reliable service. The usefulness of exhaled nitric oxide (eNO) measurements as a surrogate marker of both airway inflammation and hyper-responsiveness has been studied. The measurement of fractional eNO (FeNO) is relatively simple and noninvasive, and levels correlate well with eosinophilic airway inflammation.[29] As FeNO levels are increased in asthmatic coughers and patients with EB, the measurement of FeNO represents an attractive means of selecting patients for steroid treatment. Several studies have sought to identify baseline cutoff values most likely to identify treatment responders. In a study by Prieto and colleagues,[30] 45% of subjects responded well to 4 weeks of treatment with fluticasone (100 mcg twice daily), but their chosen baseline FeNO cutoff value of 20 parts per billion (ppb) was poor at predicting response with a sensitivity and specificity of 53% and 63%, respectively.

The inhalation of mannitol is known to cause bronchospasm and cough possibly by inducing an osmotic effect on the airway, leading to activation of inflammatory cells. Asthmatics cough more than healthy controls, and with the development of mannitol dry powder administration devices, mannitol may prove to be a practical and superior alternative to other indirect bronchial challenge methods in the identifying cough patients likely to respond to a trial of anti-inflammatory therapy.[31]

GERD

Expert opinion largely has prevailed in the development of existing recommendations for treatment of GERD-associated cough.[4,32] These have focused mainly on the treatment of acid reflux and based on fairly limited evidence have recommended high-dose acid suppression for an extended duration (3 months or longer). The future management and treatment of GERD-associated cough must extend beyond simply suppressing acid with medical therapy and consider the role of new medicines and evolving surgical techniques in the treatment of nonacid (volume) reflux.

The notion that treating GERD-associated cough with acid suppression has been disputed for some time with doubt about the efficacy of trials of acid suppression[33] and the reliability of existing diagnostic techniques (in particular 24-hour esophageal pH monitoring) in identifying those likely to respond to acid suppression having been raised.[34] Recent attention has focused on multichannel intraluminal impedance (MII-pH) monitoring, which has the advantage of identifying and characterizing both acidic and nonacidic reflux episodes.[35] In a study of healthy volunteers using MII-pH, only 25% of reflux episodes reaching the pharynx were nonacidic.[36] Recent findings suggest that nonacidic reflux episodes are strongly associated with episodes of cough.[37] The value of prokinetic agents or treatments such as baclofen (which act directly on lower esophageal tone) in managing volume reflux remains to be confirmed. More likely to have a prominent place in the future treatment of patients with cough caused by the nonacidic and volume effect reflux are surgical techniques such as laparoscopic fundoplication. There have been several open-label studies of laparoscopic fundoplication offered to patients with refractory cough that have reported promising results.[38,39] How best to identify patients likely to benefit and the exact form of intervention (especially as technological advances in endoscopic procedures emerge) are unknown.

UACS

Most patients with nasal secretions do not complain of cough,[40] and the idea that postnasal drip represents a distinct disease has been questioned.[41] Nonetheless, rhinitis or rhinosinusitis commonly features in the reported causes of cough.[42] The introduction of the term UACS, which encompasses these two upper airway conditions, has helped the move away from the reliance on a symptom profile (postnasal drip) and toward a causative factor. Current recommendations for treating UACS suggest sedating first-generation antihistamines, which although not universally available on prescription, are preferred over newer agents.[42] Intranasal corticosteroids are recommended, but there is a lack of necessary detail as to the dose and duration of therapy.

As with the asthma/airway eosinophilia syndrome, future treatment strategies would be helped greatly by noninvasive methods (ideally a point-of-care test) to identify those likely to respond to specific therapy. At present, there is no support in the literature for the routine use of sinus computed tomography (CT) scanning for patients with chronic cough, as up to 30% of asymptomatic adults will have mucosal abnormalities on imaging[43] nasal NO (nNO) has gained attention as a noninvasive technique in the diagnosis of chronic rhinosinusitis. Low nNO correlates with patients who have chronic rhinosinusitis with nasal polyps and could prove a quick, noninvasive test to identify those patients likely to benefit from medical or also surgical management of their disease.[44] An open interventional study by Macedo and colleagues[45] reports improvement in cough after 28 days treatment with fluticasone nasules, ipratropium bromide, and azelastine nasal sprays.

The future of treatment in this area will be to accurately identify likely responders and advances being made in both medical and surgical of upper airway disease.

COUGH REFLEX HYPERSENSITIVITY AND ITS ASSOCIATION WITH COMMON ACUTE AND CHRONIC COUGH SYNDROMES

The cough reflex is hypersensitive in a range of respiratory diseases including acute viral cough, asthma, chronic obstructive pulmonary disease (COPD), and pulmonary fibrosis.[46–48] It is also heightened in extrapulmonary diseases associated with cough such as GERD[49] and rhinosinusitis.[10] The physiology of the cough reflex and the pathophysiological mechanisms responsible for sensitization (peripheral and central) have been detailed elsewhere in this publication by Canning. In this section, the authors suggest that a broader appreciation of the clinical consequences of cough reflex hypersensitization and more insight into the neuroinflammatory events considered mechanistically important should be a priority in future efforts to improve the treatment of cough.

What are the Clinical Characteristics of Cough Reflex Hypersensitivity?

Patients frequently complain of bouts of coughing triggered by relatively innocuous stimuli such as exposure to aerosols and scents, change in air temperature, or when talking, laughing, or singing. These triggers are recognized by approximately two thirds of patients referred with chronic cough,[50] and because they occur during the patients' normal daily routine, this aspect of their condition is felt to be the most disruptive. In the development of the two most widely used cough quality-of-life questionnaires, items perceived as important by patients included statements such as "exposure to paint or fumes made me cough,"[51] and "I can no longer sing, for example in church".[52]

Airway hypersensitivity is not the only clinical symptom reported by cough patients, as many describe an unpleasant sensation such as the urge to cough or the feeling of an itch or choking sensation at the back of the throat, or sometimes central chest discomfort. It is likely that these clinical features arise as a direct consequence of cough reflex sensitization, as vagal anesthesia is known to inhibit them.[53] These symptoms are also absent in patients following bilateral lung transplant.[54] The areas of the cerebral cortex and brainstem that may activated by these vagal lung afferents recently have been identified by researchers using functional magnetic resonance imaging of the brain following inhalation of the tussive agent capsaicin by healthy volunteers.[55]

A more widespread appreciation among general and respiratory physicians of the symptom profile of airway sensory hyper-responsiveness reported by cough patients is required. The development of health status questionnaires that capture the impact of airway sensory hyper-reactivity more completely should be developed. These may provide a novel and clinically relevant study endpoint for therapeutic trials in the future.

Factors Associated with Cough Reflex Sensitization and the Development of Chronic Cough

The human cough reflex is in a dynamic state of activation, and several exogenous and endogenous factors may alter the degree of sensitization. One obvious example of this is the change in cough reflex sensitivity following an upper respiratory tract infection.

After a viral infection, the cough reflex becomes hyper-reactive and remains in this activated state for a variable period. During this time, the patient is symptomatic, although the cough typically subsides after 2 to 3 weeks,[56] and the hypersensitive cough reflex returns to its baseline state.[46] In some circumstances, however, this hypersensitized state persists long after the initial triggering event, leading to a chronic cough state (**Fig. 1**). It is unclear if this arises because of direct viral damage of the peripheral sensory nerves or virus-induced changes in central processing of the sensory signal. Several aggravating factors are believed to promote this transition to a chronic cough state, and a schematic of possible relationships has been outlined in the **Fig. 2**. Therefore, careful clinical assessment of the patient to identify some of these factors is recommended.[4] In some instances, simply removing the aggravant (angiotensin converting enzyme-inhibitor or cigarette smoke) is sufficient. It is suggested that the coexistence of two or more inflammatory (possibly infective) stimuli to the airway (multiple hit) may be a factor in the development of more severe airway disease.[57] In a recent study of chronic cough patients referred to otolaryngology clinics, *Helicobacter pylori* infection was detected in 86% of patients compared with 45% of controls. The cough responded to eradication therapy in 75% of cases, suggesting a role for the detection and treatment of *H pylori*.[58] It is recognized that women are over-represented at cough clinics, but it is not clear why gender has such a strong influence on the development of chronic cough. Females (both healthy and coughers) have a heightened cough reflex compared with males,[59,60] and there may be hormonal factors that influence airway inflammatory events.[61,62] On the other hand, this difference may be related to women demonstrating worse cough-related health-related

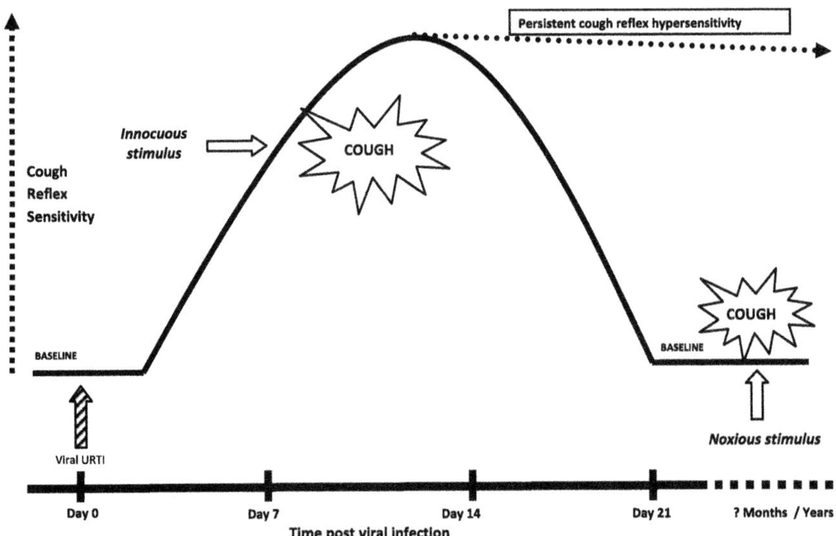

Fig. 1. Schematic of proposed changes in cough reflex sensitivity following viral upper respiratory tract infection. Following a viral infection, the cough reflex becomes hyper-reactive and remains in this activated state for a variable period of time (2 to 3 weeks), during which cough may be provoked by innocuous stimuli such as exposure scents, aerosols, and changes in air temperature. In most subjects, the hyper-reactivity diminishes, and the cough reflex responsiveness returns to its baseline state. In some circumstances, however, this hypersensitized state persists long after the initial triggering event, leading to a chronic cough state. (*From* McGarvey L, McKeagney P, Polley L, et al. Are there clinical features of a sensitized cough reflex? Pulm Pharmacol Ther 2009;22(2): 59–64; with permission.)

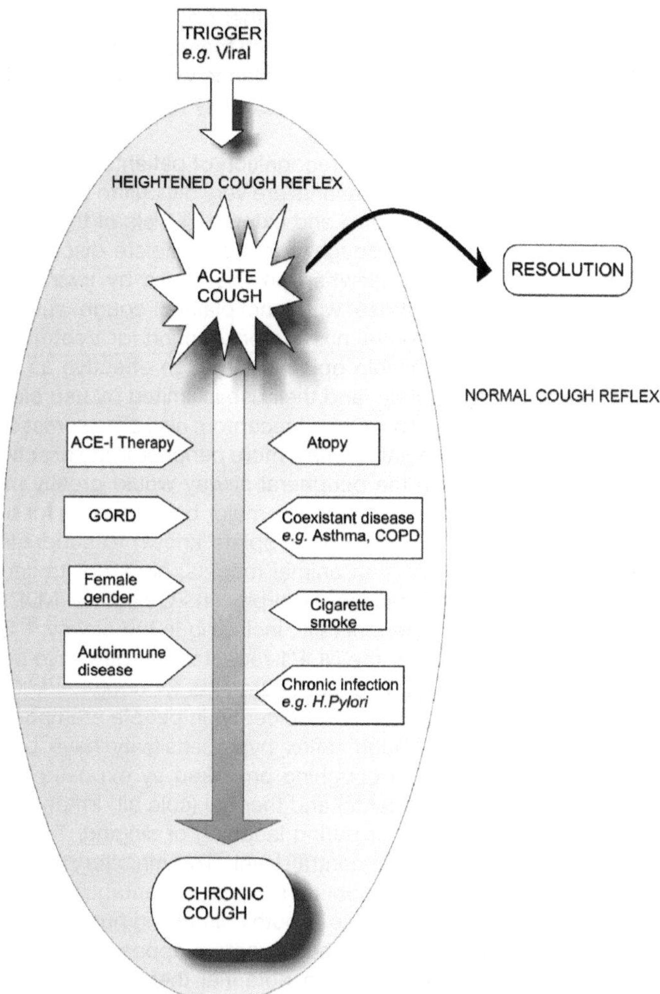

Fig. 2. Schematic of the possible triggering and maintaining of cough reflex hypersensitivity in patients with persistent cough (*From* McGarvey L, Polley L, MacMohan J. Review Series: Chronic cough: Common causes and current guidelines. Chron Respir Dis 2007;4(4): 215–23; with permission.)

quality of life than men, perhaps related to more urinary incontinence and other adverse effects. Elucidating the mechanisms responsible for this gender association will be an important advance in the development of new treatments for cough.

THE DEVELOPMENT OF NEW TREATMENTS FOR COUGH

An important factor responsible for directing efforts to develop new cough therapies has been recent concerns over the safety of existing cough medicines particularly in children. OTC cough and cold preparations are used commonly by children, particularly those 2 to 5 years of age.[63] Recent case reports detailing serious adverse events following accidental ingestion have contributed to a decision to withdraw the sale of

OTC for use in the under-5-year-old group.[9] A further obstacle to the development of new OTC treatment is the lack of evidence that such therapies provide much improvement in symptoms over placebo.[7,64] A major challenge will be to ensure that the efficacy of potential new compounds is tested adequately in carefully designed clinical trials.[65]

Another factor has been the increasing recognition of patients (usually adults) with idiopathic or unexplained cough. Such patients are very difficult to treat, having generally failed to respond to several (intensive and extended) trials of therapy directed at the commonly recognized causes of cough. A more complete discussion on unexplained cough has been provided elsewhere in this series by Irwin. Patients with persistent cough and especially those with unexplained cough suffer significant impairment in health status, and sometimes the only option for treatment is the use of regular opiates.[66] Currently available opiates, although effective as antitussives, have a centrally acting mode of action, and their use is limited by neurologic adverse effects such as sedation and addiction. Opioid receptors also are expressed on airway sensory nerves,[67] and identifying opiates with a more peripheral site of action or developing a means to deliver them to the peripheral airway would greatly minimize the systemic adverse effects and would represent a major breakthrough for the pharmaceutical industry. Nociceptin, the endogenous opiate known to suppress capsaicin and mechanically induced cough[68,69] in animal models, does not target the opioid receptors but rather the opioid-like nociceptin/orphanin FQ peptide (NOP1) receptor, which is distributed centrally and peripherally, including in the airway.[70] Several tropane derivatives with high affinity for the NOP1 receptor recently have been synthesized and have been suggested as potential treatments for cough.[71,72] Clinical trials evaluating the potential antitussive role for nociceptin in people are underway.

The clinical consequences of cough reflex hypersensitivity have been covered earlier and typically feature bouts of coughing provoked by exposure to chemicals (eg, cigarette smoke, acidic air pollutants) and thermal (cold air) irritants and the mechanostimulatory effects of inhaled air during laughing or singing. The cough reflex may be sensitized at a peripheral or central level. The inhibitory activity of novel compounds such as the selective cannabinoid 2 receptor antagonists on peripheral sensory nerve function has shown promise in both animal and human models.[73] Centrally, the release of neuropeptides from the brainstem appears to influence central cough reflex sensitization and represents a potential therapeutic target.[74] Further discussion on this area is outside the scope of this article.

Patients with chronic cough sometimes associate the onset of cough with an upper respiratory tract infection.[11] Following a respiratory virus infection, the airway reflexes responsible for cough become hypersensitive,[46,75] which may be thought of as equivalent to the hyperalgesia recognized in chronic pain syndromes. Efforts to elucidate the mechanisms of sensory hyperalgesia have resulted in the development of several promising new treatments for pain.[76] A logical strategy for the development of cough treatments in the future would be the adopt some of these pain research findings combined with a clearer understanding of the mechanisms of respiratory virus-induced cough. One particular target of importance is the novel transient receptor potential (TRP) cation channel family, which is expressed in many cell types including airway sensory nerves[77] and the bronchial epithelium.[78] Several TRP channels, in particular TRP channel, subfamily V, member 1 (TRPV1); TRP channel melastatin member 8 (TRPM8); and TRP channel, subfamily A, member 1 (TRPA1), which are activated directly by chemical, thermal, and mechanical stimuli, represent potential candidate receptors responsible for respiratory virus-induced airway hypersensitivity. Several TRP receptor antagonists are already in clinical development, and insights into the role of these receptors in virus-induced asthma exacerbations may identify new therapeutic options.[79]

Drugs that directly block sensory nerve activation may inhibit the important protective reflex function that coughing provides. Therefore, therapy directed at inhibiting the processes involved in afferent nerve sensitization seems a more logical approach to drug development. The peripheral termini of sensory nerves express receptors several mediators, including histamine, tryptase, tumor necrosis factor α, interleukin (IL)-1β, IL-6, IL-8, bradykinin, and prostaglandin E_2 (PGE_2), which induce and maintain neural sensitization and activation of nociceptors.[80] Virus infection of the respiratory epithelium is associated with release of an array of inflammatory mediators, neurotransmitters, and growth factors.[15] Experimental infection of cotton rats with respiratory syncytial virus is associated with increased airway expression of nerve growth factor (NGF) and its receptors.[81] NGF is known to up-regulate airway sensory nerve function with increased substance P expression, which can be inhibited with anti-NGF antibody. However, identifying the correct animal model in which to study the relevant respiratory viruses and accurately measure cough as an endpoint remains a challenge. To date, studies on mechanisms of virus-induced cough in people have been extremely limited. In vivo studies of human challenge with rhinovirus have offered important mechanistic insights into virus-induced exacerbations of asthma and COPD.[82,83] Similar in vivo studies are required in people with cough as a key study endpoint. Advances in antiviral chemotherapy may offer hope for the sizable population troubled with acute viral cough.

SUMMARY

There is broad agreement that new treatments for cough are needed. At present, there is considerable effort by basic science and clinical researchers, in cooperation with the pharmaceutical companies, to advance novel drug development. Recent interest has focused on cough reflex hyper-reactivity and the associated abnormal airway sensory hypersensitivity that is so troublesome for patients with cough. Treatment aimed at resetting this cough reflex sensitization to baseline or predisease levels is a key therapeutic objective.

REFERENCES

1. Irwin RS, Pratter MR, Hamolsky MW. Chronic persistent cough: an uncommon presenting complaint of thyroiditis. Chest 1982;81(3):386–8.
2. Irwin RS, Curley FJ, French CL. Chronic cough. The spectrum and frequency of causes, key components of the diagnostic evaluation, and outcome of specific therapy. Am Rev Respir Dis 1990;141(3):640–7.
3. Morice AH, Fontana GA, Sovijarvi AR, et al. The diagnosis and management of chronic cough. Eur Respir J 2004;24(3):481–92.
4. Morice AH, McGarvey L, Pavord I. British Thoracic Society Cough Guideline Group. Recommendations for the management of cough in adults. Thorax 2006;61(Suppl 1):i1–24.
5. Irwin RS, Baumann MH, Bolser DC, et al. Diagnosis and management of cough executive summary: ACCP evidence-based clinical practice guidelines. Chest 2006;129(Suppl 1):1S–23S.
6. Shields MD, Bush A, Everard ML, et al. British Thoracic Society Cough Guideline Group. BTS guidelines: recommendations for the assessment and management of cough in children. Thorax 2008;63(Suppl 3):iii1–iii15.

7. Schroeder K, Fahey T. Over-the-counter medications for acute cough in children and adults in ambulatory settings. Cochrane Database Syst Rev 2004;(4):CD001831.
8. Cough guidelines choke on evidence. Lancet 2006;367(9507):276.
9. Centers for Disease Control and Prevention (CDC). Revised product labels for pediatric over-the-counter cough and cold medicines. MMWR Morb Mortal Wkly Rep 2008;57(43):1180.
10. McGarvey LP, Heaney LG, Lawson JT, et al. Evaluation and outcome of patients with chronic non-productive cough using a comprehensive diagnostic protocol. Thorax 1998;53(9):738–43.
11. Haque RA, Usmani OS, Barnes PJ. Chronic idiopathic cough: a discrete clinical entity? Chest 2005;127(5):1710–3.
12. Pratter MR. Unexplained (idiopathic) cough: ACCP evidence-based clinical practice guidelines. Chest 2006;129(Suppl 1):220S–1S.
13. Levine BM. Systematic evaluation and treatment of chronic cough in a community setting. Allergy Asthma Proc 2008;29(3):336–42.
14. Gonzales R, Malone DC, Maselli JH, et al. Excessive antibiotic use for acute respiratory infections in the united states. Clin Infect Dis 2001;33(6):757–62.
15. Footitt J, Johnston SL. Cough and viruses in airways disease: mechanisms. Pulm Pharmacol Ther 2009;22(2):108–13.
16. Fendrick AM, Monto AS, Nightengale B, et al. The economic burden of noninfluenza-related viral respiratory tract infection in the United States. Arch Intern Med 2003;163(4):487–94.
17. Irwin RS, Boulet LP, Cloutier MM, et al. Managing cough as a defense mechanism and as a symptom. A consensus panel report of the American College of Chest Physicians. Chest 1998;114(2 Suppl 2):133S–81S.
18. Kohno S, Ishida T, Uchida Y, et al. Committee for the Japanese Respiratory Society Guidelines for Management of Cough. The Japanese respiratory society guidelines for management of cough. Respirology 2006;11(Suppl 4):S135–86.
19. Lin L, Poh KL, Lim TK. Empirical treatment of chronic cough—a cost-effectiveness analysis. Proc AMIA Symp 2001;383–7.
20. Poirier-Elliott E. Cost-effectiveness of non-physician health care professionals. Nurse Pract 1984;9(10):54–6.
21. Field SK, Conley DP, Thawer AM, et al. Assessment and management of patients with chronic cough by certified respiratory educators: a randomized controlled trial. Can Respir J 2009;16(2):49–54.
22. Dettmar PW, Strugala V, Fathi H, et al. The online cough clinic—developing guideline-based diagnosis and advice. Eur Respir J 2009;34(4):819–24.
23. Gibson PG, Dolovich J, Denburg J, et al. Chronic cough: eosinophilic bronchitis without asthma. Lancet 1989;1(8651):1346–8.
24. Brightling CE, Ward R, Goh KL, et al. Eosinophilic bronchitis is an important cause of chronic cough. Am J Respir Crit Care Med 1999;160(2):406–10.
25. McGarvey L, Heaney L, MacMahon J, et al. Eosinophilic bronchitis is an important cause of chronic cough. Am J Respir Crit Care Med 2000;161(5):1763–4 [author reply 1765].
26. Chung KF, Pavord ID. Prevalence, pathogenesis, and causes of chronic cough. Lancet 2008;371(9621):1364–74.
27. Gibson PG, Hargreave FE, Girgis-Gabardo A, et al. Chronic cough with eosinophilic bronchitis: examination for variable airflow obstruction and response to corticosteroid. Clin Exp Allergy 1995;25(2):127–32.
28. Birring SS, Parker D, Brightling CE, et al. Induced sputum inflammatory mediator concentrations in chronic cough. Am J Respir Crit Care Med 2004;169(1):15–9.

29. Chatkin JM, Ansarin K, Silkoff PE, et al. Exhaled nitric oxide as a noninvasive assessment of chronic cough. Am J Respir Crit Care Med 1999;159(6):1810–3.
30. Prieto L, Ferrer A, Ponce S, et al. Exhaled nitric oxide measurement is not useful for predicting the response to inhaled corticosteroids in subjects with chronic cough. Chest 2009;136(3):816–22.
31. Singapuri A, McKenna S, Brightling CE. The utility of the mannitol challenge in the assessment of chronic cough: a pilot study. Cough 2008;4:10.
32. Irwin RS. Chronic cough due to gastroesophageal reflux disease: ACCP evidence-based clinical practice guidelines. Chest 2006;129(Suppl 1):80S–94S.
33. Chang AB, Lasserson TJ, Kiljander TO, et al. Systematic review and meta-analysis of randomised controlled trials of gastro-oesophageal reflux interventions for chronic cough associated with gastro-oesophageal reflux. BMJ 2006; 332(7532):11–7.
34. Patterson RN, Johnston BT, MacMahon J, et al. Oesophageal pH monitoring is of limited value in the diagnosis of reflux cough. Eur Respir J 2004;24(5):724–7.
35. Sifrim D, Holloway R, Silny J, et al. Acid, nonacid, and gas reflux in patients with gastroesophageal reflux disease during ambulatory 24-hour pH-impedance recordings. Gastroenterology 2001;120(7):1588–98.
36. Oelschlager BK, Quiroga E, Parra JD, et al. Long-term outcomes after laparoscopic antireflux surgery. Am J Gastroenterol 2008;103(2):280–7 [quiz 288].
37. Patterson RN, Mainie I, Rafferty G, et al. Nonacid reflux episodes reaching the pharynx are important factors associated with cough. J Clin Gastroenterol 2009;43(5):414–9.
38. Mainie I, Tutuian R, Agrawal A, et al. Fundoplication eliminates chronic cough due to nonacid reflux identified by impedance pH monitoring. Thorax 2005;60(6): 521–3.
39. Fathi H, Moon T, Donaldson J, et al. Cough in adult cystic fibrosis: diagnosis and response to fundoplication. Cough 2009;5:1.
40. O'Hara J, Jones NS. Postnasal drip syndrome: most patients with purulent nasal secretions do not complain of chronic cough. Rhinology 2006;44(4):270–3.
41. Morice AH. Postnasal drip syndrome—a symptom to be sniffed at? Pulm Pharmacol Ther 2004;17(6):343–5.
42. Pratter MR. Chronic upper airway cough syndrome secondary to rhinosinus diseases (previously referred to as postnasal drip syndrome): ACCP evidence-based clinical practice guidelines. Chest 2006;129(Suppl 1):63S–71S.
43. O'Hara J, Jones NS. The aetiology of chronic cough: a review of current theories for the otorhinolaryngologist. J Laryngol Otol 2005;119(7):507–14.
44. Bommarito L, Guida G, Heffler E, et al. Nasal nitric oxide concentration in suspected chronic rhinosinusitis. Ann Allergy Asthma Immunol 2008;101(4): 358–62.
45. Macedo P, Saleh H, Torrego A, et al. Postnasal drip and chronic cough: an open interventional study. Respir Med 2009;103(11):1700–5.
46. O'Connell F, Thomas VE, Studham JM, et al. Capsaicin cough sensitivity increases during upper respiratory infection. Respir Med 1996;90(5):279–86.
47. Doherty MJ, Mister R, Pearson MG, et al. Capsaicin responsiveness and cough in asthma and chronic obstructive pulmonary disease. Thorax 2000;55(8):643–9.
48. Hope-Gill BD, Hilldrup S, Davies C, et al. A study of the cough reflex in idiopathic pulmonary fibrosis. Am J Respir Crit Care Med 2003;168(8):995–1002.
49. Benini L, Ferrari M, Sembenini C, et al. Cough threshold in reflux oesophagitis: influence of acid and of laryngeal and oesophageal damage. Gut 2000;46(6): 762–7.

50. McGarvey L, McKeagney P, Polley L, et al. Are there clinical features of a sensitized cough reflex? Pulm Pharmacol Ther 2009;22(2):59–64.
51. Birring SS, Prudon B, Carr AJ, et al. Development of a symptom specific health status measure for patients with chronic cough: Leicester cough questionnaire (LCQ). Thorax 2003;58(4):339–43.
52. French CT, Irwin RS, Fletcher KE, et al. Evaluation of a cough-specific quality-of-life questionnaire. Chest 2002;121(4):1123–31.
53. Winning AJ, Hamilton RD, Guz A. Ventilation and breathlessness on maximal exercise in patients with interstitial lung disease after local anaesthetic aerosol inhalation. Clin Sci (Lond) 1988;74(3):275–81.
54. Butler JE, Anand A, Crawford MR, et al. Changes in respiratory sensations induced by lobeline after human bilateral lung transplantation. J Physiol 2001; 534:583–93.
55. Mazzone SB, McLennan L, McGovern AE, et al. Representation of capsaicin-evoked urge to cough in the human brain using functional magnetic resonance imaging. Am J Respir Crit Care Med 2007;176(4):327–32.
56. Curley FJ, Irwin RS, Pratter MR, et al. Cough and the common cold. Am Rev Respir Dis 1988;138(2):305–11.
57. Pavord ID, Birring SS, Berry M, et al. Multiple inflammatory hits and the pathogenesis of severe airway disease. Eur Respir J 2006;27(5):884–8.
58. Talaat M, Gad MS, Magdy EA, et al. *Helicobacter pylori* infection and chronic, persistent cough: is there an association? J Laryngol Otol 2007;121(10): 962–7.
59. Fujimura M, Kasahara K, Kamio Y, et al. Female gender as a determinant of cough threshold to inhaled capsaicin. Eur Respir J 1996;9(8):1624–6.
60. Kastelik JA, Thompson RH, Aziz I, et al. Sex-related differences in cough reflex sensitivity in patients with chronic cough. Am J Respir Crit Care Med 2002; 166(7):961–4.
61. Mund E, Christensson B, Larsson K, et al. Sex dependent differences in physiological ageing in the immune system of lower airways in healthy non-smoking volunteers: study of lymphocyte subsets in bronchoalveolar lavage fluid and blood. Thorax 2001;56(6):450–5.
62. Mund E, Christensson B, Gronneberg R, et al. Noneosinophilic CD4 lymphocytic airway inflammation in menopausal women with chronic dry cough. Chest 2005; 127(5):1714–21.
63. Vernacchio L, Kelly JP, Kaufman DW, et al. Cough and cold medication use by US children, 1999–2006: results from the Slone survey. Pediatrics 2008;122(2): e323–9.
64. Smith SM, Henman M, Schroeder K, et al. Over-the-counter cough medicines in children: neither safe or efficacious? Br J Gen Pract 2008;58(556):757–8.
65. Birring SS. Developing antitussives: the ideal clinical trial. Pulm Pharmacol Ther 2009;22(2):155–8.
66. Morice AH, Menon MS, Mulrennan SA, et al. Opiate therapy in chronic cough. Am J Respir Crit Care Med 2007;175(4):312–5.
67. Adcock JJ. Peripheral opioid receptors and the cough reflex. Respir Med 1991; 85(Suppl A):43–6.
68. McLeod RL, Parra LE, Mutter JC, et al. Nociception inhibits cough in the guinea-pig by activation of ORL(1) receptors. Br J Pharmacol 2001;132(6): 1175–8.
69. Bolser DC, McLeod RL, Tulshian DB, et al. Antitussive action of nociceptin in the cat. Eur J Pharmacol 2001;430(1):107–11.

70. Jia Y, Wang X, Aponte SI, et al. Nociceptin/orphanin FQ inhibits capsaicin-induced guinea pig airway contraction through an inward-rectifier potassium channel. Br J Pharmacol 2002;135(3):764–70.
71. Yang SW, Ho G, Tulshian D, et al. Identification of 3-substituted N-benzhydryl-nortropane analogs as nociceptin receptor ligands for the management of cough and anxiety. Bioorg Med Chem Lett 2009;19(9):2482–6.
72. Ho GD, Anthes J, Bercovici A, et al. The discovery of tropane derivatives as nociceptin receptor ligands for the management of cough and anxiety. Bioorg Med Chem Lett. 2009;19(9):2519–23.
73. Belvisi MG, Patel HJ, Freund-Michel V, et al. Inhibitory activity of the novel CB2 receptor agonist, GW833972A, on guinea-pig and human sensory nerve function in the airways. Br J Pharmacol 2008;155(4):547–57.
74. Joad JP, Munch PA, Bric JM, et al. Passive smoke effects on cough and airways in young guinea pigs: role of brainstem substance P. Am J Respir Crit Care Med 2004;169(4):499–504.
75. Empey DW, Laitinen LA, Jacobs L, et al. Mechanisms of bronchial hyperreactivity in normal subjects after upper respiratory tract infection. Am Rev Respir Dis 1976;113(2):131–9.
76. Attal N, Bouhassira D. Translating basic research on sodium channels in human neuropathic pain. J Pain 2006;7(Suppl 1):S31–7.
77. Groneberg DA, Niimi A, Dinh QT, et al. Increased expression of transient receptor potential vanilloid-1 in airway nerves of chronic cough. Am J Respir Crit Care Med 2004;170(12):1276–80.
78. Sabnis AS, Shadid M, Yost GS, et al. Human lung epithelial cells express a functional cold-sensing TRPM8 variant. Am J Respir Cell Mol Biol 2008;39(4):466–74.
79. Adcock JJ. TRPV1 receptors in sensitisation of cough and pain reflexes. Pulm Pharmacol Ther 2009;22(2):65–70.
80. Brenn D, Richter F, Schaible HG. Sensitization of unmyelinated sensory fibers of the joint nerve to mechanical stimuli by interleukin-6 in the rat: an inflammatory mechanism of joint pain. Arthritis Rheum 2007;56(1):351–9.
81. Hu C, Wedde-Beer K, Auais A, et al. Nerve growth factor and nerve growth factor receptors in respiratory syncytial virus-infected lungs. Am J Physiol Lung Cell Mol Physiol 2002;283(2):L494–502.
82. Bardin PG, Fraenkel DJ, Sanderson G, et al. Peak expiratory flow changes during experimental rhinovirus infection. Eur Respir J 2000;16(5):980–5.
83. Mallia P, Message SD, Kebadze T, et al. An experimental model of rhinovirus induced chronic obstructive pulmonary disease exacerbations: a pilot study. Respir Res 2006;7:116.

Index

Note: Page numbers of article titles are in **boldface** type.

Otolaryngol Clin N Am 43 (2010) 213–219
doi:10.1016/S0030-6665(10)00009-5

Printed and bound by CPI Group (UK) Ltd, Croydon, CR0 4YY
03/10/2024
01040463-0004